Student Mental Health

A Guide for Psychiatrists, Psychologists, and Leaders Serving in Higher Education

Student Mental Health

A Guide for Psychiatrists, Psychologists, and Leaders Serving in Higher Education

Edited by

Laura Weiss Roberts, M.D., M.A.

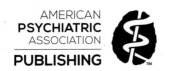

AMERICAN
PSYCHIATRIC
ASSOCIATION
PUBLISHING

If you wish to buy 50 or more copies of the same title, please go to www.appi.org/specialdiscounts for more information.

Copyright © 2018 American Psychiatric Association Publishing

ALL RIGHTS RESERVED

First Edition

Manufactured in the United States of America on acid-free paper
22   21   20   19   18   5   4   3   2   1

American Psychiatric Association Publishing
800 Maine Ave. SW
Suite 900
Washington, DC 20024-2812
www.appi.org

Library of Congress Cataloging-in-Publication Data
Names: Roberts, Laura Weiss, 1960- editor.
Title: Student mental health : a guide for psychiatrists, psychologists, and leaders serving in higher education / edited by Laura Weiss Roberts.
Description: First edition. | Washington, DC : American Psychiatric Association Publishing, [2018] | Includes bibliographical references and index.
Identifiers: LCCN 2018000212 (print) | LCCN 2018001342 (ebook) | ISBN 9781615371945 (eb) | ISBN 9781615371143 (pb)
Subjects: | MESH: Mental Health Services | Student Health Services
Classification: LCC RA440.6 (ebook) | LCC RA440.6 (print) | NLM WA 353 | DDC 362.1071—dc23
LC record available at https://lccn.loc.gov/2018000212

British Library Cataloguing in Publication Data
A CIP record is available from the British Library.

For Gabrielle, Helen, Illianna,
Kyle, Madeline, Tom, Tuli, and Willa.
You fill my heart.

Dedicated to Ira M. Friedman
for his decades of service to the students
of Stanford University

Contents

Part I
Overview

Part II
Life Transitions and the Student Experience

Part III
Caring for Students
With Mental Health Issues

Part IV
Fostering Mental Health for Distinct
Student Populations

Contributors

Molly Adrian, Ph.D.
Assistant Professor, Department of Psychiatry and Behavioral Sciences, University of Washington, Seattle, Washington

Amy Alexander, M.D.
Clinical Assistant Professor, Department of Psychiatry and Behavioral Sciences, Stanford University School of Medicine, Stanford, California

Jacob S. Ballon, M.D., M.P.H.
Clinical Assistant Professor, Department of Psychiatry and Behavioral Sciences, Stanford University, Stanford, California

Michele S. Berk, Ph.D.
Assistant Professor, Department of Psychiatry and Behavioral Sciences, Stanford University School of Medicine, Stanford, California

Victor G. Carrion, M.D.
Professor and Associate Chair, Department of Psychiatry and Behavioral Sciences, Stanford University School of Medicine, Stanford, California

Lindsay C. Chromik, M.S.
Clinical Research Coordinator, Center for Interdisciplinary Brain Sciences Research, Stanford University School of Medicine, Stanford, California

Danielle Colborn, Ph.D.

Clinical Assistant Professor, Department of Psychiatry and Behavioral Sciences, Stanford University School of Medicine, Stanford, California

Whitney Daniels, M.D.

Clinical Assistant Professor, Department of Psychiatry and Behavioral Sciences, Stanford University School of Medicine, Stanford, California

Jennifer Derenne, M.D.

Clinical Associate Professor, Department of Psychiatry and Behavioral Sciences, Stanford University School of Medicine, Stanford, California

Neir Eshel, M.D., Ph.D.

Resident in Psychiatry, Department of Psychiatry and Behavioral Sciences, Stanford University School of Medicine, Stanford, California

Rachael Flatt, B.S.

Projects Director, Center for m2Health, Palo Alto University, Palo Alto, California

Lawrence K. Fung, M.D., Ph.D.

Instructor, Department of Psychiatry and Behavioral Sciences, Stanford University School of Medicine, Stanford, California

Brenda Gonzalez-Flores, M.S.

Doctoral Candidate in Clinical Psychology, PGSP-Stanford Psy.D. Consortium, Palo Alto University, Stanford California

Michael Haberecht, M.D.

Clinical Associate Professor, Department of Psychiatry and Behavioral Sciences, Stanford University School of Medicine, and Vaden Health Center, Stanford University, Stanford, California

Inge Hansen, Psy.D.

Psychologist, Counseling and Psychological Services, and Faculty Affiliate, Program in Feminist, Gender, and Sexuality Studies, Stanford University, Stanford, California

Kate V. Hardy, Clin.Psych.D.

Clinical Assistant Professor, Department of Psychiatry and Behavioral Sciences, Stanford University School of Medicine, Stanford, California

David S. Hong, M.D.
Clinical Assistant Professor, Center for Interdisciplinary Brain Sciences Research, Stanford University School of Medicine, Stanford, California

Doris Iarovici, M.D.
Assistant Consulting Professor, Department of Psychiatry and Behavioral Sciences, Duke University Medical Center, Durham, North Carolina

James R. Jacobs, M.D., Ph.D.
Associate Professor, Department of Psychiatry and Behavioral Sciences, and, by courtesy of Emergency Medicine, Stanford University School of Medicine, Vaden Health Center, Stanford University, Stanford, California

Shashank V. Joshi, M.D.
Associate Professor, Child and Adolescent Psychiatry, Department of Psychiatry and Behavioral Sciences, Stanford University School of Medicine, Stanford, California

Megan Kelly, Psy.D.
Clinical Instructor, Department of Psychiatry and Behavioral Sciences, Stanford University School of Medicine, Stanford, California

Michael Kelly, M.D.
Clinical Assistant Professor, Department of Psychiatry and Behavioral Sciences, Stanford University School of Medicine, Stanford, California

Christina Tara Khan, M.D., Ph.D.
Clinical Assistant Professor, Department of Psychiatry and Behavioral Sciences, Stanford University School of Medicine; Research Associate, National Center for Posttraumatic Stress Disorder, VA Palo Alto Health Care System, Palo Alto, California

Eric Kuhn, Ph.D.
Clinical Assistant Professor, Department of Psychiatry and Behavioral Sciences, VA Palo Alto Health Care System, Palo Alto, California

Kyle Lane-McKinley, M.F.A.
Program Manager, Department of Psychiatry and Behavioral Sciences, Stanford University School of Medicine, Stanford, California

Anna Lembke, M.D.
Assistant Professor, Department of Psychiatry and Behavioral Sciences, Stanford University School of Medicine, Stanford, California

Ryan B. Matlow, Ph.D.
Clinical Assistant Professor, Department of Psychiatry and Behavioral Sciences, Stanford University School of Medicine, Stanford, California

Anne McBride, M.D.
Assistant Clinical Professor, Department of Psychiatry and Behavioral Sciences, UC Davis School of Medicine, Sacramento, California

Shannon McCaslin, Ph.D.
Clinical Associate Professor, Department of Psychiatry and Behavioral Sciences, VA Palo Alto Health Care System, Palo Alto, California

Lawrence McGlynn, M.D., M.S.
Clinical Professor, Department of Psychiatry and Behavioral Sciences, Stanford University School of Medicine, Stanford, California

Adriana Sum Miu, Ph.D.
Clinical Instructor, Department of Psychiatry and Behavioral Sciences, Stanford University School of Medicine, Stanford, California

Douglas L. Noordsy, M.D.
Clinical Professor, Department of Psychiatry and Behavioral Sciences, Stanford University School of Medicine, Stanford, California

Chinyere I. Ogbonna, M.D., M.P.H.
Adjunct Assistant Professor, Department of Psychiatry and Behavioral Sciences, Stanford University School of Medicine, Stanford, California

Bina Patel, M.D.
Clinical Assistant Professor, Department of Psychiatry and Behavioral Sciences, Stanford University School of Medicine, and Assistant Director, Clinical Services, Vaden Health Center, Stanford University, Stanford, California

Sujata Patel, M.D.
Clinical Assistant Professor, Department of Psychiatry and Behavioral Sciences and Staff Psychiatrist, Stanford University School of Medicine, and Staff Psychiatrist, Vaden Health Center, Stanford University, Stanford, California

Matthew Pesko, M.D.
Child and Adolescent Psychiatry Fellow, Department of Psychiatry, University of Colorado School of Medicine, Aurora, Colorado

Lisa Post, Ph.D.
Clinical Associate Professor, Department of Psychiatry and Behavioral Sciences, Stanford University School of Medicine, Stanford, California

Douglas S. Rait, Ph.D.
Chief, Couples and Family Therapy Clinic, and Clinical Professor of Psychiatry and Behavioral Sciences, Stanford University School of Medicine, Stanford, California

Laura Weiss Roberts, M.D., M.A.
Chair and Katharine Dexter McCormick and Stanley McCormick Memorial Professor, Department of Psychiatry and Behavioral Sciences, Stanford University School of Medicine, Stanford, California

Athena Robinson, Ph.D.
Clinical Associate Professor, Department of Psychiatry and Behavioral Sciences, Stanford University School of Medicine, Stanford, California

Daniel Ryu, M.S.
Doctoral Candidate in Clinical Psychology, PGSP-Stanford Psy.D. Consortium, Palo Alto University, Stanford, California

Ripal Shah, M.D., M.P.H.
Resident in Psychiatry, Department of Psychiatry and Behavioral Sciences, Stanford University School of Medicine, Stanford, California

Daniel C. Silverman, M.D., M.P.A.
Santa Fe, New Mexico

Shannon S. Sullivan, M.D.
Clinical Assistant Professor, Stanford Center for Sleep Sciences and Medicine, Department of Psychiatry and Behavioral Sciences, Stanford University School of Medicine, Stanford, California

Allison L. Thompson, Ph.D.
Clinical Associate Professor, Department of Psychiatry and Behavioral Sciences, Stanford University School of Medicine, Stanford, California

Mickey Trockel, M.D.
Clinical Associate Professor, Department of Psychiatry and Behavioral Sciences, Stanford University School of Medicine, Stanford, California

Raziya S. Wang, M.D.
Clinical Assistant Professor (Affiliated), Department of Psychiatry and Behavioral Sciences, Stanford University School of Medicine, Stanford, California

Helen W. Wilson, Ph.D.
Clinical Associate Professor, Department of Psychiatry and Behavioral Sciences, Stanford University School of Medicine, Stanford, California

Sanno Zack, Ph.D.
Clinical Associate Professor, Department of Psychiatry and Behavioral Sciences, Stanford University School of Medicine, Stanford, California

Foreword

SIMPLY put, we are experiencing an epidemic of serious psychiatric disturbances in our college and graduate student populations. Of the thousands of students completing the Fall 2016 National College Health Assessment,[1] 12% reported having been diagnosed or treated by a professional for depression and anxiety within the prior year. Even though many experts believe this is a significant underreporting of prevalence,[2] in an estimated population of 20.5 million college students,[3] this represents a cohort of nearly 2.5 million individuals without even considering other common major conditions such as substance

---

[1]American College Health Association: *American College Health Association–National College Health Assessment II: Fall 2016 Reference Group Executive Summary*. Hanover, MD, American College Health Association, 2017. Available at: http://www.acha-ncha.org/docs/NCHA-II_Fall_2016_Reference_Group_Executive_Summary.pdf. Accessed January 17, 2018.

[2]Blanco C, Okuda M, Wright C, et al: "Mental Health of College Students and Their Non–College-Attending Peers: Results From the National Epidemiologic Study on Alcohol and Related Conditions. *Archives of General Psychiatry* 65(12):1429–1437, 2008.

[3]National Center for Education Statistics: Back to School Statistics for 2017. Available at: https://nces.ed.gov/fastfacts/display.asp?id=372. Accessed January 17, 2018.

abuse, attention deficit/hyperactivity, eating, sleep, and psychotic disorders. The impact on the lives of students and their social surround of coexisting with an array of serious psychiatric disorders is profound. This effect is exacerbated by the growing gulf between the enormous need for accessible, high-acuity mental health services and the severely limited availability of such expertise and resources on college campuses.[4,5]

Adding to the overwhelming demand for mental health services for both undergraduate and graduate students is the fact that the crisis of mental illness itself and the students who suffer serious psychiatric conditions tend to be disavowed, feared, and marginalized on campus. Keeling and associates[6] have observed that the determinants that drive the vertical organization of colleges and universities into disciplines, departments, and stand-alone programs are amplified by centrifugal forces that serve to decentralize "governance, responsibility, and resources peripherally." Anyone familiar with the action-oriented environment of an emergency room is conversant with the strength and velocity of the "centrifugal forces" that propel patients presenting with mental health issues, first, from medical staff to any available mental health professional and then, as quickly as possible out the door in a phenomenon sometimes described as "turbo turfing." Having to deal with depressed, angry, and potentially dangerous students suffering from mood, anxiety, substance abuse, and eating disorders, or trauma secondary to sexual assault, or an episode of psychosis may be the example par excellence of a "responsibility" predestined to be denied, ignored, and—most dangerously of all—underresourced by college leaders, administrators, and, paradoxically at times, college medical and mental health service professionals themselves.

Rahm Emanuel, Chief of Staff in the crisis-filled days of the Obama administration's first term, is famously said to have observed, "There was *no blueprint or how-to manual* for fixing a global financial meltdown, an auto crisis, two wars and a great recession, all at the same time" (emphasis added). University leaders, student affairs staff, and college mental

---

[4]Kwai I: "The Most Popular Office on Campus." *Atlantic Monthly,* October 19, 2016. Available at: https://www.theatlantic.com/education/archive/2016/10/the-most-popular-office-on-campus/504701/. Accessed January 17, 2018.

[5]Xiao H, Carney DM, Youn SJ, et al.: "Are We in Crisis? National Mental Health and Treatment Trends in College Counseling Centers." *Psychological Services* 14(4):407–415, 2017.

[6]Keeling RP, Underhile R, Wall AF: "Horizontal and Vertical Structure: The Dynamics of Organization in Higher Education." *Liberal Education* 93(4):22–31, 2007.

health professionals responding to students struggling with suicidality, overdoses, panic attacks, acute intoxication, postrape trauma, psychotic episodes, and the ubiquitous stresses of modern college life experience daily a similar scarcity of practical, evidence-based, actionable wisdom. *Until now that is.*

Dr. Laura Roberts and her more than two score experts have begun a much-needed dialogue with college health specialists about *how to* conceptualize, diagnose, treat, and manage a comprehensive spectrum of mental disorders and age-appropriate developmental issues that touch the physical, emotional, psychological, interpersonal, and social lives of college students. It takes only a brief scan of the table of contents and essential topics covered in this valuable work to grasp the magnitude of the challenge facing mental health professionals and their colleagues in college settings.

In a more perfect higher education world, certain "horizontal" forces (i.e., the collaborative efforts and resources of university leaders; student affairs staff; faculty; academic counseling, coaching, public safety and health services professionals; students; and families; etc.) would offer some counterbalance to the powerful fear and loathing that students with personality disorders and depressed, suicidal, psychotic, and potentially violent students can evoke. Marshaling these countervailing forces and therapeutic efforts underlies the choice of subjects covered in this guide. There is also a shared set of values on the part of the authors, including an authentic desire to lessen the burden of illness on students with mental health disorders; the wish to prevent tragedy and loss of human life on campus; the reasonable hope of managing institutional risk; and a growing sense of shared responsibility among a generation of academic, student affairs, and mental health professionals committed to proactive engagement with students coping with mental disorders and developmental crises.

The authors address a set of topics all too often dreaded, disregarded, and left unaddressed (e.g., first-episode psychoses, neurodevelopmental disorders, post–sexual assault trauma, outreach to special student populations) and moves them to the center of an indispensable consideration of how to help students coexist with and remain academically active in spite of the expression of serious mental disorders and developmental crises during their college years.

Student Mental Health makes an invaluable contribution to the canon of mental health practice in higher education. It does so in three ways: First, it identifies and explicates key areas of developmental, object relations, stress management, resilience, and risk reduction theories relevant to the lives of college students. Second, it details the clinical competencies required of caregivers to diagnose and manage students with serious disorders and developmental stresses. Third, it provides philosophical and therapeutic rationales for developing programs not only intended to protect students, the academic surround, and the larger campus community from harm but also designed to give students with mental health challenges an opportunity to not merely *survive* their college or graduate school experience, but to *flourish* and *excel*.

I'll close with one final but not insignificant caveat concerning this essential guide. The clinical and programmatic expertise offered in this volume will be most powerfully effective when its *blueprints and how-to's* are applied within the context of a fully actualized campus ecology model.[7,8] An ecological approach assumes that mental and physical health and well-being are interwoven with all aspects of campus life and campus infrastructures. This perspective advances the notion that a necessary "first principle" to the understanding of and response to any particular health- or wellness-related issue is consideration of the interplay of multiple components of the campus environment. This interplay occurs in the context of and among the *inhabitants* (students, faculty, administration, nonacademic staff, alumni, trustees, parents, etc.); the nature of the *academic environment* (e.g., community college, large public institution, research university); the *physical environment* (e.g., whether the school is a residential or commuter college); the *cultural environment* (e.g., socioeconomic, gender, ethnic, and religious demography of the students, staff, and faculty); the *sociodevelopmental environment* (e.g., a "late adolescent" social structure in a traditional 4-year college and/or adult students with their own families matriculating in a community college); and *the values, norms, and traditions of the university community* (e.g., among undergrads, whether the meme of "cool" is to "Work hard, then party hard"; for the academic enterprise, whether the relative importance of preparing students to be deeply engaged citizens of the

---

[7]National Association of Student Personnel Administrators: *Leadership for a Healthy Campus: An Ecological Approach for Student Success.* Washington, D.C., National Association of Student Personnel Administrators, 2004. Available at: http://www.kvccdocs.com/KVCC/2013-Spring/FY125-OLA/content/L-18/ HealthyCampus.pdf. Accessed January 17, 2018.

[8]Moses K, Schoenfield D, Swinford P, Grizzell J: "Healthy Campus: Reintroducing the Ecological Model and Collaboration for Student Learning Outcomes" (webinar). Washington, D.C., National Association of Student Personnel Administrators, Health in Higher Education Knowledge Community, 2011. Available at: https://www.acha.org/HealthyCampus/HealthyCampus/Ecological_Model.aspx. Accessed January 17, 2018.

larger world is more or less salient than preparation for prestigious professional vocations).

The ecological perspective both assists in identification of the key stakeholders for any particular issue related to the health and well-being of the larger community and fosters recognition of potential approaches to needs assessment, policy formation, resource allocation, and programmatic responses.

Building a robust college mental health program must be based in a shared and integrated administrative structure, collaborative training of all relevant university professionals, and campus-wide outreach initiatives that facilitate regular and real-time communication between all key constituents responsible for promoting the safety, health, and well-being of students. The virtues of such a model include a collective ownership of the responsibility for creating a safe and supportive campus environment, responsiveness to emotional distress and suffering, and the ability to help students function academically while living with their mental health conditions and negotiating key developmental tasks (e.g., coping with academic stress, forming cohesive sexual and gender identities, developing capacity for intimate adult relationships).

In an ecological approach, the desired *behavioral* and *educational student success outcomes* (e.g., personal maturation, active societal engagement, academic mastery, on-time graduation) are neither exclusively nor by default the domain of the deans who deal with crises and conduct issues, the academic cohort, or university health service clinicians, but rather are "owned" by an integrated, actively communicating campus consortium of students, families, university leaders, academic staff, and mental health professionals. With the publication of *Student Mental Health*, that coalition of key campus stakeholders now have an invaluable set of *"blueprints"* and *"how-tos"* to guide their deliberations, decisions, and actions.

Daniel C. Silverman, M.D., M.P.A.

Santa Fe, New Mexico, 2017

Preface

THE lives of university students are filled with immense promise. These young people have access to educational resources and opportunities, as well as access to teachers, mentors, counselors, and staff. These students become part of an academic community dedicated to learning and, often, to social change. Yet, while engaging in this community, university students often struggle. They struggle to be healthy. They struggle to find and grow into themselves during a time of remarkable emotional and physical development. They struggle to begin their adult lives in a complex world with a sense of self-knowledge, competence, belonging, and well-being. They struggle as they make decisions that will affect their future as well as the futures of others. Typically, they do all of this during a short period of life, roughly between ages 16 and 30, when potential vulnerability to mental illness and distress is heightened. It is not easy for these young people or for those who are entrusted with educating them and supporting them through their university experience.

This book has been created to help psychiatrists, psychologists, and campus leaders—who may be students themselves or senior administrators—as they work to build a university culture that supports the health, resilience, and maturation of students. The book is organized into four parts: an overview, life transitions and the university student experience, caring for university students with mental health issues, and fostering mental health for distinct university student populations. Unless specified otherwise, the terms *college, university,* and *school* will be used interchangeably and are meant to be inclusive of most campus-based institutions of higher education. The descriptions of people in the book are hypothetical. Any resemblance to actual people is completely by chance, and names in the case examples were chosen randomly.

Overall, the book covers topics related to safety, respect, conflict, and connection on campus, as well as students' evolving relationships with family, friends, and romantic partners. Positive self-care activities that students may adopt in relation to sleep, nutrition, and exercise are an important emphasis of this work and are offered with the hope that these activities will become lifelong habits and self-management strategies toward optimal health. The topics of self-care and the prevention of emotional exhaustion in clinicians who work closely with students are also covered in the text.

Because the needs of young people today are quite different from the needs of young people even 5 years ago, this book pays great attention to the specific issues encountered in caring for today's students who experience distress or develop significant mental health conditions. Some of these issues are quite difficult, including responding to students who are experiencing suicidality, newly emergent psychosis, problems associated with substance misuse, the health risks of eating disorders, and the devastation of sexual assault.

This book also focuses on experiences and concerns of individuals who belong to distinct and vitally important student populations. Examples include student athletes, graduate students, students of color, LGBTQ students, students who are among the first generation in their families to attend college, students who are veterans or active military personnel, and medical students. Along with the chapter authors, I hope that this additional material will be helpful in overcoming a common problem on many university campuses—that is, that students who do not identify with mainstream campus populations may be overlooked, and their mental health and well-being needs may not be properly addressed.

Student Mental Health: A Guide for Psychiatrists, Psychologists, and Leaders Serving in Higher Education is the result of a sustained collaboration of scholars, leaders, clinicians, educators, and learners based primarily out of Stanford University, an institution of higher education that is deeply committed to student health and well-being. The authors come from many different disciplines and perspectives, which will, I hope, greatly enrich and strengthen the contribution that the text may make.

My intent in developing a book of this nature is informed by many aspects of my life. It is inspired by my clinical work as a psychiatrist and my role as a university leader responsible for clinical, educational, research, and community-based programs in the service of students. It is enriched by my nearly 30 years of teaching and of research on student health and professionalism. And it is grounded in my experiences as a mother, aunty, and mentor to many, many young people. I feel such compassion for these remarkable young people who must shoulder so much, both for themselves and for us, and who are so unprotected from the hardships and distorting influences that seem to be shaping everyday life at this precise moment in history. The prevalence of dystopian literature suggests that I am not alone in this concern, yet one need only spend an hour on any university campus to feel inspired, reassured, and hopeful for the future. Our faith in young people is well placed. Even so, our responsibilities to nurture students and create a constructive community to sustain and support them are also greater than in the past. This book is one small gesture toward these aims.

Laura Weiss Roberts, M.D., M.A.
Stanford, California, 2017

Acknowledgments

I wish to express my heartfelt appreciation to John Etchemendy, Ph.D., Ira Friedman, M.D., and Stephanie Kalfayan, Ph.D., of Stanford University, for their extraordinary service and their dedication to students on our campus and elsewhere throughout the world.

I also thank Kendra Dority, Ph.D., Katie Ryan, M.A., Ann Tennier, E.L.S., and Gabrielle Termuehlen, members of my team who engage in every scholarly project with utmost professionalism and invaluable expertise. The wonderful team at American Psychiatric Association Publishing, Books Division, whom I also consider to be "my team," has made this book far better, and I thank them too. It is my great fortune to have the privilege to work with such very fine colleagues each day.

PART I

Overview

CHAPTER 1

Student Mental Health

Douglas L. Noordsy, M.D.
Laura Weiss Roberts, M.D., M.A.

Transition-Age Youth at the Intersection of Stress and Vulnerability

This book is inspired by the experiences of students and parents who have embarked on college journeys that have been disrupted by mental health problems. Our culture views college as a time of transition and a rite of passage, a time of discovery and a step toward a life of purpose—and possibly a paycheck. The college years are a period of bonding with peers, strengthening one's sense of self, and practicing roles of increasing responsibility and independence.

For some young people, early experiences on a college or university campus can inspire confidence, but for other students, the early experiences are quite the opposite. Some students struggle to get out of bed, miss class, fail to complete assignments, and get lost in thought, substance use, disordered eating, and destructive behaviors toward themselves and communal property. Some do not return for the next term. Others take longer to graduate. Some drop out. Some engage in dangerous behaviors that put their lives at risk. These students are not getting off track for direct academic reasons; they are talented, intellectually capable individuals who have been selected by their colleges and universities for their achievements. Moreover, young people at this moment in history are highly, perhaps overwhelmingly, connected and exposed through social media and digital communication—they are saturated with images and messages of varying origins, and their lives are highly shaped by these influences that are rapidly and powerfully communicated. Students on university and college campuses may experience heightened racial, socioeconomic, and political division, which at times produces unprecedented distress and mistrust toward institutions, elders, and one another. All of these young adults—students who have clear strengths but who face extraordinary and new challenges—are in the midst of the highest-risk period of life for the onset of psychiatric disorders.

THE STRESS-VULNERABILITY MODEL

The onset of psychiatric disorders is best understood using the stress-vulnerability model. None of the major psychiatric disorders results from a singular genetic mutation or inheritance. As individuals, we acquire vulnerability to the development of psychiatric disorders through the accumulation of polygenic risk (Duncan et al. 2017). Thus, the accumulation of variation in single-nucleotide polymorphisms throughout our genome creates some level of risk for developing specific psychiatric disorders for each of us. In other words, it is normal to have one of two, three, or four possible amino acids at specific locations throughout one's DNA, and this variability either raises or lowers an individual's risk for developing major depression, addiction, or schizophrenia. Each of these variations changes one's risk by a small amount, but that risk adds up with variability at other sites to create an individual's overall risk, or vulnerability, for developing a psychiatric disorder. The risk for developing a specific psychiatric disorder is highly correlated with risk for other psychiatric disorders and moderately correlated with some general medical disorders and some physical and personality traits

(Duncan et al. 2017). However, genetic factors account for only about half of the likelihood of developing a psychiatric disorder.

Most psychiatric disorders are quiescent during early childhood, and most people are unaware of their vulnerability to developing a disorder. It is only as people grow and develop that psychiatric disorders begin to emerge, most commonly during their teens and twenties. The brain is changing rapidly during this time period, pruning synapses and neurons and myelinating axons. Our brains are designed to be broad networks when we are young, capable of absorbing a wide range of material and developing in many directions. We might call this a horizontal emphasis in early childhood. As we transition to an adult brain, there is a shift toward making the circuits that we use regularly as efficient as possible and pruning out unused capacity. We might call this a vertical emphasis in the adult brain. However, this transition can be disruptive, as evidenced in the tumult of the typical adolescent development process. It has been hypothesized that in those who develop psychiatric disorders, either the pruning process may be dysregulated or the normal pruning process uncovers vulnerabilities.

Stress commonly triggers or hastens the expression of biological and psychosocial vulnerability—and it is clear that stress is dramatically increasing in the lives of transition-age youth. The stakes get higher as a young person moves through high school to college as a young adult. University students who are individuating are attempting to navigate social and academic pressures with less reliance on others. They experience intense romances that sometimes fail. They attempt to join social groups that sometimes let them down. Their families are changing and growing older, and they may experience losses. Substance use becomes more common and more intense as students congregate in university settings. Head injuries are common in sports and accidents. Time pressures lead to sleep deprivation, poor nutrition, and lack of self-care. All of these environmental factors have been associated with triggering the onset of psychiatric disorders.

THE PERFECT STORM

The university is an immersion experience designed to maximize opportunities for engagement, stimulation, and growth, which carries with it inherent stress on the individual who is trying to take it all in. Students embark on their college journey just as their vulnerability to onset of psychiatric disorders is peaking, family supports are fading, and their brains are undergoing transformation. This intersection of individuation and maturation explains both why the college experience is so powerful for those who make it through, and why it is such a "perfect storm" for those who experience onset of a psychiatric disorder.

Shifting Center of Support

Attending a university is typically the most concrete step for transition-age youth in moving from childhood into adult life. For many families, this step represents the beginning of offspring leaving home. Students shift from living with their parents to living in a dorm, with roommates or alone. Transition-age youth are already in the midst of shifting their primary alliances from family to friends, and the move from family home to university dorm consolidates that process. This shift means that parents are at a distance, and students revel in the freedom from parental supervision. However, with that freedom often comes the loss of daily contact with those who provided unconditional caring and support.

DECISION VALIDATION

Students attending a university join a community of similar age individuals who live, work, and play together. Daily decisions about self-care that may have been largely in the background, determined in part by structured schedules and family routines, are now up to the student to figure out. Students affiliate with friends in their dorm, sorority, or team, and daily rhythms are driven in part by the group. Sleep is commonly compromised by late nights studying and socializing, roommates' activities, and the constant presence of peers. Substance use is influenced by peer pressure, and experimentation with both quantities of substances and types of substances is common. Nutrition may not be first in mind as students eager to affiliate join their friends in finding cheap food and late-night pizzas. Physical exercise facilities are generous on most campuses, with a range of casual and organized sports options typically available, and yet, only a small number of students find themselves part of an organized sports team that provides a training schedule. Exercise may fall to the wayside when time is pressured and when academic, club, and social activities take center stage.

FRIENDS, FOR BETTER AND FOR WORSE

One of the most compelling aspects of the university experience is forming deep and lasting friendships with classmates. The opportunities for social engagement and affiliation on college campuses are great. These peer relationships can provide tremendous support and encouragement, and they can foster a sense of belonging and value, filling the student's reservoir of strength and self-esteem. But these peer relationships also have potential to be transient, volatile, or even destructive. At a minimum, the reference group shift from nuclear family to peers leaves students relying on others at a similar stage of maturation for support and decision validation. Unfortunately, some campus social groups encourage unhealthy behaviors and may normalize or facilitate excess substance use, poor sleep habits, and procrastination. In the worst instances, these groups may also reinforce negative alliances in which some students are in the "in crowd" and others are not, some students are devalued or objectified, and some even become victims of student-on-student violence. Although students may naturally enjoy the freedom of their newfound independence from home, they soon may find that it is challenging to maintain healthy habits and a positive mind-set in an environment where everyone else seems to be making different decisions.

Identity Change, Experimentation, and Pushing the Limits

Transition-age youth are in the midst of robust identity adaptation and revision. Trying on various identities and learning one's limits support the maturational process. College is a time of identity change, experimentation, and pushing the limits. This process may be exhilarating precisely because it is emotionally and physically "dangerous." As students join the campus environment, they have an opportunity to shed who they were and find out who they can become. These young adults are defined less by their family of origin and more by their interests, skills, and relationships. Students might stay up all night, drink to blackout, go to wild concerts, try out rock climbing, engage in campus protest, or find out how they respond to a psychedelic drug. Even those students who are not doing these things are hearing about them because others are engaging in and talking about these behaviors.

MIND-BODY HEALTH

Student mental health is naturally embedded in student health, both individually and institutionally. Maintaining a healthy body supports a healthy mind. University student health centers take care of the common health conditions of young adults, such as upper respiratory infections, sexually transmitted diseases, and injuries. These largely preventable conditions are made more prevalent by the extreme lifestyles of students. An injury or an infectious disease can precipitate a spiral of missing class, getting behind on assignments, and feeling overwhelmed. Maintaining physical health will support maintaining mental health. Most universities take steps to support wellness on their campuses, but these messages struggle to penetrate the student culture of experimentation. Psychiatrists and other mental health professionals serving students play an important role in helping students to understand mind-body health during this critical developmental phase of young adult life.

SELF-CARE, NUTRITION, EXERCISE, SUBSTANCE USE, AND SLEEP

As decision making about daily routines shifts and supervision declines in the residential university environment, self-care habits become a juggling act. Students repeatedly set targets for sleep, exercise, and substance use, only to have them disrupted by the next big event, such as when everyone is going out for the night or the university team is playing a big game out of town. Engagement with social media and use of online resources that are seemingly endless further threaten self-care. Students' schedules also may change substantially each term, and within a term, students may have one day with many classes and the next with few or none. Academic work shifts from supervised, classroom-based instruction to discussion-based classes paired with voluminous reading assignments and longitudinal projects. The "flipped" classroom approach puts even more responsibility on learners to manage their out-of-class time effectively. This freedom ideally contributes to the development of robust lifelong learning habits, but it also creates a lot of opportunity for students to get behind and feel overwhelmed. Managing personal health, sleep, nutrition, and exercise in a low-structure environment can be challenging on two extremes: students commonly describe the problem of having too much time, which leads to distraction, procrastination, and substance use, alternating with having too much to do, leading to cramming, sleep deprivation, eating junk food, and inactivity. Self-care suffers during both extremes.

Challenges of Early Identification

Initial symptoms of a psychiatric disorder are often vague or hard to discern. These symptoms may be difficult for individuals and those around them to distinguish from their usual life variation. For students, sleep, energy, and motivation may be constantly in flux, and transition-age youth have yet to set ingrained routines. Change is normal in the college environment, and there is plenty of social encouragement to keep a person seemingly functional by outward appearance. The good news about these less established symptoms is that they are more amenable to prevention and treatment. The bad news is that they are harder to recognize.

Students live in a subculture somewhat isolated from the authority figures around them. Protecting one's friends with problems from detection by the adults remains the predominant developmental mind-set. When students skip class or end up sobbing after drinking too much, who wants their friends telling teachers, dormitory heads, or administrators? Students are confused by the changes they are experiencing in themselves and the behaviors of those around them. In this fast changing, dramatic, and often chaotic environment, students are struggling to keep up with the demands of their academic program and social lives, and their relationships with faculty and administrators have an inherent element of judgment about performance. Taking time to carefully consider their own psychological health and that of their peers often may not make it to the top of their list of concerns.

Students and university staff also lack knowledge about the signs and symptoms of psychiatric disorders. Early signs are often nonspecific or amorphous, and even well-trained mental health professionals may not be versed in recognizing prodromal or initial symptoms of common psychiatric disorders such as mood, anxiety, and psychotic disorders. Sleep disruption, for example, strongly predicts onset of a psychiatric disorder. Fatigue is a common symptom of depression in male individuals, whereas dysphoria is more common in female individuals. Depression, anxiety, and impairment in attention and concentration are common initial symptoms of schizophrenia. These indicators, so obvious in retrospect, are hard to differentiate from the very wide spectrum of more normative experiences and behaviors of young adult students.

Universities also struggle with striking a balance between respecting students as adults and communicating with families. Parents and caretakers become frustrated when they find out that a pattern of academic and functional changes has gone on for months without intervention or notification. Parents are often in the best position to support a student in arranging care, but universities do not ask students for their preferences regarding release of information about their functioning or medical care to their family. When friends are confused and families unaware, the burden typically falls on students and the student health service to identify the onset of a disorder. For students who are developing psychiatric symptoms for the first time, this is a tall obstacle to overcome.

When students do identify a mental health problem, gaining access to care remains a substantial barrier. Stigma surrounding psychiatric disorders leads many students to dismiss their symptoms or to try to resolve them on their own. If they do seek care, locating a clinician while at school can be daunting. Many student health programs are woefully understaffed and underresourced. Students with experience using mental health care or families willing to seek out a clinician have a relative advantage, but identifying a clinician who accepts an individual's insurance is often difficult in the best circumstances. University student health services are typically oriented toward crisis management and brief interventions, and they usually refer students outside the university for ongoing care. This orientation toward crisis and brief intervention services followed by referral means that there can be discontinuities in care. Moreover, off-campus referral for longitudinal care can be a challenge for students who may not have access to transportation or who may be struggling to manage their schedules. Finding a clinician who is both accessible and an expert in early identification, prevention, and treatment for transition-age youth can be an even greater, and in some circumstances nearly insurmountable, obstacle to appropriate mental health care.

Psychiatric disorders are very common. Over a quarter of the U.S. population will experience a psychiatric disorder in a given year, with about half experiencing a psychiatric disorder at some point during their lifetime (Kessler et al. 2005). Psychiatric disorders are currently the second leading cause of disability worldwide, and they are expected to become the leading cause by 2020 (Demyttenaere et al. 2004). However, these disorders begin much earlier in life than is often recognized (Insel and Fenton 2005). Half of all psychiatric disorders have onset by age 14 and three-quarters by age 25 (Kessler et al. 2005). Psychiatric disorders are currently the leading cause of disability for transition-age youth (Gore et al. 2011). Tragically, the Centers for Disease Control and Prevention (2013) identified suicide as the second leading cause of death for adolescents and young adults, emphasizing the mortality risk associated with mental disorders in this period of life.

Although there is some evidence for an increase in prevalence of psychiatric disorders in adolescence (McGorry et al. 2007), the high prevalence of psychiatric disorders in transition-age youth is not new. Nearly 20% of young adults ages 18–25 report experiencing a psychiatric disorder, and nearly 30% report a psychiatric or substance use disorder in the prior year (Center for Behavioral Health Statistics and Quality 2015). This age group represents the highest incidence, prevalence, and burden of psychiatric disorders across the lifespan (McGorry 2005; Murray et al. 2013). However, 18- to 25-year-olds are significantly less likely than other adults to receive mental health services (Kessler et al. 2005). Young adults often may be uninsured, have few resources, and have significant debt (Collins et al. 2012). It is also increasingly recognized that there is a large population of homeless students who lack family or economic resources but who are seeking to improve their situation despite extraordinary stress and living in conditions of tremendous adversity (Goldrick-Rab et al. 2017). These individuals are among the most vulnerable and least likely to be able to access necessary mental health services.

Psychiatric disorders have represented a silent epidemic in young adults for far too long. The problem is based not in a sudden explosion of psychiatric disorders in college students, but rather in the recognition that psychiatric disorders have been quietly disrupting the progress, productivity, and achievement of bright, talented young people for far too long. To address this epidemic, many efforts are needed to engage the systems in which young people live, work, and learn to build the capacity to more effectively identify and treat their psychiatric disorders. Moreover, the aim of such care should be far more than mere symptom reduction; it should be true recovery that allows affected individuals to maintain their social and vocational networks and prevent this massive loss of productive life years.

Role of the University

UNIVERSITY CULTURE

University culture is based on selectivity. The value of a university degree is based on the premise of passing the tests. Universities amass talented faculty to teach and to evaluate. University graduates have been evaluated by a series of accomplished professors who certify their capability. Assisting students to get higher scores on a graduate entrance examination or grades in a class would in most circumstances be viewed as cheating. Universities must live up to families' trust in stewarding their children while upholding rigorous standards that support a strong reputation with graduate schools and employers. Acutely aware of the problem of low graduation rates, universities have typically concentrated on academic support for struggling students. Like most institutions, universities focus on their expertise: academics and learning. Most universities have traditionally held the position that their responsibility has been to maintain a rigorous academic environment and that students who are struggling should take leave until they are prepared to perform in that environment. It is up to the student to get well enough to return to the challenges of academia.

The uncomfortable truth that the primary cause of disability in people ages 15–25 is psychiatric disorder has not entered into university discourse until recently. From a public health perspective, these transition-age youth also face the greatest barriers to access to mental health services. A basic tenet of public health efforts is to identify the onset of a progressive, relapsing disorder and initiate treatment as soon as possible in order to prevent accumulation of disability and improve treatment response. However, university service systems do not deliver screening and early intervention for psychiatric services well, and universities are not leading the charge.

This problem is embedded in the larger context of the U.S. health care system. The fee-for-service model struggles broadly to embrace primary and secondary prevention efforts that make sense at a population health level but do not yield direct revenues to support clinical services. University student health centers and wellness campaigns uncomfortably straddle population health and fee-for-service sector models as they attempt to meet the needs of students during their time on campus. Universities, like other U.S. institutions, cringe at the financial risks of taking responsibility for the health outcomes of people in their community.

HIDDEN CURRICULUM

Students experience a hidden curriculum within universities: the need to excel in multiple domains related to their future career opportunities. There is a palpable expectation of success; stories abound of the accomplishments of recent graduates. Students feel pressure to achieve high marks in their courses; engage in clubs, sports, and social organizations; arrange study abroad; prepare for graduate entrance examinations; and line up internships and summer jobs that will strengthen their career path. In short, they feel a need to be perfect. Social media appear to reinforce this view. Students may panic when they fall short of perfection and experience feelings of failure and a rupture from their peer group or social milieu that can lead to suicidal thoughts. Students experiencing psychiatric disorders often find their distress compounded by failure to achieve important benchmarks and can quickly fall behind in preparing for a career.

Universities bear the responsibility of balancing the obligation to support and educate while at the same time ensuring standards of excellence. The hidden curriculum is a natural consequence of the desire of universities to demonstrate the value they bring to students' lives. Universities are grappling with the reality of psychiatric disorders as a major cause of disruption in their students' lives, including the students' ability to remain in school and to be academically successful. University leaders find that they must figure out how to help students continue in school while actively managing a psychiatric disorder and how to address the hidden curriculum so that the university can acknowledge and support various paths to success. Some universities have begun to organize seminars and events, such as the Stanford Resilience Project, that focus on the value of failure in personal and career development to combat the perception that the only route to life accomplishment is unblemished success (Stanford University 2016).

A Call to Action

Every one of us, no matter our circumstance, is touched by the personal and societal impact of mental illness.

Laura Weiss Roberts (2017)

This book is designed to bring together thought leaders from throughout psychiatry and university health to respond to the challenge of changing the status quo. Centuries of tradition are embedded in the undergraduate and graduate education systems—traditions of setting high standards and then evaluating, weeding out, and bestowing degrees on those who pass the test. The higher education community is already engaged in assessing the value of these pedagogical traditions in preparing people for careers in the modern world. Mental health professionals and university leaders have a responsibility to advance similar engagement in evaluating the role of student mental health as a major contributor to disrupted educational achievement and to foster a sense of responsibility for the outcomes of sons, daughters, brothers, sisters, and classmates who experience these unfortunate barriers to linear progress. These individuals deserve consideration as members of the university community, and they deserve the opportunity to complete their education.

When the White House used the clout of federal funding in the mid-2010s to force universities to attend to the uncomfortable issues around sexual assault on campus, it created a shift in the dynamics of responsibility for student health outcomes. This moment in U.S. history opened an opportunity for identifying the range of mental health needs among university students and for designing new approaches to meet those needs.

We, the contributors to this volume, seek to support the efforts of psychiatrists and other mental health professionals who serve in university mental health programs to help their students to do well. We also wish to provide evidence and wise practices that may inform novel approaches that ensure greater mental health on our college and university campuses. Finally, we hope to stimulate a much-needed conversation about how to maximize the value of university education through incorporating thoughtful, sophisticated approaches to optimizing student mental health.

KEY CONCEPTS

- University students are living at the intersection of substantial stress and peak lifetime vulnerability to developing psychiatric disorders.

- University students are developmentally in the midst of a shifting center of support, identity change, and experimentation, all of which increase their risk for health problems.

- Psychiatric disorders are difficult to detect because of amorphous, gradual onset; lack of knowledge; and stigma.

- Mental health services are least accessible to transition-age youth despite psychiatric disorders being the leading cause of disability in this age range.

- Leaders in higher education and mental health professionals have an opportunity to come together to improve outcomes for students with psychiatric disorders.

Discussion Questions

1. Why should universities pay particular attention to student mental health?

2. What is the most common age at onset for psychiatric disorders?

3. Why are early identification and treatment of a psychiatric disorder important?

4. Why are university campuses important places to identify transition-age youth who are developing psychiatric disorders?

5. Why is student mental health such a big problem now?

Suggested Reading

McGorry PD: 'Every me and every you': responding to the hidden challenge of mental illness in Australia. Australas Psychiatry 13:3–15, 2005

References

Center for Behavioral Health Statistics and Quality: Behavioral Health Trends in the United States: Results From the 2014 National Survey on Drug Use and Health (HHS Publication No SMA 15-4927, NSDUH Series H-50). Rockville, MD, Center for Behavioral Health Statistics and Quality, 2015

Centers for Disease Control and Prevention (CDC): Web-Based Injury Statistics Query and Reporting System (WISQARS), 2013. National Center for Injury Prevention and Control, CDC (producer). Available at: https://www.cdc.gov/injury/wisqars/index.html. Accessed July 20, 2017.

Collins SR, Robertson R, Garber T, Doty MM: Young, uninsured, and in debt: why young adults lack health insurance and how the Affordable Care Act is helping: findings from the Commonwealth Fund Health Insurance Tracking Survey of Young Adults, 2011. Issue Brief (Commonw Fund) 14:1–24, 2012 22679639

Demyttenaere K, Bruffaerts R, Posada-Villa J, et al; WHO World Mental Health Survey Consortium: Prevalence, severity, and unmet need for treatment of mental disorders in the World Health Organization World Mental Health Surveys. JAMA 291(21):2581–2590, 2004 15173149

Duncan LE, Shen H, Ballon JS, et al: Genetic correlation profile of schizophrenia mirrors epidemiological results and suggests link between polygenic and rare variant (22q11.2) cases of schizophrenia. Schizophr Bull Dec 27, 2017 [Epub ahead of print]

Goldrick-Rab S, Richardson J, Hernandez A: Hungry and Homeless in College: Results From a National Study of Basics Needs Insecurity in Higher Education. Madison, WI, Wisconsin HOPE Lab, March 2017. Available at: http://wihopelab.com/publications/Hungry-and-Homeless-in-College-Report.pdf. Accessed July 20, 2017.

Gore FM, Bloem PJN, Patton GC, et al: Global burden of disease in young people aged 10–24 years: a systematic analysis. Lancet 377(9783):2093–2102, 2011 21652063

Insel TR, Fenton WS: Psychiatric epidemiology: it's not just about counting anymore. Arch Gen Psychiatry 62(6):590–592, 2005 15939836

Kessler RC, Berglund P, Demler O, et al: Lifetime prevalence and age-of-onset distributions of DSM-IV disorders in the National Comorbidity Survey Replication. Arch Gen Psychiatry 62(6):593–602, 2005 15939837

McGorry P: 'Every me and every you': responding to the hidden challenge of mental illness in Australia. Australas Psychiatry 13(1):3–15, 2005 15777406

McGorry PD, Purcell R, Hickie IB, Jorm A: Investing in youth mental health is a best buy. Med J Aust 187:S5–S7, 2007

Murray CJL, Atkinson C, Bhalla K, et al; U.S. Burden of Disease Collaborators: The state of U.S. health, 1990–2010: burden of diseases, injuries, and risk factors. JAMA 310(6):591–608, 2013 23842577

Roberts LW: A message from the Chair. Stanford, CA, Department of Psychiatry and Behavioral Sciences, Stanford University School of Medicine, n.d. Available at: http://med.stanford.edu/psychiatry.html. Accessed May 2, 2017.

Stanford University: The Resilience Project, 2016. Available at: https://vptl.stanford.edu/resilience-project. Accessed May 2, 2017.

Creating a Culture of Belonging, Respect, and Support on Campus

Kyle Lane-McKinley, M.F.A.

A great deal of research points to the benefits of creating a culture of belonging, respect, and support throughout society, particularly on college campuses. Beyond the seemingly obvious and commonsensical group benefits of fostering such a culture, such as increasing group cohesion while accommodating a greater diversity of opinions, a culture of belonging has substantial mental health benefits for individuals as well. Thomas Joiner's interpersonal theory of suicidal behavior maintains that alongside the self-perception of being a burden on others, a thwarted sense of belonging is the major contributor to a desire to take one's own life (Joiner 2005). Similarly, as philosopher John Rawls convincingly argued almost half a century ago, "respect" is a primary good of human society, and we might usefully think of "justice" as merely the

17

public expression of people's respect for one another (Rawls 1971). Examined in this light, the frequently reiterated request of young people to be "shown respect" takes on the contours of a personalized demand for social justice and is a crucial component in the creation of a successful learning environment.

The numerous functions that college campuses fulfill in contemporary society necessarily present numerous, overlapping, routes toward creating a greater culture of belonging on college campuses. These routes reflect the different populations who live and work at college campuses and the variety of roles they play there. For students living on campuses, initiatives to establish the college residential setting as a site of home have an important role in producing a welcoming environment. For nonacademic staff, efforts to valorize and respect those staff members play an important role in recognizing such labors as important contributions to knowledge. For researchers, reflecting critically on the manner in which women and people of color have been historically excluded from many fields serves as a reminder of the ways that such exclusions predetermine the outcomes of inquiry by shaping the epistemological horizon of possibilities.

Role of Cultural Centers on Campus

Since the 1970s, one of the most frequent and successful attempts to create a culture of belonging for racial or ethnic minorities on college campuses has been the construction of cultural centers (Hurtado and Carter 1997). In "Latina/o Culture Centers: Providing a Sense of Belonging and Promoting Student Success," Lozano (2010) makes the case for the particularly important role that campus cultural centers can provide to Latinx students,[1] given the specific challenges that these students en-

---

[1]Throughout this chapter, I have used "Latinx" to refer to people of Latin American descent rather than the more conventional "Latina/o" that Lozano used in the 2010 work referenced here. I have done so not only because the term is more in keeping with efforts to be more inclusive of gender minorities referenced elsewhere in this chapter but also because it is in keeping with Lozano's more recent work focused specifically on the emergence of Latinx as a term (see Salinas and Lozano 2017). Indeed, the rapid shifts in preferred ethnonyms that Salinas and Lozano note there, and the contested field of race, ethnicity, language, and politics on which those shifts are playing out, is a perfect case study in the need for college educators to remain attentive to the ways in which their students and colleagues identify themselves.

counter in finding a sense of belonging elsewhere on campus. Lozano's approach is holistic, coming at the problem of low retention rates among Latinx students in terms of the wide breadth of campus culture—from institutional assumptions to dorm life. Ultimately, she concludes, quite reasonably, that Latinx cultural centers can serve an important function of providing a site for students to socialize with other members of a shared culture and for out-of-class discussion of course themes, both of which are long-held tenets in efforts to increase student retention and produce a sense of belonging on campus.

Such centers have been under threat of late, both from legislative attacks on funding for higher education and rhetorical attacks on the very idea of "safe spaces." Lozano (2010, p. 16) describes a dynamic in which budgetary pressures on higher education broadly have dramatic impacts on cultural centers and ethnic resource centers, as reduced staffing leaves such centers appearing less relevant or less vital to campus life and, consequently, vulnerable to further cuts. In an essay defending the importance of such cultural centers, Okeke (2016) highlights the role that such spaces can play in anticipating and accommodating the needs of students who suffer from conditions associated with adversity and traumatic experience. In so doing, Okeke provides useful insights into the obstacles that colleges face in attempting to create a culture of belonging across the physical spaces of campuses and offers anecdotal accounts of the manner in which cultural centers can help overcome these obstacles. The fact that such spaces are under attack should be of serious concern to anyone seeking to build a culture of belonging and inclusion on college campuses.

At the same time, if we limit our understanding of the possibilities of a culture of belonging to the confines of cultural centers and student affairs offices, we risk marginalizing these strategies from the central experience of undergraduate education: that of the college classroom. The task of creating an atmosphere of belonging and inclusion within the college classroom is something that I myself have struggled with and found some success in. These struggles and successes directly inform the strategies that I have developed or gleaned from others for effective and supportive environments of belonging and inclusion.

The Classroom as a Site of Belonging

Centering the classroom as a site of belonging has a number of advantages, foremost being the long, if uneven, history of pedagogical practices that attempt to forge a sense of belonging for a variety of types of students. The classroom also has the advantage of already being a place in which dialogue and debate are the expected norm, which means that students are relatively open to having a meta-debate about the manner in which learning and dialogue take place and thus about how we might better foster a culture of belonging in the classroom. It has been my experience that fostering such a culture within the classroom can result in binding the core teaching function of colleges to the practices of inclusivity. When we do so, we create the possibility for these practices to radiate outward from the classroom to include other aspects of college life as well.

The following strategies can be used in various ways by college educators to create a culture of belonging in the classroom. It is important to note that these are not cookie-cutter solutions; the effective application of these strategies will necessarily vary across disciplines, across geographic locations, and indeed from one educator to the next. Rather, the list is provided as a framework that includes some specific tactics that have proven helpful in my own classroom.

STRATEGY 1: ACKNOWLEDGE THE PROBLEM

The first challenge to creating a culture of belonging in the classroom is recognizing that such a culture probably does not exist already. Educators, and college professors in particular, have undergone a process of self-selection, and they very likely have experienced a sense of belonging in the classroom both now and as young scholars themselves. That experience, however, is far from universal. College instructors might *intend* for their classrooms to be welcoming and inclusive environments, but these intentions do not in themselves account for the prior experiences of students. Assumptions about who is to speak and who is to listen quietly are ingrained at a very early age and are disproportionately likely to train women, people of color, and poor or working-class students that their voices are not needed or that their perspectives are peripheral. Interrogating the assumption that the classroom is a safe space for "everyone" is therefore an important step in creating a culture of belonging in the classroom.

STRATEGY 2: ENCOURAGE DIALOGUE

The desire for dialogue is a wish to belong in the conversation. The pedagogical model of many classrooms is one of transmission of information: the teacher stands at the front of the class and broadcasts information to the many students seated in a crowd. Not only does this model fail to recognize important distinctions between the transmission of information and the shared production of knowledge, but it also overlooks the important role that speaking and being heard can have for an individual student's sense of belonging in the classroom. While it is certainly the case that the instructor, by virtue of expertise in the area of study, will speak a great deal more than the students will, increasing the role of dialogue and discussion in classrooms has a number of positive benefits, from increased sense of belonging to improved learning outcomes.

STRATEGY 3: RESPECT STUDENTS AS INDIVIDUALS

Students are individuals, with their own names, cultures, and expectations. This may seem obvious, but it bears stating, specifically because in so many college lecture halls the instructor has limited opportunity to get to know the students. Learning the names and pronouns of students can be a first step toward learning what their expectations and desires for the class might be and how the instructor can best serve those needs. Even in the context of large lecture hall teaching assignments, I have found that when I introduce myself, I can include something about how I would like to be addressed (simply by my first name, in my case) and what I prefer as my own personal pronouns (either he/him or they/them, in my case). Doing so, and attempting to learn the names of as many students as possible, sends the message that each of us belongs in the classroom and that we all are deserving of autonomy and respect.

A Frank Discussion About Gender

Mental health professionals will no doubt be familiar with the updated diagnosis of gender dysphoria in DSM-5 (American Psychiatric Association 2013) and the broader shift in thinking about gender identity and expression that it reflects in our society. It is not always obvious, however, how to effectively apply these social and clinical changes to the pedagogical practices of the classroom. The relation that students have with teachers is not the same as that between patients and clinicians. Although certain features of the two pairings may be analogous, the differences are elided at great peril. Such questions of how to create a culture in which transgender and gender-nonconforming students feel that they belong in the classroom are particularly vexing when we consider the uneven distribution of power within pedagogical spaces: the instructor's actions can go a great way to either set a tone of respect and support or to create a model of dismissiveness and derision.

Many of the strategies elaborated in this chapter have their origins in activist or community-organizing contexts and have been variously modified to better fit the context of the college classroom. Such activist milieus might be structurally characterized as embracing a high degree of horizontalism and a distaste for formal hierarchy, with a stated purpose of fostering a sense of belonging and inclusion. Because of this, and because of the outspoken presence of lesbian, gay, bisexual, transgender, and queer/questioning (LGBTQ) activists within such organizations, a number of strategies for acknowledging and respecting gender-nonconforming individuals have developed. Foremost among these is the suggestion that when individuals introduce themselves at the beginning of a meeting or event, they include a statement about their pronouns. Typically stylized as "preferred gender pronouns" or "preferred personal pronouns," the suggestion is that all individuals in the room state the pronouns that they are most comfortable with, such as he/him, she/her, or the gender-neutral singular pronouns they/ them or ze/zir. In addition to providing an opportunity to learn how to refer to everyone in the room, this practice is intended to denaturalize or call into question the assumption that gender expression is the outcome of biological sex.

Attempts to apply such strategies to the classroom are necessarily contingent on the size of the classroom. In small classes, it can work well to ask students to introduce themselves on the first day, including saying a bit, perhaps, about their cultural background and pronouns. However, even in such relatively intimate learning environments, instructors may find that students default to opting out of the request to provide personal pronouns. This can be a sticky situation: Some students may feel shy in general about talking about themselves in front of a group or an authority figure. Other students may find the request to provide personal pronouns novel or uncomfortable. Still others might be quiet on the subject because they may be grappling internally with their own questions about gender identity and gender performance. Instructors attuned to the culture of belonging will find that they need to tackle these situations on a case-by-case basis.

It is of course important to take care to avoid "outing" someone's transgender identity without their permission and to prevent gender-nonconforming individuals from being singled out in having their gender called into question. The goal is to normalize the experience of declaring pronouns for everyone, not to put special attention on transgendered or genderqueer/gender-nonconforming students. If the instructor does not know a student's pronoun, it is perfectly acceptable to ask privately and use it when referring to the student. When earnest mistakes happen, an instructor might acknowledge the misgendering, apologize, and move on, effectively sending a message of respect without making a big deal about it. Maybe most importantly, if a student misgenders another student, the instructor has the opportunity to correct the mistake either in public or one on one, either of which can provide openings for ongoing conversation.

In contrast to previous diagnoses such as gender identity disorder, the diagnosis of gender dysphoria in DSM-5 is intended to emphasize that the harm to the patient stems from the distress of the experience of dysphoria and from the social prejudices that surround transgender identity rather than from the identity itself. Therefore, it seems reasonable that those harms can be reduced by creating a culture of belonging on college campuses that is inclusive and welcoming of a variety of gender expressions and experiences.

STRATEGY 4: USE PEOPLE-FIRST LANGUAGE

One way to emphasize the shared humanity of marginalized groups is to use terms that put the personhood of individuals or groups out front, such as "people of color" or "a person who uses a wheelchair." Anecdotally, in teaching classes about race and ethnicity, I have had numerous experiences in which students confuse "people of color" with "colored people." Some of this confusion stems from an unfamiliarity with the history of derogatory language in the United States, but explaining that background can be confusing and seemingly contradictory and may entail an understanding of American history that exceeds the scope of the class. Instead, students can often understand, empathize with, and remember that anyone would want to be thought of as a person first, rather than having the whole of their identity reduced to one aspect, which is what happens when minorities are referred to as "the blacks," "the gays," "the disabled," and so on.

STRATEGY 5: STEP UP, STEP BACK

The strategy of stepping up and stepping back derives from groups that use consensus processes for decision making and encapsulates a view of the responsibilities that all participants in a conversation have to recognize the ways in which they have been socialized and to push beyond their comfort zones. In essence, the idea is that some people (disproportionately women and people of color) have been trained in school and elsewhere to keep their thoughts to themselves. These folks are encouraged to resist this training by "stepping up." At the same time, discussion in such situations tends to be dominated by folks—disproportionately white men—who have been trained that their views are always the most important. These folks are encouraged to resist that training by "stepping back" and self-monitoring how often they contribute to conversations. Ideally, this ongoing process has an effect of retraining everyone involved and creating a greater capacity for both speaking and listening. Although this strategy emerges from nonpedagogical contexts such as workers' collectives and activist groups, it has a particularly strong track record, in my experience, of conveying to students the responsibilities that we have to one another in the classroom. Moreover, I have had students come back to me years later claiming that this strategy has helped them in professional and personal contexts—for some people, it can prove a useful mantra to live by.

Reaching Out

In an article about how to support undocumented students in a political climate in which they have been threatened or targeted, Ferrera and Sanchez (2017) conclude their remarks with a suggestion to reach out to affected students, explaining that instructors "can maintain a healthy and appropriate boundary with students while still being human with them as an educator." Although Ferrera and Sanchez are providing advice that is specific to undocumented students, the general principle can be helpfully expanded to include all manners of interactions on college campuses. All too often instructors assume that students who are struggling (whether with academic problems or otherwise) will feel comfortable coming to office hours or seeking help through formal mechanisms. It has frequently been my experience that the students most in need of support need a bit of prompting to feel comfortable reaching out.

The potential importance of reaching out to students who are struggling is reinforced by what researchers refer to as "role morality." *Role morality* is the idea that we act differently depending on the role we are playing in a situation. Witnesses to inappropriate behavior in a public setting might feel a duty to respond in their role as fellow-citizens, yet, somewhat paradoxically, those same individuals might not feel a duty to respond when witnessing similar behavior in the workplace, because it is not part of their job description. Creating a culture of belonging is only possible in a campus environment of safety and community. Threats to physical safety are perhaps unlikely in the classroom itself, yet educators have a role to play there as well; by modeling behaviors that make it clear that all members of the campus community have a duty to respond to inappropriate behavior, educators can set the tone for the campus climate.

STRATEGY 6: DO NOT TAKE THE TOOLS OUT OF SOMEONE'S HANDS

When I teach sculpture classes, I often reflect on experiences I had as a young artist and of feeling ashamed and embarrassed when an instructor took a tool out of my hands to show me how to use it "correctly." This experience is one that women are disproportionately likely to have and one that is particularly likely to be replicated in technical fields that are dominated by men. I have attempted to intervene in this experience by making a rule in my classes that we never take tools out of someone else's hands without talking about it first. I might say, "Yes, that's good. Can I try it out on this area over here to demonstrate a technique?" Deploying the idea of "tools" more metaphorically, we can expand this notion to think about the ways that the instructor's attitude about how to apply a lesson may have unintended consequences on the sense of belonging in the classroom. Constructing pedagogical situations in which students are given the opportunity to deploy their knowledge or skills, without stepping in to correct imperfect responses, provides numerous benefits in the classroom: the instructor is better able to ascertain what students are learning and what they are failing to understand, the students can model their practices on each another, and individual students receive the message that their success matters.

STRATEGY 7: SPEAK FOR ONESELF

In the role of college instructor, many educators may often find it helpful to defer to discursive or institutional authority while making claims about the subjects they teach. In attempting to create a culture of belonging, however, educators are likely to be speaking outside their areas of expertise and not necessarily about the specific subjects of course instruction. When doing so, it is helpful to speak for oneself rather than on behalf of the institution. Instructors who are attuned to the emotional tenor of the classroom find that they try to use "I" statements to explain when something makes them uncomfortable, rather than projecting that discomfort onto other students or some abstract or institutional authority. In my own teaching, I frequently find that I rely on pedagogical authority when conveying technical knowledge or historically objective facts, but I attempt to switch to the first-person singular when relating an interpretation or analysis. I might, for example, demonstrate how to weld steel in a metal sculpture class with an attention to safe use of tools to create objectively strong welds, but when it comes to discussing the meaning of the artwork, my opinion is merely one voice among many, and not necessarily the most important one. Once supplied context and tools for analysis, all members of a classroom community are thus supplied equal right to form and articulate their own opinions. This strategy has the double benefit of grounding the concerns of instructors in their own individual experience and of signaling to students that their own individual experiences are worthy of respect and inclusion.

STRATEGY 8: KNOW THE AUDIENCE

The particular ethnic demographic of a given college or university may reflect geographic as well as economic factors. Similarly, the gender makeup within classrooms may vary dramatically from department to department within an institution. However, it appears uncommon that college educators think about how to customize their teaching to better match specific demographics. By learning about the life experiences of their students, college instructors may learn new lessons about their area of teaching, or even open up new research questions. At the University of California, Santa Cruz, where I taught from 2011 to 2017, diversity and inclusion efforts in recent years have resulted in a substantial increase in the percentage of the undergraduate student body that identifies as Latinx or Hispanic. I do not identify as either Latinx or Hispanic, and I am far from an authority on the art histories or visual cultures of these ethnic identities, yet my training as a digital artist has helped me to perceive those aspects of these cultures that are particularly relevant to discussions of contemporary art and cyberculture, such as the influence that Mexican mural painting and Latinx street art have had on contemporary ideas of graphic design. Valorizing such aspects of Latinx cultures in a university classroom not only provides unique inroads to the material for students who do identify as Latinx or Hispanic, but it also provides an opportunity for all of my students to think about the legacy of Latinx visual culture throughout California. Following up on these lessons with students who identify as Latinx or Hispanic has helped me hone a pedagogy that serves their needs while challenging their assumptions, even as these conversations have helped me to identify new themes and research questions for my own work.

STRATEGY 9: CREATE SAFER SPACE THROUGH CONFLICT MEDIATION

Setting aside debates about the pros and cons of so-called safe spaces on college campuses for now, it is clear that educators who are committed to a culture of belonging aspire to establish classroom environments in which all students feel safe enough to share their thoughts and to challenge one another. I refer to that atmosphere as a "safer space." One strategy for creating a safer space is to model the notion that conflict does not have to be a crisis. Despite the large and growing body of scholarship and policy dedicated to conflict mediation in K–12 educational contexts, relatively little has been written about how to mediate conflicts that occur in college classrooms. Likely, this stems from a belief that the disruptive behaviors common in compulsory K–12 education do not exist at the college level, where students attend by choice because "they want to be there." What college instructor, however, has not had a conflict with a student who is chronically late or does not pay attention because that student really does not want to be there? Conflicts arise in every classroom, and they are particularly likely to occur when instructors are effective at generating student participation by forging a culture of belonging. How an instructor responds to these conflicts will determine whether students continue to feel safe and included in future discussions. As I discussed above with regard to speaking for oneself (see strategy 7), there can be a strong impulse for instructors to rely on institutional or disciplinary authority to quash conflicts, particularly when students call into question something that the instructor presents. Yet, a reliance on external authority tends to skip over an opportunity to hear and respect the thoughts and experiences of the students in the classroom and can tend to come off as dismissive or even disrespectful. Effective mediation between students who disagree can often be as simple as repeating what the students say back to them. When an instructor listens to the position a student takes and restates it to the class, maybe pausing to note factual corrections, the student's experience is validated even as that student has the opportunity to perceive inconsistencies or problems with the position that are made more obvious by externalization. Such strategies do not necessarily resolve the conflict or result in everyone agreeing, and that is usually just as well. Real and substantive conflicts and disagreements will and should exist in college classrooms; however, when educators can act as mediators in good faith, they facilitate a process by which everyone involved can feel heard and respected, which are crucial ingredients for a culture of belonging.

Safe Space

Recent critiques of safe spaces (and of the closely related phenomena of "trigger warnings," through which instructors warn students that certain content might be emotionally challenging or may even reactivate responses to traumatic experiences) center on their supposed potential to inhibit debate or to censor controversial materials. This position is maybe best typified by a story featured in *The Atlantic* by Lukianoff and Haidt (2015). The authors' central contention is that trigger warnings and other strategies are unnecessary because "classroom discussions are safe places to be exposed to incidental reminders of trauma" in the sense that students are unlikely to be the victims of physical violence in the classroom. In other words, Lukianoff and Haidt believe that classrooms already are safe spaces, without making any changes to the historical pedagogical arrangement. It is thus worth noting that critics and advocates of safe spaces appear to be in agreement that the classroom *should* be a space in which all students are safe to learn and debate. Yet, many students, particularly women, students of color, and gender minorities, profess to feeling unsafe engaging in precisely the sorts of classroom academic debates that critics of safe spaces perceive to be under threat.

Setting aside for now the debate about the pros and cons of safe spaces, it is clear that creating a culture of belonging in the classroom entails strategies for making the classroom a *safer* space, with an acknowledgment that no shared space of learning can be safe for everyone. Although the idiom of *safe space* seems to have initially emerged within 1960s and 1970s gay and lesbian communities to refer to neighborhoods and particular bars and other establishments within them, as Hanhardt (2013) highlights in *Safe Space: Gay Neighborhood History and the Politics of Violence*, the language became fairly widespread within trauma-informed discourses of mental health by the late 1990s. The terminology gained wide acceptance in social justice organizations as well, where it signaled a commitment of participants to examine the ways they have internalized systems of oppression, as well as a desire for inclusion and a culture of belonging. More recently, however, a number of such groups have shifted to the language of "safer spaces" to recognize that, despite good intentions and best practices, triggering or retraumatizing events may happen within most any group. This logic is perhaps best typified by the language deployed by the Bluestockings Bookstore and Activist Center in New York (http://bluestockings.com/about/ safer-space), which highlights the anti-oppression framework through which their collective talks about relative safety and relative power and paints an accurate portrait of the aspirational, rather than prescriptive, character that safer space policies aim to establish. Of course, the context and power dynamics within a college classroom are quite distinct from those of an activist organization and entail a different set of strategies for envisioning and creating a safer space.

STRATEGY 10: REMEMBER THAT THE EXPERIENCE OF INCLUSIVENESS IS NOT UNIVERSAL

Educators frequently believe that it is their duty to teach to an amorphous "everyone." The notion of such an undifferentiated everyone may well stem from antiracist and antisexist impulses, yet the effect can often be to recenter the experiences of whiteness and maleness. By taking up curricula that reflect the specific cultural experiences of particularly marginalized groups, college educators can provide cultural breadth for the majority of students while specifically supporting minority students. This is a particularly important strategy for white and male educators to adopt, in recognition of the fact that they are unable to provide cultural mirrors for women and people of color: if we cannot look like or share the experiences of all of our students, we can at least make an effort to teach specifically to those whom we do not look like and with whom we do not share all experiences.

Conclusion

Creating a real culture of belonging, respect, and support on university and college campuses involves changes at many different levels—from lived experience in the dorms to federal policy. Teachers in higher education can advocate for all of those changes even as they recognize the relative autonomy that they have within their own classrooms to bring about change now. Effective strategies for creating a culture of belonging, respect, and support in the classroom are historically and geographically specific and will reflect the instructor's specific disciplinary expertise as well. Some general themes emerge, however: recognizing the problems that exist, encouraging dialogue, respecting students, and reflecting on personal experiences and teachers in higher education fostering an atmosphere of inclusion and belonging in the classroom, which will have far-reaching effects on college campuses and beyond.

KEY CONCEPTS

- Acknowledge that a culture of belonging, respect, and support does not occur automatically in a classroom.
- Encourage dialogue with students and between students.
- Respect students as individuals.
- Use people-first language.
- Step up and step back by encouraging people to share their views and, in turn, to listen to the perspectives of others.
- Do not take the tools out of someone's hands: give students the opportunity to deploy their knowledge or skills without stepping in to correct any imperfections.
- Speak for oneself rather than on behalf of the institution or an abstract authority.
- Know the demographic, geographic, and economic factors of the audience.
- Create safer space through conflict mediation.
- Remember that the experience of inclusiveness is not universal and make an effort to understand the individual experiences of students.

Discussion Questions

1. How does the culture of belonging, respect, and support surface in your work on campus?
2. What unique experiences do today's students face? How do these experiences present new challenges for today's educators, clinicians, and leaders who serve in higher education settings?
3. What are the communities in need of greater inclusion in your institution? How can you go about creating a greater culture of belonging?

Suggested Readings

Boice B: Classroom incivilities. Research in Higher Education 37:453–486, 1996

Ferrera M, Sanchez B: We have your back: how educators can support undocumented students. Diverse: Issues in Higher Education, February 13, 2017. Available at: http://diverseeducation.com/article/92592. Accessed July 20, 2017.

Hallsett M, James K: Creating a Culture of Belonging (Web site). Available at: https://cultureofbelonging.wordpress.com. Accessed July 20, 2017.

Harris M: What's a 'safe space'? A look at the phrase's 50-year history. Fusion Magazine, November 11, 2015. Available at: http://fusion.kinja.com/what-s-a-safe-space-a-look-at-the-phrases-50-year-hi-1793852786. Accessed July 20, 2017.

Meyers SA, Bender J, Hill EK, Thomas SY: How do faculty experience and respond to classroom conflict? International Journal of Teaching and Learning in Higher Education 18(3):180–187, 2006

References

American Psychiatric Association: Diagnostic and Statistical Manual of Mental Disorders, 5th Edition. Arlington, VA, American Psychiatric Association, 2013

Ferrera M, Sanchez B: We have your back: how educators can support undocumented students. Diverse: Issues in Higher Education, February 13, 2017. Available at: http://diverseeducation.com/article/92592. Accessed July 20, 2017.

Hanhardt CB: Safe Space: Gay Neighborhood History and the Politics of Violence. Durham, NC, Duke University Press, 2013

Hurtado S, Carter DF: Effects of college transition and perceptions of the campus racial climate on Latino college students' sense of belonging. Sociol Educ 70(4):324–345, 1997

Joiner T: Why People Die by Suicide. Cambridge, MA, Harvard University Press, 2005

Lozano A: Latina/o culture centers: providing a sense of belonging and promoting student success, in Culture Centers in Higher Education: Perspectives on Identity, Theory, and Practice. edited by Patton L. Sterling, VA, Stylus, 2010 pp 3–25, 2010

Lukianoff G, Haidt J: The coddling of the American mind. The Atlantic, September 2015. Available at: https://www.theatlantic.com/magazine/archive/2015/09/the-coddling-of-the-american-mind/399356/. Accessed July 20, 2017.

Okeke C: I'm a black UChicago graduate. Safe spaces got me through college. Vox, August 29, 2016. Available at: https://www.vox.com/2016/8/29/12692376/university-chicago-safe-spaces-defense. Accessed July 20, 2017.

Rawls J: A Theory of Justice. Cambridge, MA, Belknap Press of Harvard University Press, 1971

Salinas C Jr, Lozano A: Mapping and recontextualizing the evolution of the term *Latinx*: An environmental scanning in higher education. Journal of Latinos and Education Nov 16, 2017

CHAPTER 3

Strategies for Excellence in Student Health Programs

James R. Jacobs, M.D., Ph.D.

ALTHOUGH classically attributed to Amherst College in 1861, the first recognized campus-based student health service in the United States was at the U.S. Military Academy at West Point, beginning in 1830 (Christmas 2011). It was not until 1910 that Princeton University became the first to add a designated mental health service for its students (Kraft 2011). Today, most of the 4,000 or so colleges and universities in the United States, including many community colleges and professional schools, provide some combination of medical, mental health, and wellness services for their students, but the structure, scope, and quantity of services offered under the rubric of student health vary tremendously from campus to campus.

The focus of this guide is college student mental health, but the purpose of this chapter is to introduce college health more broadly and, specifically, to highlight strategies for excellence and success in the delivery of health services for college students. In this regard, and unless specified otherwise, the terms *college*, *university*, and *school* will be used interchangeably and are meant to be inclusive of most campus-based institutions of higher education. Although the terms *school health* and *student health* are often associated with school-based services for K–12 students, in this chapter *student health* and *college health* will be used interchangeably to refer to clinical and preventive health care services overseen by the institution for the college's students on the grounds of the campus.

Wherefore College Health?

An editorial appearing in the *American Medical Association Bulletin* in 1927 suggested that "[a] school…is under no more obligation to supply medical care…than it is to supply clothing, food, or any other necessities.… It should supply first aid and suitable advice in the selection of physicians when the student needs medical service. Further than this the school should not go" ("School and College Contracts" 1927, p. 137). The author of this editorial appears to be bemoaning the fixed rather than fee-for-service salary received by college health physicians. Similar concerns persist today in some quarters, nearly a hundred years later, but now the much louder voice urges provision of more and more services, particularly resources supporting student mental health and well-being. Most of the rhetoric in these regards concerns improving the safety, efficiency, and richness of the collegiate experience, but importantly, there is also an effort to distinguish the university's appeal in the ever-intensifying competition for students and benefactors.

Provision of primary care medical and mental health services for students, which the institution subsidizes to a greater or lesser extent, is justified largely on the basis of efficiency: it should be quicker and easier for students to obtain health care through an on-campus resource than they might routinely be able to accomplish by attempting to negotiate health care in the adjacent community, especially for younger students. The on-campus resource should ideally reduce cost barriers for an ill student to seek needed health care and thus make it more likely that the student will actually seek care. Further to this point, blithely expecting students to navigate use of health insurance to access health care in the community can be a morass, especially when many students are covered by a health insurance policy that provides few or no in-network benefits in the proximity of the college. For funded graduate students, access to the on-campus health services might be further subsidized by the graduate department, as a perk of sorts. Additional motivations for the institution to support on-campus student health services include public health interventions and prevention, outreach and health promotion, and a ready resource for consultation or referral by faculty and staff when a student is known or suspected to be in distress.

Student Health Program Structure

Although there is a vast clinical literature pertaining to health and wellness of college students and other young adults, there have been few scholarly efforts addressing implementation of college health services. Examples include one textbook (Turner and Hurley 2002), several textbook chapters (e.g., Van Orman and Jacobs 2016), and rare peer-reviewed articles (e.g., Patrick 1988; Prescott 2011). Importantly, the American College Health Association has published multiple relevant guidelines, including "Framework for a Comprehensive College Health Program" (www.acha.org/ACHA/Resources/Guidelines/ACHA/Resources/Guidelines.aspx; American College Health Association 2016). Also, many of the standards promulgated by the Council for the Advancement of Standards in Higher Education (www.cas.edu/standards) are applicable to student health and wellness services. The strategies for excellence in student health programs discussed in this chapter are informed by several of these guidelines but are not evidence based per se; rather, they are derived largely from the author's long-standing experience and observations.

Units of a prototypic college health service include, in broad terms, medical (as used here inclusive of nursing services), mental health (as used here inclusive of psychiatry and counseling services), auxiliary, administrative, and wellness (or health promotion), with the director of each of these units reporting to an executive director, who reports to a senior university official, such as the vice president for student affairs. In practice, there are so many variations that suggesting any prototypic arrangement is hyperbole, and, most notably for this text, it is not uncommon for the medical and mental health units to have wholly separate reporting structures and separate medical records, even if the two units reside within the same building. Integration of medical and mental health services is a topic of considerable ongoing national debate with respect to college health services (American College Health Association 2010).

Student health *medical* services are specifically oriented around primary care, although for this relatively healthy patient population the subtle differences between primary care and episodic care can be argued, especially for students who maintain relationships with physicians at home. The medical clinic ideally offers some capacity for walk-in or urgent care services, and a robust capacity for triage is required. Additional medical services might include allergy and immunization clinics, immunization compliance monitoring, and travel medicine. Some centers are able to offer on-site access to specialists, such as those in acupuncture, chiropractics, dentistry, dermatology, optometry, orthopedics, and sports medicine.

Mental health services generally include crisis intervention, assessment and referral, short-term therapy (and in rare instances long-term therapy), outreach, case management, group therapy, and postvention. In the preferred arrangement, there is a team approach involving psychologists, master's-trained therapists and social workers, and psychiatrists. It is important to appreciate, however, that many small- to medium-size college health services (and increasingly even some large organizations) have little or no psychiatric coverage, resulting in increased reliance on referral for medication management and increased demands on primary care clinicians for psychotropic prescribing.

The medical and mental health services should offer some form of year-round after-hours coverage, which increasingly is outsourced to third-party telemedicine vendors, with on-call student health services clinicians as backup.

Auxiliary services might include laboratory, radiography, pharmacy, and physical therapy services. Administrative components might include human resources, budget and finance, facilities, contracts, reception and customer service, health information management, information technology, quality management, and others. Historically, many schools have also provided front-end management of a customized student health insurance plan, but this is currently in flux.

Wellness services potentially include education and intervention around nutrition, sexual health, alcohol and other drugs, gambling, accident prevention, and increasingly—and of particular relevance to this text—elements of positive psychology, such as stress management, resilience, happiness, mindfulness, and self-compassion. Clinical and nonclinical resources around issues of sexual and relationship violence prevention and response have expanded markedly in the past 10 years and are often incorporated, at least in part, into the portfolio of student health services.

College health programs have been implemented on a spectrum that ranges from a solo nurse with a few hours per week of physician and therapist coverage up to a 200-staff multispecialty practice with 24/7 infirmary capacity for both medical and psychiatric observation. Determinants of the scale of student health services offered on a particular campus include funding, space, commuter versus residential student population, mix of undergraduate and graduate programs, proximity of primary and tertiary health care resources in the community, relationship (if any) to the institution's academic medical center, and the culture of the university. Of interest, most schools have eliminated any infirmary beds that they might have once operated, because of concerns of expense and liability, although Harvard University and Dartmouth University are notable exceptions at the time of this writing.

Strategies for Excellence

Success of a student health program is nearly assured when a thoroughly diverse and exquisitely competent staff provides a vast array of services at times and places convenient to all students, with immediate access and no out-of-pocket expense. Acknowledging that this ideal will rarely be achieved, the remainder of this chapter enumerates multiple broad and narrow strategies toward excellence in college health programs. Some of these strategies are germane to a variety of ambulatory medical practices, but each is presented in the context of college health.

It is presumed that the reader is new to, or relatively unfamiliar with, college health. For the sake of brevity, the emphasis in this section is on clinical services, but the role of wellness services is asserted at several junctures. The strategies listed below do not provide a recipe for running a student health service but rather are offered to provide context for the more focused mental health chapters that follow.

STRATEGY 1: MAXIMIZE ACCESS TO SERVICES

Although the health care sands have shifted and continue to change, the ultimate currency (the paramount measure of value) of outpatient medical and mental health practices remains the one-on-one encounter with a clinician. Short of clinical catastrophes (which do happen) and salacious scandals (which do happen), a college health service's reputation (perception of excellence) among students and their families is influenced primarily by the accessibility of services. Students want to be seen when they want to be seen, and angst emerges when the supply does not meet the demand. Additional urgency is fueled by parents, caretakers, and family members, who, many miles away, are appropriately concerned for the health, wellness, and success of their loved ones. In this pressured environment, the student health service is charged by the university with maximizing the quality and quantity of care provided to students. Excellent student health programs will weigh every policy change, every budget request, every staffing accommodation and incentive package, the scheduling of every administrative meeting or other nonclinical assignment, and every strategic initiative against the anticipated effect on student access to the services that they offer.

Medical Services

For medical services, the access challenge in student health is often about perceived need for same-day or walk-in options, but, depending on the setting, access can be more about student desire for ever-expanding evening and weekend clinic hours. Short of 24/7 operation (which only a very few college health services continue to provide), there will always be complaints. Resources are not unlimited, and there will always be mathematical limits to appointment availability, but the excellent health service will manage the schedule daily and dynamically to maximize patient access and will be ever vigilant to recognize and dismantle obstacles to optimal care.

Mental Health Services

For college mental health services, access is almost universally characterized by wait time, usually understood to be the time between initial screening (often done by phone) and the first one-on-one meeting with a therapist. A now-famous article appearing in the *Chronicle of Higher Education* (Wilson 2015) was titled "An Epidemic of Anguish." The subtitle, "Overwhelmed by Demand for Mental-Health Care, Colleges Face Conflicts in Choosing How to Respond," reflects in large part the fiscal and philosophical challenges of employing a counseling staff large enough to ensure that the wait time never exceeds some arbitrary duration. Opaque to many observers is the fact that the wait time for routine assessments and therapy is occurring in a milieu where the counseling staff is responding immediately and daily to crisis interventions, hospitalizations, and acute case management.

For college mental health services, the International Association of Counseling Services (2017) recommends an aspirational staffing ratio of "one F.T.E. [full-time-equivalent] professional staff member (excluding trainees) to every 1,000 to 1,500 students." The observation, however, is that centers that have achieved even more luxuriant staffing ratios, such as 1:750 and better, continue to confront wait times deemed unacceptable by their constituencies, and thus the "epidemic of anguish" persists. Moving forward, excellent student counseling services will maximize access by continuing to advocate for funding mechanisms that enable staffing ratios of at least 1:1,000, but these services will also maximize use of group therapy, develop novel context-appropriate treatment models such as micro-term therapy (the vast majority of students seeking care do not need even short-term duration of therapy [Center for Collegiate Mental Health 2017]), leverage emerging virtual approaches to screening and intervention, and partner with wellness professionals to provide outreach and education (e.g., resilience training) that achieves prevention or intervention for students who are struggling but who do not need clinical intervention.

Communicating the Access Message

> A student has had a sore throat for several days. The student's mother, 500 miles away, has been imploring the student to "go to student health to get checked out to make sure you don't have strep." The student walks in to the health center at 5 minutes prior to closing and is seen briefly by a triage nurse, who schedules him for an appointment at 8:30 A.M. the next day. Before the student has even exited the building, he is texting his mother that student health refused to see him, just as his roommate had predicted. The mother is frustrated and frightened, instructs her son to go immediately to an urgent care clinic 2 miles from campus, and calls university administration the next day angrily asking why her son was turned away from the student health center.

When students are in distress and when parents (who may be at a distance) are concerned, there is a natural expectation that student health needs will be met immediately. The idea of being "turned away" can become a volatile problem, leading to complaints to university administration. The excellent student health service will engage in continuous staff development related to serving student-patients and balancing students' health needs, reasonable access constraints, and students' wishes to be seen immediately.

STRATEGY 2: PROVIDE CLARITY OF SCOPE

By definition, the mission of a student health service is to provide health care services to the college's students, but the interconnectivity of scope and funding can be remarkably nuanced. Both of these topics are worthy of their own treatise but will be introduced only briefly here. Excluded here is discussion of the additional complication that a minority of student health services actually provide care to a broader university population, which might include faculty, staff, dependents (including infants and children), and others.

Scope of Services

Does the student health service's scope include suturing of extremity lacerations but not facial lacerations? Colposcopy but not biopsy? Stimulant prescribing but not psychoeducational testing? Administration of IV fluids but not of IV medications? Individual cognitive behavioral therapy for anxiety but not dialectical behavioral therapy groups for personality disorder? Medication and psychological support for gender transitioning? And so forth.

University administrators will usually be poorly equipped to mandate a scope of services, so a strategy regarding scope typically evolves from within the health service. In general, however, the more resources the unit has, or is perceived to have, the broader the scope is expected to be. Another way of thinking about scope is to consider the services to which the student is reasonably entitled in return for paying the mandatory health fee (if there is one; see subsection "Funding" below). A fee of $10–$25 per term probably does not entitle students to a very broad scope, but $200–$350 per term probably does. An excellent student health service will apply scope consistently, market its scope accurately and effectively, ensure staffing with sufficient expertise to execute its scope, and routinely revise scope based on evolving best practices and student demographics.

Funding

Student health services are funded through one or a hybrid of multiple mechanisms. In the most transparent approach, students pay a mandatory "health fee" each academic term, which, in the absence of other revenue sources, provides a fully capitated budget within which the health service must operate. Often the institution subvenes the health fee with additional funding or, in the absence of a designated health fee, subvenes most of the health service budget with base funding. Most centers are supplemented by a small revenue stream from purchase for resale (e.g., margins on in-clinic administration of certain medications or retail sale of crutches) and designated fees for certain specialized services (e.g., allergy shots). In general, when there is a health fee or significant subvention, health insurance is not applicable for most or any of the services provided by the health service. A small, but growing, minority of student health services do, however, operate in a traditional fee-for-service model, with billing to third-party insurance carriers, but it is virtually impossible to contract with all of the insurance carriers represented by a large or diverse student body, leaving pockets of students without in-network benefits. Further, and even under the most productive of circumstances, some amount of subvention will be required, because of the multitude of non-billable services (e.g., emergency preparedness or mental health outreach) expected of the health services staff. Regardless of the student health center's scope and funding mechanisms, to receive an appropriate standard of care, some students will likely need additional health insurance to cover services (e.g., emergency department, CT scan, specialists, care while traveling domestically or abroad) for which robust health insurance is required.

Health Insurance

In the current era, there are few topics as thorny and labile as health insurance, but for the purposes of this discussion, there are two basic considerations:

1. Does the institution require that all students have health insurance coverage? From an institutional perspective, uninsured students pose a liability to themselves and to the institution. One university, for example, started requiring proof of insurance after an undergraduate student experiencing flu-like symptoms with high fever and a rash but without health insurance chose not to go to the emergency department because of cost and then died of meningococcal meningitis. A more difficult task is safeguarding that all students have insurance that provides reasonable benefits in the local area.
2. Does the institution sponsor a student health insurance program (SHIP)? Current federal regulations distinguish SHIPs from individual and employer-sponsored health insurance plans in that SHIPs are generally designed to be benefit rich, student centered, and exquisitely matched to the local health care environment. A significant advantage of a SHIP is that health service staff will be expertly familiar with the plan's benefits and provider networks and thus will be well positioned to guide student-patients in utilizing their insurance benefits. Because a SHIP is often subsidized for graduate students, the percentage of graduate students covered by a SHIP is almost always higher than that of undergraduates. The excellent student health service will vehemently advocate that all students have health insurance that is locally useful and, where appropriate, will

unabashedly extol the benefits (literal and figurative) of the SHIP to students and parents.

STRATEGY 3: BE STUDENT CENTERED

If a college's student health services are not elegantly student centered, then they might just as well be outsourced to the family medicine practice down the street. It is not adequate to provide excellent health care; the care must be student centered and campus specific.

Young Adult Medicine

The overwhelming majority of patients seen by a student health service are ages 18–28. Practitioners of college health must be, or must be willing to become, expert in transitional-age and young adult medicine and mental health. Some college health services, however, will have responsibility to care for young teens participating in summer camps and special programs or for octogenarians who have returned to school as adult learners, and these services must accordingly ensure that expertise, policies, and realistic expectations are in place to provide safe and effective treatment or triage.

Ease of Care

It is specious and dangerous to assume that caring for a college student is "easy." Although most student-patients are reasonably healthy and will present with mild illness, injury, or situational distress, others will present with malignancy, thrombosis, undiagnosed congenital malformations, new-onset metabolic disorders, surgical emergencies, history of significant emotional trauma, acute suicidality, and so forth. For example, the routine sore throat, the simple cough, or straightforward anxiety might well be a peritonsillar abscess, non-Hodgkin's lymphoma, or emerging psychosis, respectively.

Student Body

At a small liberal arts college, the functional lifestyle of most of the student body might be relatively uniform, but at larger institutions the demographics might include graduate students, professional students, visiting students, and others. For example, if medical students are served, the student health service might consider offering some evening hours to accommodate those medical students who feel that social pressures to avoid missing time in clinical rotations prohibit them from seeking their own care during usual business hours.

Programs

Student health programs should provide services that align with the special needs of the academic programs. Because, for instance, many programs now require at least one academic term spent studying abroad, student health should offer robust and compelling travel medicine services. If the institution includes a dance program, there should be ready access to foot specialists. If there is a dental or medical school, there should be ready access to evaluation for sharp instrument exposure. If scuba courses are popular, there should be ready access to preparticipation scuba physicals.

Cultural Competence

Students are increasingly demanding that health care professionals be both culturally competent and identity sensitive. For example, the credibility of the student health service will be threatened with transgender and gender-fluid students if pronouns are not used consistently. An institution may have recruited American Indian and first-generation students, but if there is the reality or perception of insufficient cultural competence among the counseling staff, these students might feel disenfranchised from needed services. Excellent student health services will continuously recruit as diverse a staff as possible and will provide regular professional development, and accountabilities, to advance cultural competence and understanding of implicit bias.

Privacy

Clinical services provided by student health centers are similar to other health care settings in their ability to preserve the confidentiality of patients. Every effort must be made to familiarize clinicians with the nuances of the Family Educational Rights and Privacy Act (FERPA) in serving student patients. Deliberate efforts must also be made to educate students about the legal, ethical, and philosophical commitment to clinical confidentiality. Students, and sometimes administrators and family members, need to understand that campus health clinicians work for the college or university but that does not mean that they share information with the institution.

Academic Calendar

Somewhat unique to college health is the seasonality of the academic calendar, providing both welcomed lulls (e.g., the week of spring break) and obligations for student-centered staffing (e.g., accommodating the assured surge in patient volume during the week following spring break). Staffing patterns, programs, and treatment plans should antici-pate the academic calendar and concomitant student migrations. There will also be predictable seasonality in demand for certain services, such as for travel medicine appointments in advance of program deadlines and urgent counseling consultations in the days following high-stakes examinations and other stressful events in the lives of students.

Referral Coordination

Student health cannot, and should not, be all things to all students. It is inevitable that some percentage of patients will be referred to specialists, to imaging centers, and to community clinicians. The excellent student health program will provide referral coordination, including insurance consultation, so that patients are not left to their own devices to navigate the referral. Similarly, for mental health cases involving crisis response, hospitalization, involuntary commitment, split care, law enforcement, or academic or enrollment status jeopardy, student health services should provide case management.

Continuity of Care

For present purposes, *continuity of care* takes on two meanings. First, stu-dent-patients generally value timeliness of access for episodic care over continuity of clinician for primary care, and thus it can be rather un-productive to try to enforce continuity. Keep in mind also that younger students might well have an ongoing relationship with a health care professional at home with whom there is a greater sense of continuity. Continuity also references desired follow-up with students known to have been in the emergency department, who have had surgery, or who have had other urgencies. The excellent student health service will en-courage students to seek a continuity relationship with one or two stu-dent health clinicians, but the service will work to meet students where they are in this regard and will designate a continuity of care profes-sional to follow up with higher-risk patients as appropriate.

Community Health

Community health as used here is distinct from public health (see "Public Health" in discussion of strategy 4 below) and is a reference to identifi-able communities of students, examples of which might include Asian American students, international students, STEM (science, technology, engineering, and mathematics) graduate students, LGBTQ (lesbian, gay, bisexual, transgender, and queer/questioning) students, residential stu-dents, commuter students, students who are veterans, and so forth. It takes a village to raise a well university student, and student health should be a partner in engaging with the campus community outside the walls of the health center. Such engagement will usually take the form of wellness education events, sponsorship for peer educator programs, and mental health outreach. In some settings, it is appropriate for the student health service to assign liaisons to several of the identified communities.

Health Care Consumerism

I recall a case (prior to electronic prescribing) when I handed my young patient a written prescription. He responded, "What do I do with this?" I explained how to get a prescription filled, which involved explaining many words he did not know, such as, prior authorization, copay, deductible, and out-of-network. All staff working with student-patients should enter every interaction assuming that the student is not yet an erudite consumer of health care, especially first- and second-year undergraduate students who might not have ever previously navigated health care without parental involvement and, most especially, international students and first-generation college students. It is the obligation and privilege of student health staff to coach young adult student-patients to become effective consumers of health care.

Benchmarks

National benchmarking studies are available, are cited widely, and should be utilized in ongoing and strategic ways. Examples include the American College Health Association's National College Health Assessment (www.acha-ncha.org/overview.html) and the Healthy Minds Study (http://healthymindsnetwork.org). These anonymous survey-based instruments generate data that assist the student health service to better understand the demographics, health care concerns, health habits, and utilization and perceptions of health care resources of the institution's students, including options for subpopulation analysis and benchmarking against other institutions.

Prematriculation Consultation

Although the concept of a required precollege physical examination has largely been abandoned, most schools still require prematriculation submission of some sort of health history form. The excellent student health service will have a mechanism for clinical review of these forms and will reach out (even if just in the form of a link to a Web page offering campus-specific advice regarding the particular condition) to prospective

students with certain health conditions, such as insulin-dependent diabetes, inflammatory bowel disease, bipolar disorder, history of prior suicide attempts, attention-deficit/hyperactivity disorder, and a few select
others. Likewise, the student health service should make it easy for prospective students, parents or family members, or the home clinician to
contact student health for prematriculation consultation (Van Orman
and Jacobs 2016).

STRATEGY 4: ENGAGE EFFECTIVELY AS A CITIZEN OF THE GREATER INSTITUTION

Even if affiliated with a behemoth academic medical center, a student
health service is ultimately only one of many units (e.g., dormitories,
dining halls, recreation facilities, libraries) deployed by the institution to
support students. An excellent student health program will deftly acknowledge and navigate its position as a citizen of the greater institution.

Reputation

College health has been disparaged as the "backwaters of medicine" and
"has, in the estimation of many, lacked a real identity and a positive image"
(Patrick 1988, p. 3304). In prior eras, there probably were some student
health services of dubious quality. Now, college health is a destination
workplace for many qualified professionals; there are accreditation agencies and other forms of oversight; and there is increased institutional
awareness of the need for, and value of, strong medical and mental health
services for students. Nevertheless, medicine is a messy business, and
bad stuff happens. Most missteps are avoidable and should serve as an
opportunity for organizational learning and process improvement. Some
missteps will result in a noisy complaint to the office of the university
president, and some might jeopardize the very existence of the service. A
student health service must engage in a continuous and rigorous process
of becoming ever more excellent, in an effort to be truly deserving of the
outstanding reputation it desires. In parallel, student health leadership
must be intentional in fostering trusted relationships with key university
officials, both to inform these officials of the work of student health and to
create brand equity.

Marketing

Student health schedules tend to stay 100% busy 100% of the time
during most weeks of the academic year (less so during the summer), so
marketing in college health is rarely about attracting new patients.
Rather, excellent student health services will engage in marketing to en-

sure that students, and to some extent faculty and administrators, are aware of the services offered and, when pertinent, any accomplishments and distinctions. There is an urban legend about the senior who "didn't even know there was a health center on campus."

Accreditation

The Joint Commission and the Accreditation Association for Ambulatory Health Care offer designated accreditation services for college health centers. The International Association of Counseling Services also offers an accreditation specific to collegiate counseling services. All but the tiniest of college health centers should reasonably be expected to achieve and maintain accreditation. Accreditation does not guarantee clinical excellence, organizational success, or a satisfactory outcome for any particular patient interaction, and for colleges, health accreditation is rarely needed to satisfy third-party payers or regulatory officials. Accreditation does, however, provide senior university officials—and the parents or family members of current and prospective students—the reassurance of knowing that student health services are routinely scrutinized by a trusted independent agency. Frankly, continuous accreditation readiness also helps to frame and motivate certain administrative controls, quality initiatives, and other best practices that might slide if not for the next looming accreditation cycle.

Academic Medical Centers

Less than 3% of the colleges and universities in the United States share a campus with an academic medical center. Even where there is a colocated academic medical center, it is typical for student health services to report through the university side of the organization rather than through the health care side of the organization. Regardless of reporting lines, student-patients are the beneficiaries when there is a close and functional relationship between student health and multiple departments of the school of medicine and medical center, including credentialing through the medical staff office.

Public Health

The excellent student health service plays a visible and critical role in public health advocacy and intervention and maintains close relationships with local and state public health agencies. At a minimum, there is advocacy around infectious diseases, including sexually transmitted infections; annual flu vaccination programs; consultation for food-borne illnesses; tuberculosis screening; enhancement of skateboard and bicycle safety; and more. The role for college counseling centers in public health response is evidenced all too often in providing postvention following campus suicides and homicides. The value of postvention activities has been demonstrated in supporting students and the campus community after national tragedies such as 9/11 and federal policy changes affecting students.

Emergency Preparedness

The severe acute respiratory syndrome (SARS) pandemic of 2003, H5N1 flu fears of 2005–2008 (and ongoing), and the H1N1 flu pandemic of 2009 thrust college health services into the forefront of emergency preparedness and disaster response, thereby expanding their public health responsibilities. Excellence in college health mandates a close and capable partnership with the institution's emergency management offices. Successes in these regards will do much to establish student health's broad credibility and indispensability. Scope of activity includes business continuity planning, participation in drills, mass casualty medical responses, and disaster mental health response.

Legal Guidance

Leadership of an excellent student health service will maintain a collaborative and robust relationship with the institution's offices of general council and risk management. There will be regular consultation regarding forms, policies, eligibility for services, treatment of minors, the Health Insurance Portability and Accountability Act (HIPAA) versus FERPA, high-risk cases, audits and compliance, and so forth. These collaborations will enhance and protect student health and will provide the institution with transparency regarding the health service's compliance and quality assurance efforts.

Information Technology

In today's clinical environment, there are often more computers than staff. Although desktop application support (e.g., Microsoft Word, Excel) can be managed, if necessary, by institutional (e.g., division of student affairs) resources, an excellent health service will insist that the electronic health record and associated interfaces will be managed by one or more dedicated health care information technology professionals.

Staffing

Finally, it is self-evident that excellence of a student health service is most critically dependent on the quality of its staff. If the institution is not able and willing to recruit and retain professionals of uncompromising quality, then it should not attempt to dabble in the business of college health.

Conclusion

In this chapter, a brief tour of selected strategies needed to build or sustain excellence in clinical student health programs is provided. There are many additional tactics and recommendations, some macro and some nuanced, that are worthy of consideration, and many more that will be specific to the particular campus, but space does not permit discussion of all of these. As you read the following chapters—whether from the point of view of an administrator with oversight for student health services, a student health clinician, or a clinician who receives referrals from and otherwise interfaces with a college health service—consider how assessment and treatment of particular mental health challenges intersect with the student health service's position in the landscape of local health care resources and its objectives of access, student centeredness, and responsibilities to the campus community.

KEY CONCEPTS

- Campus-based, institutionally sponsored primary care and mental health services are available on most college campuses, but there is tremendous variability in how student health services are implemented, scoped, and funded.

- Student health is a form of corporate medicine, serving the needs of both student-patients and the greater institution.

- Excellence in college health service requires relentless emphasis on access, elegant student centeredness, continuous reassessment of mission and scope, and leveraging of many other campus resources.

Discussion Questions

1. Discuss the scope of student health services available on your campus. How is scope determined and assessed? Might a small change or redirection of priorities facilitate meaningful student-friendly expansion of scope?

2. Are the primary care and counseling/psychiatric services available for students on your campus aligned to maximize scope, efficiency, safety, and access?

3. Are there subsets of students who are effectively disenfranchised from the services being offered?

4. Is your student health service deserving of the reputation you want or deserving of the reputation that it has? What are the areas of weakness or vulnerability? What are the strengths that drive positive reputation?

5. Who are some of your student health service's key on-campus partners (e.g., office of risk management, dean of students office, campus housing department, academic medical center, the provost) and off-campus partners (e.g., emergency medical service agencies, local public health department, private practices in the community), and how might these relationships be leveraged even further in the service of student health and wellness?

Suggested Readings

American College Health Association: Considerations for Integration of Counseling and Health Services on College and University Campuses. Hanover, MD, American College Health Association, March 4, 2010. Available at: http://acha.org/documents/resources/guidelines/ACHA_Considerations_for_Integration_of_Counseling_White_Paper_Mar2010.pdf. Accessed April 12, 2017.

Balon, R, Beresin, EV, Coverdale, JH, et al: College mental health: a vulnerable population in an environment with systemic deficiencies. Acad Psychiatry 39: 495–497. doi.org/10.1007/s40596-015-0390-1 2015

International Association of Counseling Services: Statement regarding recommended staff to student ratios, 2017. Available at: http://www.iacsinc.org/staff-to-student-ratios.html. Accessed April 12, 2017.

Prescott HM: Student bodies, past and present. J Am Coll Health 59(6):464–469, 2011

Wilson R: An epidemic of anguish. The Chronicle of Higher Education, August 31, 2015

References

American College Health Association: Considerations for Integration of Counseling and Health Services on College and University Campuses. Hanover, MD, American College Health Association, March 4, 2010. Available at: http://acha.org/documents/resources/guidelines/ACHA_Considerations_for_Integration_of_Counseling_White_Paper_Mar2010.pdf. Accessed April 12, 2017.

American College Health Association: Framework for a Comprehensive College Health Program. Hanover, MD, American College Health Association, 2016

Center for Collegiate Mental Health: 2016 Annual Report. Publ No STA-17-74. University Park, PA, Center for Collegiate Mental Health, Penn State University, January 2017. Available at: https://sites.psu.edu/ccmh/files/2017/01/2016-Annual-Report-Final_2016_01_09-1gc2hj6.pdf. Accessed July 20, 2017.

Christmas WA: Campus-based college health services before the Amherst program (1860): military academies lead the way. J Am Coll Health 59(6):493–501, 2011 21660804

International Association of Counseling Services: Statement regarding recommended staff to student ratios, 2017. Available at: http://www.iacsinc.org/staff-to-student-ratios.html. Accessed April 12, 2017.

Kraft DP: One hundred years of college mental health. J Am Coll Health 59(6):477–481, 2011 21660801

Patrick K: Student health: medical care within institutions of higher education. JAMA 260(22):3301–3305, 1988 3054192

Prescott HM: Student bodies, past and present. J Am Coll Health 59(6):464–469, 2011 21660799

School and college contracts (editorial). AMA Bulletin 22(6):137, 1927

Turner HS, Hurley JL (eds): The History and Practice of College Health. Lexington, University of Kentucky Press, 2002

Van Orman S, Jacobs JR: College health, in Neinstein's Adolescent and Young Adult Health Care: A Practical Guide, 6th Edition. Edited by Neinstein L, Katzman DK. Philadelphia, PA, Wolters Kluwer, 2016, pp 622–633

Wilson R: An epidemic of anguish: overwhelmed by demand for mental-health care, colleges face conflicts in choosing how to respond. Chronical of Higher Education, August 31, 2015

CHAPTER 4

Burnout and Self-Care of Clinicians in Student Mental Health Services

Jennifer Derenne, M.D.

IN the helping professions, *burnout* is defined as emotional exhaustion, feelings of inadequacy or worthlessness, and depersonalization (Beresin et al. 2016). Physicians, residents, fellows, and medical students may be at particularly high risk of developing burnout for a number of reasons. Medicine is a demanding profession, one in which practitioners bear witness to joy and happiness, as well as to unspeakable pain and tragedy. The human condition is intense. Physicians, psychologists, and other health professionals must deal with uncertainty and with the fact that things can sometimes go wrong, even when every effort is made to prevent a bad outcome. In addition, medical and graduate education is long and expensive. Work hours may make it difficult to remain connected to family and friends. Trainees delay gratification for years, and then they may find themselves in a specialty that they do not love as much as they thought they would, but they feel pressured to work long hours to pay back loans and have a "doctor lifestyle" (Balch et al. 2009). It can be difficult to maintain good boundaries between work and leisure time. Some estimates suggest that 20%–25% of medical students have been depressed (Rosenthal and Okie 2005). One study of medical residents demonstrated that 25%–35% had four or five symptoms of depression (Collier et al. 2002). Another revealed that 76% of medical residents met criteria for burnout on the Maslach Burnout Inventory (Shanafelt et al. 2002). Among 740 interns in various specialties, rates of depression (defined as a score of >10 on the nine-item Patient Health Questionnaire) increased from 3.9% prior to starting an internship to 26.6% after 12 months (Sen et al. 2010).

Psychiatrists may be at even higher risk of burnout than colleagues in other medical specialties. Gratitude can be scarce in psychiatry, and psychiatrists are often the target of negative emotion and transference reactions. At times, patients are incredibly ill, with chronic illnesses that do not yet have great treatments. Many patients have stories that are difficult to hear and that may actually result in secondary traumatization to the clinician (Maslach and Leiter 2016). Despite best efforts, some patients die by suicide. Others struggle to make sustained behavior change. Still other patients need firm limits and consistency that make them angry. Poorly managed anger, impulsivity, and even psychosis can lead to threats of harm and may result in actual assault (Coverdale et al. 2005). Family members of patients and physicians in other medical specialties may have unrealistic expectations of what can be done with medications and psychotherapy. Psychiatrists themselves may be frustrated with the limits of the craft (Maslach and Leiter 2016). There is a significant shortage of mental health professionals, which forces clinicians to expand patient panels, to schedule more patients each day, to see increasingly complex patients, and to decrease the amount of time spent with each patient. To raise revenue-generating patient contacts, psychiatrists are sometimes encouraged to shift their caseloads to primarily psychopharmacology and to split patient management with psychotherapists with doctoral and master's degrees. The vast majority of trainees who choose psychiatry are interested in learning and providing psychotherapy, but it is often not what most of them end up doing in their daily lives.

Medical education has long valued going "above and beyond" in patient care. Indeed, the Accreditation Council for Graduate Medical Education (ACGME) states in the milestone competency for professionalism in patient care that residents must demonstrate the following: respect, compassion, integrity, and a responsiveness to the needs of patients and society that supersedes self-interest (Accreditation Council for Graduate Medical Education 2017). To its credit, the ACGME has explicitly stated that physician well-being is important and, as a result, has introduced modifications to duty hours and added training for faculty to recognize sleep deprivation and physician impairment in trainees. However, language like the ACGME's above makes it challenging for residents to feel as though they can speak up when they are struggling to manage. Nevertheless, it is in everyone's best interests that clinicians learn to recognize burnout. Patient satisfaction and patient outcomes are correlated with physician well-being (Beresin et al. 2016).

Physicians, psychologists, and trainees tend to have perfectionistic temperaments, are prone to overworking, and may internalize pressure to solve problems themselves, without asking for help. Many also minimize their own distress, to sometimes tragic consequences. Physicians have double the suicide rate of the general population (Center et al. 2003). In addition, they have higher rates of depression, anxiety, and substance use. They are more likely to divorce (Rollman et al. 1997) and to experience isolation from family and friends due to long work hours. In addition, documentation requirements in medical licensing that include disclosure of mental illness and treatment may deter physicians from seeking appropriate mental health care (Louie et al. 2007). Even if disclosure were not a concern, many physicians and trainees cite busy work schedules and worries about privacy and confidentiality as compounding reasons contributing to their reluctance to seek care. This is especially true if they are to see clinicians within their own work setting or if they need to fill prescriptions at the same pharmacies that their patients use.

The Changing Landscape of College Mental Health

Mental health treatment on college campuses has changed in recent years. At one time, college counseling centers focused primarily on helping students manage academic stress and relationship issues, but counseling center clinicians are now needing to care for students with more complex diagnoses. High numbers of students report elevated stress, anxiety, and depression that affect their functioning. According to the most recent iteration of the biannual American College Health Association National College Health Assessment, 86% of students reported feeling overwhelmed by all they had to do over the past 12 months, and 38.2% reported feeling so depressed at some time in the past 12 months that it was difficult to function (American College Health Association 2017). Increasing numbers of students matriculate with a history of previous treatment for mental illness. The 2016 Association for University and College Counseling Center Directors survey reports that 57% of counseling center directors believe that the severity of student mental health concerns and related behavior on campus has risen in the last year (Reetz et al. 2016). In many ways, this increase speaks to the significant advances that have been made in reducing stigma, as well as improving identification and treatment of mental illness. Students who would not previously have been well enough to attend college are now applying and accepting offers of admission, often at schools far from home. In addition, many severe mental health disorders have an onset in the young adult years, which may coincide with the time typically spent at college and graduate school (ages 18–24).

Colleges and universities do not always have the resources and staffing to adequately meet the needs of this changing population. Further, there is no standardization to the services offered. Many counseling centers limit students to a few sessions each semester and refer students to mental health professionals in the community when more intensive or longer-term treatment is necessary. Current figures estimate staffing ratios at one full-time psychiatrist per 10,000 students (Chan et al. 2016).

Transition to college is exciting, but it can be challenging for even the most well-adjusted individuals. The vast majority of young people feel intense pressure to "stay in step" with their peers, even when they may have different needs. College students are faced with more autonomy and less parental oversight of schedules, class attendance, outside activities, and homework. They are also in the position of navigating new platonic and romantic relationships, negotiating roommate conflicts, and managing laundry, budgets, and self-care tasks (Derenne 2013). This process of increasing independence can be fraught with stress that may trigger relapse in vulnerable individuals with prior mental health issues. Child and adolescent psychiatrists are becoming increasingly aware of the importance of well-thought-out transfer-of-care plans that encourage students to start practicing independence with life skills, illness management, and health advocacy well in advance of high school graduation. They are also encouraging some families to consider alternative plans, which may allow students the chance to experience independence in more carefully calibrated ways, such as taking a gap year, or starting at a community college and transferring to a 4-year college after 1 or 2 years.

Despite these efforts, many students arrive at college with poor preparation to live independently and inadequate connection to necessary resources (Derenne and Martel 2015). Even in those cases where a proper transition care plan has been developed, students may avoid connecting to treatment. There is often a hope that the "fresh start" afforded by the transition to college will negate the need for accommodations and therapeutic interventions. These services are voluntary, and students must be willing to advocate for themselves to access them. Clinicians in student health services often do not get involved until a student has a relapse or crisis.

Student well-being is of major concern to universities; they want their students to be healthy, happy, and able to earn their degrees within a reasonable time frame. Universities also do not want to be held responsible for negative outcomes, such as violence, accidental overdoses, and completed suicide. Universities are responsible for more than just higher education; they also act in loco parentis and have a duty to protect students as well as the campus at large. At the same time, administrators need to respect autonomy and confidentiality, and they cannot discriminate against students based on diagnosis or disability. These competing duties introduce tension into the offices responsible for student mental health. Clinicians are faced with the pressure to rapidly identify and adequately treat mental illness, while also respecting the individual's right to seek or refuse treatment. They listen to intense stories of trauma, abuse, neglect, and loss. Students die by suicide despite the best efforts of clinicians, administrators, faculty, and staff.

Unfortunately, many college counseling centers and student health centers are inadequately staffed. Clinicians are often young and inexperienced and may have limited opportunities for ongoing supervision. At the same time, they are expected to provide services to students struggling to balance academics and relationships, as well as to identify and treat (or refer) those experiencing more serious mental health issues. Those clinicians with more experience and clinical wisdom are not immune to the chronic stresses of their work. They are saddled with providing cost-effective outreach and prevention, as well as high-quality, evidence-based interventions. Midterms and finals are especially high-stress times for students and can trigger mental health decompensation and crisis. The chronically stressful environment can be taxing on clinicians as well as students, and providing good care in this setting may feel like a daunting task.

Burnout in College Mental Health Centers: Prevention and Intervention

The culture of medical training, the nuances and difficulty of providing behavioral health treatment, and the unique stresses of caring for college students put clinicians on college campuses at particularly high risk of burnout. As defined by Maslach and Leiter (2016), burnout results from chronic interpersonal job stresses, which lead to emotional exhaustion, cynicism, detachment, and a sense of ineffectiveness or lack of accomplishment. These stresses may be amplified by the amount of work one is expected to accomplish, whether there is a sense of agency and control over that workload, and whether there is the belief that expectations are fair and equal. Burnout can be "contagious" and lead to a culture of demoralization and discontent among colleagues. It may manifest as changes in mood and behavior, such as irritability, poor communication, agitation, and avoidance. Clinicians suffering from burnout may appear fatigued or may exhibit noticeable changes in grooming and self-care. They may also be more frequently absent as well as less productive during work hours. Obsessive and perfectionistic traits can exacerbate the problem. See Table 4–1 for a list of the signs of burnout. There has been much discussion about the difference between burnout and depression, with the consensus that the two are different entities, although they may be interrelated. When not properly identified and appropriately managed, burnout may lead to depression.

In contrast, working within a community that is aligned with one's values may offer rewards that mitigate job stresses and facilitate employee engagement. University administration plays an essential role in creating a supportive and responsive work environment. Student mental health centers need to prioritize campus wellness. This can be achieved by employing an adequate number of clinicians to prevent long waits for services; adjustments to student health fees and working with health insurance may alleviate some of the financial burdens that can keep services understaffed.

Employers can help further by providing adequate administrative support and by allowing mental health professionals to diversify their clinical activities to keep things interesting. Particularly high-acuity cases should be evenly distributed among team members so that no one person is overburdened. Time should be protected for regular supervision and peer support. In addition to performing clinical work, some clinicians like to introduce more variety into their workday by taking on administrative, research, teaching, or outreach responsibilities. Cer-

TABLE 4–1. Signs of burnout

Emotional exhaustion

Physical fatigue

Poor self-care

Irritability, agitation, and mood lability

Poor communication and avoidance behaviors

Suboptimal clinical care and medical errors

Detachment from clinical work and depersonalization

Absenteeism and decreased clinical productivity

Lack of enjoyment

Poor sleep

Depression

tainly, it is important not to be overly ambitious, which negates the spirit of trying to "change up" the workload.

To prevent burnout, clinicians often find it helpful to focus on improving work-life balance by modifying work schedules, achieving better boundaries between work and leisure time, and making sure to take vacations at reasonably spaced intervals (see Table 4–2). Meaningful engagement, personal connection, and joy are all important, and it can be helpful to compare one's values with the lifestyle one is actually leading. It can also help to devote time to promoting self-awareness through counseling, therapy, or job coaching. Clinicians should have the opportunity to seek help (covered by their insurance) outside of their own work environment. Developing and refining communication skills, coping strategies, and time management skills may increase interpersonal effectiveness and improve work flow (Beresin et al. 2016). Although asking for assistance from colleagues, family, or friends may be challenging, it can be incredibly important. Maintaining healthy habits such as adequate sleep, proper nutrition, and balanced exercise provides a foundation that is essential for maintaining well-being and resiliency in times of high stress. In many ways, it helps for clinicians to focus on the same advice that they impart to their college-age patients to get them through the ups and downs of a busy semester.

Obviously, completely preventing burnout would be ideal but may not always be possible. When exhibiting signs of burnout, clinicians should address their situations promptly to optimize their personal well-being, while taking care to make sure that clinical care is not adversely affected. Clinicians should be encouraged to review their caseload, to delegate or defer nonessential tasks to a less stressful time, and to prioritize self-care.

TABLE 4–2. Strategies for preventing burnout

Maintain good boundaries between personal and professional life.

Invest in hobbies and relationships to increase meaningful engagement and joy.

Practice good self-care, including proper sleep, good nutrition, and moderate, healthy exercise.

Improve self-awareness, interpersonal effectiveness and assertiveness, cognitive restructuring, time management, and organizational skills.

Diversify work, when possible, to include administrative, research, and teaching tasks.

Engage in regular supervision and peer support.

Take regular vacations at appropriately spaced intervals.

Resiliency is not only a trait that some people are lucky enough to possess. It can be learned and may be used in both preventive and corrective manners (Beresin et al. 2016). The long-held attitude that medical "professionalism" is synonymous with selflessness and deprivation needs to be changed. Patient outcomes and satisfaction are correlated with physician well-being and professional satisfaction. Shifts in attitude will only occur through explicit changes in ACGME language, and faculty modeling of good work-life balance for trainees and early-career clinicians.

Case Examples

EXAMPLE 1

Dr. Smith has been working as the consulting psychiatrist at a medium-sized liberal arts college for the past 25 years. Historically, his colleagues at the counseling center and student health clinic referred to him any patients who were experiencing garden-variety anxiety and depression that were not responding to supportive and expressive psychotherapy. He was able to evaluate students over the course of 1 or 2 hours and began seeing them for regular psychotherapy, while also prescribing an antidepressant or anxiolytic. He found that students often improved quickly in the course of his work with them, and he continued to manage their medications and therapy over the course of their time at the college. He also ran a peer supervision group for the therapists in the counseling center, provided consultation to clinicians at the student health medical clinic, and participated in outreach activities such as anxiety and depression screening. He served as the faculty advisor for the Active Minds advocacy group on campus as well. He has always felt that his position was satisfying and fulfilling.

In the last few years, Dr. Smith has noticed that the counseling center has been much busier than previously. He has been invited to participate in outreach efforts frequently, because the counseling center administration wanted to free up his schedule for new evaluations. There is a 3-week wait for new intake, and he finds himself prescribing more mood stabilizers and antipsychotics than ever before. It is not uncommon for him to see students in the walk-in clinic with new-onset psychosis and mania. One student has asked him to prescribe buprenorphine and naloxone for treatment of opioid dependence.

The director of the counseling center has pressured him to give up his psychotherapy practice, because it is much less costly to hire master's-level psychotherapists and psychology interns to provide psychotherapy. The director wanted to prevent having to hire another psychiatrist if at all possible. Dr. Smith has agreed to the changes in his schedule, because he has worked at the college for a long time and does not want to find another job. Over time, he has been asked to schedule more and more new intakes and medication follow-up appointments each week. He initially had 30 minutes for a follow-up medication management appointment, but he has been asked to cut down to 15 minutes so that he can squeeze in more patients.

Dr. Smith has been anxious about the change in his work. He has found himself up late each night reading medical journals to keep current on new psychopharmacological treatments. He canceled his family vacation so he can attend a conference to improve his skills. He has found himself questioning his decision making, which has resulted in his always running behind schedule. His family has been irritated that he is never available for activities and that he does not seem like himself anymore. Dr. Smith's colleagues at the counseling center have noted that he seems distracted and disheveled and has avoided eye contact in the hallway. He recently lost his temper with the office staff after a patient was double-booked in his schedule during finals week, a behavior that was not in line with his usual temperament.

EXAMPLE 2

Dr. Jones is finishing her first semester of a college student mental health fellowship at a large public university. She has a special interest in providing treatment, including trauma-focused cognitive-behavioral therapy (CBT), to survivors of sexual trauma and has made that the focus of her work during training. Dr. Jones loves working with young adults and initially enjoyed her fellowship but over the course of the semester notes that she is becoming troubled and overwhelmed by the content of the stories she hears each day. She feels honored that students are willing to share such personal details of their lives with her, yet she yearns for a break from the intensity. She is doing her best not to take her work home with her but is often up at night replaying the sessions and worrying about the well-being of the students she saw that day. Because she is not sleeping well, she finds that she is short-tempered and easily annoyed with her partner, who does not work in health care. She spends the weekends trying to catch up on sleep.

She meets with her clinical supervisor each week to review cases, but she finds their sessions rushed because there is much to discuss in a short period of time. Dr. Jones would like to talk about how to manage her reactions to her caseload but worries that she will be thought "weak" if she tries to discuss her feelings during supervision. She notices that everyone at the counseling center works long hours during the semester and seems very busy. As a trainee, she wants to be sure that she is being a team player and is managing her share of the workload.

Conclusion

Working in mental health can be both fulfilling and incredibly challenging. College student mental health centers have been particularly stressed by increased demand for mental health services on campus. Despite this need, staffing at many centers has not increased, which has led to larger and more acute caseloads for many clinicians. Attention to clinician well-being and work-life balance are essential in order to maintain professional longevity and improve patient outcomes and satisfaction with services.

KEY CONCEPTS

- Clinicians in the behavioral health professions are at risk of burnout due to the nature of the work, the culture of medical training, personal qualities of perfectionism, and reluctance to ask for help.
- Burnout leads to professional dissatisfaction and poor patient outcomes.
- Clinicians experiencing burnout may be at risk for developing depression. Physicians already have higher rates of sub-

stance dependence, anxiety, depression, and suicide than the general population.

- College student mental health services may be chronically stressful due to inadequate staffing, students experiencing higher crisis levels during exam time, and increasing demands for clinicians to care for students with more significant mental health issues.

- Burnout can be prevented by facilitating a workplace culture that values adequate self-care, reasonable boundaries between personal and professional life, and diversification of clinical, research, and educational activities.

Discussion Questions

1. What can training programs do to reverse the previous belief that professionalism equates with selflessness and, instead, to facilitate a culture of well-being and adequate self-care among clinicians?

2. How can child and adolescent mental health professionals best communicate to students and their families the importance of having a thoughtful transfer-of-care plan and relapse prevention strategy in place to optimize transition? Are there ways for colleges and universities to also stress the importance of this planning during the college application, interview, acceptance, and orientation processes?

3. What can college student mental health centers do to meet the rising demand for adequate psychotherapy and psychiatry services on campus, rather than referring the treatment of chronic or severe mental health conditions to local community clinicians?

4. Is it possible to standardize the availability of wellness and mental health services on college campuses? Students, families, and child and adolescent health professionals are currently in the position of trying to navigate college choice and appropriate care planning based on the information about mental health services that is available on a Web site or in a brochure.

5. How can clinicians take responsibility for maintaining adequate self-awareness, engaging in clinical supervision, and developing better time management and communication skills? What can employers do to create a culture that values wellness and encourages healthy boundaries between excellent clinical work and a fulfilling personal life?

Suggested Readings

Beresin E, Milligan T, Balon R, et al: Physician wellbeing: a critical deficiency in resilience education and training. Acad Psychiatry 40(1):9–12, 2016

Corbett BA, Love L, Yellowlees PM, Hilty DM: Taking care of yourself, in Handbook of Career Development in Academic Psychiatry and Behavioral Sciences, 2nd Edition. Edited by Roberts LW, HIlty DM, Arlington, VA, American Psychiatric Association Publishing, 2017, pp 373–383

Gabel S: Demoralization in mental health organizations: leadership and social support help. Psychiatr Q 83(4):489–496, 2012 22415227

Gengoux GW, Roberts LW: Enhancing wellness and engagement among healthcare professionals. Acad Psychiatry 2018 Jan 2. doi: 10.1007/s40596-017-0875-1.

Jennings ML, Slavin SJ: Resident wellness matters: optimizing resident education and wellness through the learning environment. Acad Med 90(9):1246–1250, 2015 26177527

Johnson S, Osborn DP, Araya R, et al: Morale in the English mental health workforce: questionnaire survey. Br J Psychiatry 201(3):239–246, 2012 22790677

Maslach C, Leiter M: Understanding the burnout experience: recent research and its implications for psychiatry. World Psychiatry 15(2):103–111, 2016

Rossi A, Cetrano G, Pertile R, et al: Burnout, compassion fatigue, and compassion satisfaction among staff in community-based mental health services. Psychiatry Res 200(2-3):933–938, 2012 22951335

Seritan AL: How to recognize and avoid burnout, in The Academic Medicine Handbook: A Guide to Achievement and Fulfillment for Academic Faculty. Edited by Roberts LW. New York, Springer, 2013, pp 447–453

Trockel M, Miller MN, Roberts LW: Clinician well-being and impairment, in A Clinical Guide to Psychiatric Ethics. Edited by Roberts LW, Arlington, VA, American Psychiatric Association Publishing, 2016, pp 223-236

Vicentic S, Gasic MJ, Milovanovic A, et al: Burnout, quality of life and emotional profile in general practitioners and psychiatrists. Work 45(1):129–138, 2013 23324671

Volpe U, Luciano M, Palumbo C, et al: Risk of burnout among early career mental health professionals. J Psychiatr Ment Health Nurs 21(9):774–781, 2014 25757038

Yoon JD, Daley BM, Curlin FA: The association between a sense of calling and physician well-being: a national study of primary care physicians and psychiatrists. Acad Psychiatry 41(2):167–173, 2017 26809782

References

Accreditation Council for Graduate Medical Education: The Psychiatry Milestone Project, July 2015. Available at: www.acgme.org. Accessed July 29, 2018.

American College Health Association: American College Health Association–National College Health Assessment II: Fall 2016 Reference Group Executive Summary. 2017. Available at: http://www.acha-ncha.org/docs/NCHA-II_Fall_2016_Reference_Group_Executive_Summary.pdf. Accessed January 22, 2018.

Balch CM, Freischlag JA, Shanafelt TD: Stress and burnout among surgeons: understanding and managing the syndrome and avoiding the adverse consequences. Arch Surg 144(4):371–376, 2009 19380652

Beresin EV, Milligan TA, Balon R, et al: Physician wellbeing: a critical deficiency in resilience education and training. Acad Psychiatry 40(1):9–12, 2016 26691141

Center C, Davis M, Detre T, et al: Confronting depression and suicide in physicians: a consensus statement. JAMA 289(23):3161–3166, 2003 12813122

Chan V, Feliciano E, Mitchell T: A decade of observations from within the U.S. college mental health psychiatry listservs. Journal of Psychiatry and Mental Health 1(1), 2016 doi http://dx.doi. org/10.16966/jpmh.101

Collier VU, McCue JD, Markus A, Smith L: Stress in medical residency: status quo after a decade of reform? Ann Intern Med 136(5):384–390, 2002 11874311

Coverdale JH, Louie AK, Roberts LW: Protecting the safety of medical students and residents. Acad Psychiatry 29(4):329–331, 2005 16223893

Derenne JL: Successfully launching adolescents with eating disorders to college: the child and adolescent psychiatrist's perspective. J Am Acad Child Adolesc Psychiatry 52(6):559–561, 2013 23702442

Derenne JL, Martel A: A model CSMH curriculum for child and adolescent psychiatry training programs. Acad Psychiatry 39(5):512–516, 2015 25895628

Louie A, Coverdale J, Roberts LW: Balancing the personal and the professional: should and can we teach this? Acad Psychiatry 31(2):129–132, 2007 17344452

Maslach C, Leiter MP: Understanding the burnout experience: recent research and its implications for psychiatry. World Psychiatry 15(2):103–111, 2016 27265691

Reetz D, Bershad C, LeViness P, Whitlock M: The Association for University and College Counseling Center Directors Annual Survey. Indianapolis, IN, Association for University and College Counseling Center Directors, 2016

Rollman BL, Mead LA, Wang NY, Klag MJ: Medical specialty and the incidence of divorce. N Engl J Med 336(11):800–803, 1997 9052662

Rosenthal JM, Okie S: White coat, mood indigo—depression in medical school. N Engl J Med 353(11):1085–1088, 2005 16162877

Sen S, Kranzler HR, Krystal JH, et al: A prospective cohort study investigating factors associated with depression during medical internship. Arch Gen Psychiatry 67(6):557–565, 2010 20368500

Shanafelt TD, Bradley KA, Wipf JE, Back AL: Burnout and self-reported patient care in an internal medicine residency program. Ann Intern Med 136(5):358–367, 2002 11874308

PART II

Life Transitions and the Student Experience

CHAPTER 5

Student Self-Care, Wellness, and Resilience

Athena Robinson, Ph.D.

THE transition into and tenure at college represent a unique time in a young person's life. Ideally, students optimize their experience throughout college in all life arenas, including social and personal development, academic performance, future endeavor readiness, and physical and mental health. Such optimization requires that the student, academic institution, and national associations and/or governing bodies of colleges and universities consider how to best address student self-care, wellness, and resilience. In this chapter, I discuss the constructs and interrelatedness of self-care, wellness, and resilience among today's college youth; outline specific self-care areas and strategies recommended for students' attention; and address future directions, including research and implementation of prevention and intervention programs, campus-wide initiatives, and technology-based considerations.

Core Concepts: Self-Care, Wellness, and Resilience

The constructs self-care, wellness, and resilience (defined in Table 5–1) are interrelated and interdependent. *Self-care* refers to actions taken by oneself to benefit oneself and can manifest in a wide variety of ways (e.g., maintaining good dental practices, engaging in safe sexual health behaviors, getting sufficient sleep, eating a healthy and balanced diet). *Wellness* refers to being in a good-quality state of health or being, typically subsequent to purposeful, consistent self-care behaviors. Both self-care and wellness directly contribute to *resilience*, the ability to manage challenges efficiently without depleting one's resources entirely. As both the breadth and intensity of student needs continue to rise, college campuses and their staff, in addition to the students themselves, are challenged with how to facilitate self-care and wellness in order to bolster and sustain students' resilience and ability to thrive.

Risks to the Self-Care, Wellness, and Resilience of the College Population

Approximately 19.1 million students were enrolled in college in the United States in 2015 (United States Census Bureau 2016), demonstrating that the national college student body is indeed a sizable population of consumer need. It follows that the demands on campus-based student health services, for all mental and physical needs, are high and consistent throughout the academic year.

Analysis of traditional risk behaviors (e.g., alcohol and tobacco use, risky sexual behavior) and lifestyle characteristics (e.g., physical activity, diet) of 2,026 college students showed that students were in need of improvement in physical activity and dietary behaviors, but that there was variability in traditional risk behaviors (Laska et al. 2009). For example, compared with their female peers, male college students had higher prevalences of adverse behaviors such as more frequent fast food

TABLE 5–1. Self-care, wellness, and resilience definitions

Construct	Definition
Self-care	Care of oneself; providing adequate attention to one's own physical and psychological wellness
Wellness	Quality or state of being in good health, body and mind, particularly as the result of purposeful effort
Resilience	One's ability to solve one's own problems, make responsible decisions, and effectively handle stress; one's ability to handle pressures and bounce back more quickly

consumption, cigarette smoking, high-risk alcohol use, and risky sexual behavior.

Mental health concerns are becoming increasingly prevalent among college youth. In a survey of 400 college counseling center directors, 95% said the number of students with significant psychological problems is a growing concern in their center or on campus, and 70% believed that the quantity of students with severe psychological problems has increased within the past academic year (Mistler et al. 2012). Relatedly, an American College Health Association (ACHA) survey of more than 123,000 students at 153 colleges found that more than one-half of students experienced overwhelming anxiety and approximately one-third felt deep depression during the academic year (American College Health Association 2013). In addition, while institutional enrollment grew by an estimated 5%, the average level of counseling center utilization grew by 30% (American College Health Association 2016).

Indeed, a wide variety of factors can contribute to the lack of student wellness and resiliency. In a survey of nearly 80,000 college students from 140 institutions, 54% of students indicated that they were diagnosed or treated by a professional within the previous 12 months for a wide variety of physical and mental health concerns, including, but not limited to, allergies (19.7%), urinary tract infection (10%), psychiatric condition (6.7%), and sexually transmitted disease (3.3%) (American College Health Association 2014). As expected, experiencing, seeking care for, and coping with these conditions or concerns can impact resiliency and academic performance.

In particular, impaired academic performance, herein defined as receiving a lower grade (on an exam, project, and/or course) or experiencing a notable disruption in work, can be a natural consequence of poor self-care, poor wellness, and/or a lack of resiliency. Students report a wide variety of factors impacting academic performance, ranging from stress and anxiety to finances and alcohol use (see Table 5–2; American College Health Association 2014). Decreased academic performance likely exacerbates the cycle of poor self-care and wellness and over time lowers students' resiliency threshold.

Common Self-Care Areas

In an effort to address their students' needs, many universities across the nation have developed handbooks on self-care, wellness, and resilience. To my knowledge, there are no data regarding how much said handbooks are used, distributed, and/or referred to by students and/or staff. Self-care areas commonly addressed by some of these handbooks are summarized briefly in Table 5–3. This list is not intended to be comprehensive; students and clinicians should seek out additional resources and options that would work best for them. Nonetheless, the broad range of listed areas highlights the need for self-care, wellness, and resilience programs.

Programs Targeting Self-Care, Wellness, and Resilience

Given both the rise in numbers of students in need and the complexity of their needs, thoughtfulness in programmatic development, evaluation, and implementation is warranted. Programs that address the self-care, wellness, and resilience needs of students must simultaneously consider the potential for other developmentally based factors that may influence the students' readiness to integrate such programming. Specifically, many first-year students struggle with procrastination, preparedness for intense academic demands, defining long-term physical and mental health and/or career goals and lack mastery of critical skills (e.g., time management, planning, organization, consideration of short- and long-term consequences of behavior).

Importantly, data demonstrate that outcomes for college youth can improve. For example, psychological well-being is positively correlated with consistent engagement in academic endeavors and performance. A recent study of 206 mostly female college students found that four self-care practices—seeking social support, good sleep hygiene, healthful food habits, and mindful acceptance—uniquely predicted well-being (Moses et al. 2016). A randomized controlled trial (RCT) of a resilience and coping in-

TABLE 5–2. Some reported factors impacting academic performance over the previous 12 months

Factor	Percentage of students who cite the factor
Stress	30.3
Anxiety	21.8
Sleep difficulties	21.0
Cold/flu/sore throat	15.1
Work	13.8
Depression	13.5
Internet/computer use	11.6
Extracurricular activities	10.5
Relationship difficulties	9.5
Finances	6.2
Alcohol use	4.1

Source.   Data from American College Health Association 2014.

tervention with college students found that students randomly assigned to the intervention condition (which included three 45-minute sessions) reported significantly more hope as well as less depression and stress after intervention compared with before intervention (Houston et al. 2017).

Online prevention and intervention programs for self-care, wellness, and resilience may provide a readily accessible and practically integrated platform for a mobile device–savvy generation. For example, a study of 476 college students from six universities throughout the United States tested the effectiveness of MyStudentBody-Nutrition (MSB-N), an Internet-based nutrition and physical activity education program for college students (Franko et al. 2008). Results indicated that students in the MSB-N group increased their fruit and vegetable intake by 0.33 servings, relative to the attention placebo control group, at postintervention. Moreover, the MSB-N group had statistically significant improvements in motivation to change eating behaviors and likelihood to increase social support and self-efficacy for dietary change. Similarly, multiple RCTs have demonstrated the efficacy of Student Bodies, an online eating disorder prevention program that targets poor body image and dietary practices. Indeed, Student Bodies significantly improved body satisfaction, eating attitudes and behaviors, and weight and shape concerns among college students compared with control subjects, and findings are sustained through follow-up (Saekow et al. 2015).

TABLE 5–3. Common self-care areas recommended for college students

Self-care area	Data brief	Specific recommendations for students' self-care health behavior
Sleep	About 27% of students reported that sleep difficulties were "traumatic" or "very difficult" to handle over the previous 12 months (American College Health Association 2014).	Acquiring adequate and regular sleep and maintaining sleep hygiene are important for all aspects of students' lives, including their cognitive and physical development, mental health and stress levels, and management of physical illness. Students are encouraged to have a routine so that bed and wake times remain relatively consistent, aiding in their ability to fall asleep readily and rise refreshed at relatively the same times each day; to have a bedtime routine that is inherently relaxing to help prepare the body for rest; to limit caffeine consumed and avoid "all-nighters"; and to engage in activities during the day.
Stress management	The emotional health of students in their first year of college is at its lowest point in 25 years (Pryor et al. 2010).	College life can be inherently stressful in a wide variety of ways. Students often overextend themselves (academically, physically, socially), which may risk their wellness. Being realistic about course loads, study hours, and degree of academic achievement, as well as employing practical study and organizational skills are important factors for students to consider. Students may have had significant assistance from their parents during high school in managing busy schedules, timeliness, and responsibilities, which they are no longer afforded in college. Campuses are encouraged to provide core education on stress management and burnout prevention techniques.
Financial stress	A survey of over 200,000 first-year students at 279 colleges and universities (Pryor et al. 2010) found that a large source of stress is financial stress, with 2010 representing the highest level of financial stress since 1971.	Many students apply for and use loans and/or grants to fund their college education—a process that is likely novel and that they may not fully understand initially. The Higher Education Research Institute survey (Pryor et al. 2010) demonstrated that students' expectations for their own employment prospects were quite hopeful.

TABLE 5–3. Common self-care areas recommended for college students *(continued)*

Self-care area	Data brief	Specific recommendations for students' self-care health behavior
Nutrition and exercise	Research consistently documents the numerous health benefits associated with good nutrition and exercise, including, but not limited to, decreased risk for longer-term health consequences and potentially improved sleep, gastrointestinal functioning, and mood and stress level. Only 6.5% of students reported eating the recommended amounts (at least five servings daily) of fruits and vegetables (American College Health Association 2014).	Recommendations for a healthful diet include eating three meals and two to three snacks at regular intervals throughout the day, as well as not skipping meals. Students often cite class schedules as reasons for failing to eat a meal or snack, and thus college campuses are encouraged to be creative with how and where food is available to the student on the go. Personal refrigerators and storage spaces in dorm rooms or apartments are ideal for students to seek food after dining halls are closed. In addition to eating regularly, eating sufficient quantities of fruit and vegetables, limiting emotional eating, and drinking plenty of water are also recommended. Students who are struggling with disordered eating behaviors are encouraged to follow up with their doctors or seek services through their campus counseling centers. Students are encouraged to walk or bike to class, make activity fun by engaging with a friend, and perhaps consider playing an intramural sport on campus.
Self-efficacy and self-compassion	Studies show that self-efficacy and self-compassion contribute to overall well-being.	*Self-efficacy* (confidence in one's ability to accomplish a particular task) and *self-compassion* (treating oneself kindly despite perceived inadequacy; moderating levels of disappointment by tempering the degree of self-berating and catastrophizing) have been shown to be related to college students' well-being. Students are encouraged to reduce the extent to which they self-berate if they are unable to meet or fall short of achieving academic goals and to work to reorient themselves toward alternative accomplishable goals in realistic iterations.

TABLE 5–3. Common self-care areas recommended for college students (continued)

Self-care area	Data brief	Specific recommendations for students' self-care health behavior
Sexual health	Of students who reported engaging in vaginal intercourse within the past 30 days, slightly over half (56%) reported using a method of contraception (American College Health Association 2014). First-year students self-identifying as gay, lesbian, bisexual, and queer reported higher levels of depression than heterosexual students (Eagan et al. 2015).	Sexual health considerations are of notable importance among college students. Students are encouraged to have open communication with their doctor and partner about birth control, condom use, and testing for sexually transmitted infections. Women are encouraged to have regular pelvic and breast exams. Web sites with readily available, medically sound information are available and ideal for students who want an anonymous way to get educated (e.g., https://www.bedsider.org/studentsexlife). Additional resources include the Centers for Disease Control guidelines on a case-based approach to management of sexually transmitted diseases among young adults (https://www.cdc.gov/mmwr/preview/mmwrhtml/rr5912a1.htm) and the Sexual Health Education and Clinical Care Coalition of the American College Health Association (http://www.acha.org/ACHA/Networks/Committees/Sexual_Health_Coalition.aspx).
Body image/disordered eating	Body image concerns, dieting, and disordered eating are prevalent among college youth.	Nationally available body image programs, such as Student Bodies (Saekow et al. 2015) or Body Positive (https://www.thebodypositive.org/), are available for implementation on college campuses. Campus administration is encouraged to offer such courses as a method of improving body positivity and reducing body image and disordered eating tendencies among their student population. Counseling centers must have staff with specialty training in eating disorders so that appropriate and timely detection, intervention, and triage occur.

TABLE 5–3. Common self-care areas recommended for college students (*continued*)

Self-care area	Data brief	Specific recommendations for students' self-care health behavior
Physical illness	Sinus- and cold-related symptoms are among the most common reasons students make an appointment at a student health care center.	Prevention, such as washing hands, avoiding sharing beverages, getting a regular flu shot, and drinking plenty of liquids, is quite helpful in reducing the risk of illness. Easy-access appointments at the student health center will facilitate students' ability to follow through with physician and wellness visits. Students are encouraged to follow their doctors' recommendations and to consider missing class as needed to get plenty of physical and cognitive rest.
Mental health	Data document the rise in students seeking mental health services. Significant numbers of students endorsed feeling that things were hopeless (46%), feeling so depressed that functioning was difficult (32%), overwhelming anger (37%), or having seriously considered suicide (8%) over the previous 12 months (American College Health Association 2014).	Students nationwide struggle with a wide array of mental health concerns. Depression and anxiety tend to be the most frequently occurring and most common prompts for students seeking aid. Knowing the signs of depression and anxiety facilitates students' early recognition in themselves or their peers. Signs of depression include trouble sleeping (too much or too little), irritability or low mood, notable procrastination and lack of motivation, and sadness and frequent crying. Signs of anxiety include feelings of being overwhelmed, panic attacks, and difficulty controlling the degree and frequency of worry. Campuses need to have staff at the ready to provide assessments, triage, and intervention for mental health concerns.

TABLE 5–3. Common self-care areas recommended for college students (continued)

Self-care area	Data brief	Specific recommendations for students' self-care health behavior
Safety	Although 88% of college students reported feeling very safe on their campus during the daytime, only 39% reported feeling very safe at nighttime, and 17% reported receiving a verbal threat of violence within the past 12 months (American College Health Association 2014).	Safety on college campuses has increasingly become an area of concern. Students are advised to avoid exercising and walking alone at night, to let others know where they are, and to be mindful of their surroundings. Reporting suspicious activity promptly can aid campus police in enforcing safety. Data support the use of the Culture of Respect and Engagement (CORE) Blueprint Program (Korman and Greenstein 2016), which works with institutions to provide them with a framework for how to respond to and prevent sexual violence on campus.
Alcohol/ substance use	When asked about the past 30 days, 66% of college students reported drinking alcohol, 14% reported using prescription medications not prescribed to them, and 21% endorsed driving after having any alcohol (American College Health Association 2014).	Alcohol and substance abuse is a complex and multifaceted area of concern across colleges nationwide. Serious consequences are related to underage college drinking, including injury, death, assault, and sexual assault. Campuses are encouraged to consult *Planning Alcohol Interventions Using NIAAA's College AIM Alcohol Intervention Matrix* (National Institute on Alcohol Abuse and Alcoholism 2015). This resource, developed by expert researchers, is a comprehensive guide designed to assist institutions in selecting interventions appropriate for their campuses. Students are advised to avoid binge drinking, defined as drinking enough to raise the blood alcohol concentration to 0.08 (approximately 4 drinks for women and 5 drinks for men consumed within about 2 hours).
Leisure activities/ hobbies	Pleasant leisure activities and hobbies can contribute to mood stability and general life enjoyment and enrichment.	Often, students are faced with scheduling challenges that make engaging in their favorite pastimes unlikely. Students are encouraged to do pleasant leisure activities when their schedule allows. Such leisure activities and hobbies may help relieve stress. Campuses can offer leisure activities in addition to time and schedule management education resources.

TABLE 5–3.   Common self-care areas recommended for college students (continued)

Self-care area	Data brief	Specific recommendations for students' self-care health behavior
Effective interpersonal communication	Effective communication skills are essential for a college student's ability to successfully navigate academic demands, develop personal and professional relationships, and become prepared for future endeavors.	Building communication, assertiveness, and problem-solving skills may help students address concerns as they arise rather than waiting until they have built up and increased stress and feelings of ineffectiveness. Some classes offered on campus may address interpersonal communication skills. *Resident assistants* (advanced students who live in the dorms alongside first-year students) may also help in moderating and facilitating effective interpersonal communication in the residential environment.
Building a community	Integrating students into the fabric of the campus community is key to helping them feel welcomed and understood and to fostering their resolve to stay and succeed on campus.	It can be beneficial for students' resilience to build a community on their campus. Such communities may be study groups, roommates, teammates, friends, and academic or intramural sports or clubs. Students are encouraged to establish and maintain positive professional working relationships with teaching assistants, professors, and classmates.
Mindfulness	College students reported reduced stress and improved academic performance and mood after receiving mindfulness meditation training (Caldwell et al. 2010; Dundas et al. 2016).	Mindfulness is the practice of bringing awareness to the present moment. Mindfulness practice can increase awareness that one is feeling depleted or in need of self-care efforts and thus create motivation for change. Many college campuses offer classes on mindfulness. Online resources, such as Koru Mindfulness (http://korumindfulness.org), offer evidence-based mindfulness training and certification for college campus instructors across the nation.

Another online program readily available to college students is CU Thrive (https://www.naspa.org/focus-areas/mental-health/cu-thrive), put forth by a collaboration between ACHA, Life Advantages, and the National Association of Student Personnel Administrators. CU Thrive partners with a campus to offer students a tailored platform to socialize, connect, garner support, find information, and learn in a way that fosters their wellness and resiliency on campus while capitalizing on the peer-to-peer relationship. It is designed to be a prevention program for health and wellness. To my knowledge, no systematic studies on the feasibility or effectiveness of CU Thrive have been conducted, although qualitative data have been gathered from student users who expressed their enthusiasm for the program. These examples demonstrate the viability of Internet-based interventions to impact positive health behavior change among college students.

Colleges are faced with making a decision about whether to mandate self-care and wellness curricula on their campuses. A recent study of a random sample of 310 undergraduate programs across the United States found that although a majority (55%) offered a personal health course, a minority (10%) required students to take the course (Henry et al. 2017). College administrators are encouraged to consider the potential benefit of requiring such self-care and wellness curricula on their campuses.

Some self-care, wellness, and resilience programs can address the student directly, whereas others target campus culture as a whole. For example, the Culture of Respect and Engagement (CORE) Blueprint Program, which engages institutions and provides them with a framework for how to respond to and prevent sexual violence, demonstrated successful programmatic changes over the course of a year and across 14 institutions (Korman and Greenstein 2016). Indeed, leveraging stakeholders to participate in and establish campus-wide initiatives may fuel rapid integration of self-care, wellness, and resilience programs.

Assessments

Colleges and universities are encouraged to consider the viability and utility of administering routine screening tools and/or full measures of student behavior in order to understand and intervene as needed to bolster student self-care, wellness, and resilience. Such assessments may facilitate identification of students in need and appropriate triage.

A self-care assessment used by Center for Collegiate Mental Health–affiliated counseling centers is the Counseling Center Assessment of

Psychological Symptoms (CCAPS), a multidimensional mental health assessment (Locke et al. 2011). On either a short version (34 items; 2–3 minutes administration time) or a long version (62 items; 7–10 minutes administration time), students indicate their responses on a 5-point Likert scale, ranging from 0 (not at all like me) to 4 (extremely like me). Both the short and long versions of CCAPS yield scores on eight subscales: depression, generalized anxiety, social anxiety, academic stress, eating concerns, family distress, hostility, and substance use. Available CCAPS norms are based on over 230,000 students who voluntarily sought assistance from college counseling centers nationwide.

ACHA provides the National College Health Assessment (NCHA; www.acha-ncha.org/). Data garnered from this assessment are notably broad and include student self-reports on sleep; mental health; nutrition and exercise; sexual behavior; tobacco, alcohol, and marijuana use; violence, abusive relationships, and personal safety; academic impacts; and disease and injury prevention. Participating campuses will receive an Institutional Executive Summary and Institutional Data Report. In addition, data from the participating campuses will be included in comprehensive reports for all schools involved, including the Reference Group Executive Summary and Reference Group Data Report. Institutions must be ACHA-NCHA members in order to participate.

The Cooperative Institutional Research Program Freshman Survey (https://heri.ucla.edu/cirp-freshman-survey/) is a widely administered survey provided to incoming first-year students prior to the start of their first term. This is another broad assessment that examines academic readiness, college expectations, student values and goals, and concerns about financing college.

Case Example

Nadine, a university sophomore, was feeling fairly drained and disinterested in her schoolwork and thus was skipping several classes per week. She also felt disconnected from campus culture and often stated, "I'm not sure I belong here." This was a complete turnaround from Nadine's engagement in and approach to her first year when she was enthusiastic about her classes and assignments, received good grades, and participated in a few clubs and other social events on campus.

Nadine's therapist first assessed for and ruled out a depressive disorder and then, upon further exploration, learned that Nadine was taking five more units than was needed to fulfill full-time student status during the current semester. Given this increase in academic load, Nadine had disengaged from her club sport, stopped spending time at the American Indian Center on campus, and decided not to apply to be a resident assistant for the following year, which was one of her long-standing goals for her time at college. Nadine also reported some interpersonal tension between herself and her roommate ("She's just so messy!"). Together, Nadine and her therapist discussed the benefits of increasing her self-care activities and thereby overall wellness. First, after meeting with her academic advisor, Nadine agreed to reduce her current academic course load. This afforded Nadine extra time to increase her investment in previously meaningful extracurricular activities, such as participating in the American Indian Center events and returning to a club sport. Sessions also focused on the pros and cons of Nadine's reconsideration of application to serve as a resident assistant and on role-playing and assertiveness training with the goal of better communication with her roommate. As Nadine worked toward these goals, she reported improved interest in and energy for her overall campus experience, as well as increased resilience in her ability to manage academic stress, especially during finals time.

Conclusion

It is clear that the self-care, wellness, and resilience needs of today's college students are broad and significant. Several factors and health behaviors can be conceptualized as part of self-care. Adoption of and consistent practice of self-care behaviors contribute to one's overall wellness, and self-care combined with wellness increases students' resiliency, the ability to effectively manage stress and problems without thoroughly depleting oneself. While programmatic efforts to date have demonstrated the potential viability of successful self-care, wellness, and resilience programs among college youth, there is a need for additional research in several areas.

First, although many college and university campuses have taken the initiative to develop and publish self-care manuals for distribution to their student bodies, the utility, uptake, and systematic implementation of these manuals have not been researched. Moreover, it appears that national collegiate associations have not issued broad recommendations for the content of such self-care and wellness manuals. A second area of potential research is the utility of mandating self-care, wellness, and resiliency programs as course work required for graduation, thereby ensuring that the entire student body is exposed to the curricula. A third area in need of significant attention is how gender and sexual orientation and identity, in addition to race and ethnicity, formulate a student's approach toward and conception of self-care, wellness, and resilience. Self-care, wellness, and resilience programs may need to be tailored accordingly. Last, research on stepped-care programs, based on a student's level of need, is also warranted and attractive, given consideration of limited campus and student resources.

Importantly, developers of self-care, wellness, and resiliency programs need to consider modality of delivery. Internet- or application-based programs have significant viability among a mobile-and-Internet-integrated generation. Moreover, the ease of anytime access in an anonymous format may entice students who otherwise would not be inclined to participate.

Finally, colleges and universities are encouraged to engage stakeholders and rouse interest and investment in the self-care, wellness, and resilience of their students. Campus-wide initiatives may build momentum toward development and research of such programming efforts.

KEY CONCEPTS

- Self-care, wellness, and resilience are all interrelated and interdependent constructs. *Self-care* refers to actions taken by oneself for oneself and can manifest in a wide variety of ways. *Wellness* refers to being in a good-quality state of health or being, typically subsequent to purposeful, consistent self-care behaviors. Both self-care and wellness directly contribute to *resilience*, the ability to manage challenges efficiently without depleting one's resources entirely.

- Online delivery of prevention and intervention programs for self-care, wellness, and resilience may provide a readily accessible and practically integrated platform for a mobile device–savvy generation. Further research on online programs is warranted.

- Campus-wide initiatives (e.g., the Culture of Respect and Engagement [CORE] Blueprint Program) may be necessary to fuel rapid integration of self-care, wellness, and resilience programs.

Recommendations for Psychiatrists, Psychologists, and Counselors

1. Note that the demands on student health services on campus, for all mental and physical needs, are high and steady throughout the aca-

demic year, and thus many students may be unable to consistently acquire the level of support they need and/or want.

2. Thoughtfully consider how gender and sexual orientation and identity, in addition to race, ethnicity, and culture, formulate a student's approach toward and conception of self-care, wellness, and resilience.

3. Be familiar with the broad array of self-care behaviors that may impact student wellness and resilience (see Table 5–3).

4. Use screening and assessments to facilitate early identification of need, and triage accordingly.

5. Students nationwide struggle with a wide array of mental health concerns. Depression and anxiety appear to be the most frequently occurring and most common prompts for students seeking aid. Know the signs of depression and anxiety to facilitate early recognition.

6. Have appropriate and thorough on- and off-campus triage referrals and resources at the ready.

Discussion Questions

1. Given the conflicting time, energy, and resource demands on today's students, what are some ways that colleges and universities can ensure that students are engaged in self-care, wellness, and resilience programs? What are some considerations (e.g., mode of delivery, subject matter) such programs should address?

2. What do observable data trends demonstrate in regard to students' use of consistent self-care behaviors? What do you find to be some of the most important self-care areas for the current-day college student?

3. How could self-care, wellness, and resilience programs and/or colleges and universities leverage technology to their advantage? Consider screening, assessment, implementation, and research purposes.

Suggested Readings

Jan J: A college student's convictions on self-care. The Huffington Post, March 23, 2017. Available at: http://www.huffingtonpost.com/jane-jun/take-care-student-culture_b_9512994.html.

Reetz DR, Mistler BJ, Krylowicz B: The Association for University and College Counseling Center Directors Annual Survey (September 1, 2013–August 31, 2014). Indianapolis, IN, Association for University and College Counseling Center Directors, 2014

References

American College Health Association: American College Health Association–National College Health Assessment II: Spring 2013 Reference Group Executive Summary. Hanover, MD, American College Health Association, 2013. Available at: http://www.acha-ncha.org/docs/ACHA-NCHA-II _ReferenceGroup_ExecutiveSummary_Spring2013.pdf. Accessed January 12, 2017.

American College Health Association: American College Health Association–National College Health Assessment II: Spring 2014 Reference Group Executive Summary. Hanover, MD, American College Health Association, 2014. Available at: http://www.acha-ncha.org/docs/ACHA-NCHA-II _ReferenceGroup_ExecutiveSummary_Spring2014.pdf. Accessed January 12, 2017.

American College Health Association: National College Health Assessment II: Fall 2015 Reference Group Executive Summary. Hanover, MD, American College Health Association, 2016. Available at: http://www.acha-ncha.org/docs/NCHA-ii%20Fall%202015%20Reference%20Group%20 Executive%20Summary.pdf. Accessed January 12, 2017.

Caldwell K, Harrison M, Adams M, et al: Developing mindfulness in college students through movement-based courses: effects on self-regulatory self-efficacy, mood, stress, and sleep quality. J Am College Health 58(5):433–442 2010 20304755

Dundas I, Thorsheim T, Hieltnes A, Binder PE: Mindfulness based stress reduction for academic and evaluation anxiety: a naturalistic longitudinal study. J College Stud sychother 30(2):114–131 2016

Eagan K, Stolzenberg EB, Bates AK, et al: The American Freshman: National Norms, Fall 2015. Los Angeles, CA, Higher Education Research Institute, UCLA, 2015

Franko DL, Cousineau TM, Trant M, et al: Motivation, self-efficacy, physical activity and nutrition in college students: randomized controlled trial of an Internet-based education program. Prev Med 47(4):369–377, 2008 18639581

Henry DS, Aydt Klein N, Kempland M, et al: Status of personal health requirement for graduation at institutions of higher education in the United States. J Am Coll Health 65(1):50–57, 2017 27661542

Houston JB, First J, Spialek ML, et al: Randomized controlled trial of the Resilience and Coping Intervention (RCI) with undergraduate university students. J Am Coll Health 65(1):1–9, 2017 27559857

Korman AT, Greenstein S: The Culture of Respect and Engagement: CORE Blueprint Program: Findings From a National Pilot Study.National Association of Student Personnel Administrators (NASPA), 2016. Available at http://archive.naspa.org/files/NASPA_CoR_PilotProgramReport_FINAL.pdf. Accessed January 2018.

Laska MN, Pasch KE, Lust K, et al: Latent class analysis of lifestyle characteristics and health risk behaviors among college youth. Prev Sci 10(4):376–386, 2009 19499339

Locke BD, Buzolitz JS, Lei PW, et al: Development of the Counseling Center Assessment of Psychological Symptoms-62 (CCAPS-62). J Couns Psychol 58(1):97–109, 2011 21133541

Mistler BJ, Reetz DR, Krylowicz B, Barr V: Association for University and College Counseling Center Directors Annual Survey: September 1, 2011 through August 31, 2012. Indianapolis, IN, Association for University and College Counseling Center Directors, 2012. Available at http://files.cmcglobal.com/Monograph_2012_AUCCCD_Public.pdf. Accessed January 2018.

Moses J, Bradley GL, O'Callaghan FV: When college students look after themselves: self-care practices and well-being. J Stud Aff Res Pract 53:346–359, 2016

National Institute on Alcohol Abuse and Alcoholism: Planning Alcohol Interventions Using NIAAA's College AIM Alcohol Intervention Matrix (NIH Publication No. 15-AA-8017), Bethesda, MD, National Institute on Alcohol Abuse and Alcoholism, 2015. Available at: https://www.collegedrinkingprevention.gov/CollegeAIM/Resources/NIAAA_College_Matrix_Booklet.pdf. Accessed February 1, 2017.

Pryor JH, Hurtado S, DeAngelo L, et al: The American Freshman: National Norms Fall 2010. Los Angeles, CA, Higher Education Research Institute, UCLA, 2010

Saekow J, Jones M, Gibbs E, et al: StudentBodies-eating disorders: A randomized controlled trial of a coached online intervention for subclinical eating disorders. Internet Interv 2(4):419–428 2015

United States Census Bureau: School enrollment in the Unites States: 2015. Release number: CB16-TPS.142. CB16-TPS.142, October 16, 2016. Available at https://www.census.gov/newsroom/press-releases/2016/cb16-tps142.html. Accessed January 2018.

CHAPTER 6

Adaptation and Stress

Sanno Zack, Ph.D.
Megan Kelly, Psy.D.

STRESS is widespread within the college population, with 80% of students reporting they regularly experience daily stress (mtvU/Associated Press 2009). In a national survey of more than 80,000 undergraduates, 33% endorsed having impairing levels of stress (American College Health Association 2016). Given that stress is also a common experience in the general adult population (80% of surveyed Americans endorse experiencing at least one symptom of stress in the previous month [American Psychological Association 2017]), it might be tempting to approach student stress as a normative, expectable, or even inevitable part of growing up and the college experience. However, several concerning trends suggest that college student stress ought to be taken more seriously.

First, although the American Psychological Association's annual report on stress has found a general trend toward stress reduction in adults over the past decade (American Psychological Association 2017), the exception to this trend has been in the youngest set surveyed. Millennials were more likely to report an *increase* in their day-to-day stress over the past year than any other age group. Second, coping strategies employed by college students often include problematic approaches, such as the attempt to suppress stress through avoidance (Mattlin et al. 1990), and even though young adults seem more aware of the need for stress management, they are also more likely to report that they are not doing enough to manage their stress (American Psychological Association 2017). Additionally, although the majority of college students state that they know they could get support for stress or mental health concerns, more than three-quarters would talk to a friend, and less than 20% would access professional support such as campus mental health services (mtvU/Associated Press 2009), suggesting that there is much more that could be done to enhance student coping and access to resources.

A large body of research demonstrates that stress is linked to an array of short- and long-term physical and mental health consequences, including contributing to disease onset such as high blood pressure and heart and kidney disease and worsening of existing chronic health conditions (American Psychological Association 2017). Studies by the Center for Collegiate Mental Health (2017) suggest that for college students, stress is often the precursor to common mental health concerns including anxiety, depression, and suicidality. In addition to affecting health and wellness, stress also affects the academic mission more directly. In fact, surveyed students endorse stress as the number one factor negatively impacting academic performance, surpassing specific physical health, mental health, or major life events (American College Health Association 2016; Iarovici 2014), with more than half endorsing having been at times so stressed that they could not get their work done (mtvU/Associated Press 2009). These findings suggest that stress is not a challenge faced by a few vulnerable students; rather, it is a widely experienced phenomenon. Whether viewed from a perspective of enhancing the wellness of the whole person or from an educational outcomes standpoint, stress in the college student population clearly has a broad impact, influencing adaptation to college, and therefore, it is important to understand, prevent, and treat.

Explanations for the elevated and increasing rate of stress among college students are multifaceted, and both population- and individual-level impacts are considered. At the level of the student body as a whole, the most frequently cited external factors contributing to stress vulnerability during the college years include developmental tasks of this age group; changing expectations for academic performance and postcollege prospects; cultural shifts leading to emerging adulthood as a developmental period; changes in child-rearing practices that prepare the adolescent for college; and changes in the makeup of the student body nationally. At the level of individual difference, the college student's ability to cope in the face of stress is impacted by internal capacities involving specific cognitive, behavioral, and emotion regulation skills, such as self-efficacy beliefs; time management; flexibility of thinking; and tolerance for uncertainty, imperfection, and negative affect. This chapter provides a brief overview of the more common influences, both internal and external, contributing to student stress, with an eye toward colleges' roles in supporting students, enhancing coping, and mitigating the negative impacts of stress on health, well-being, and academic performance.

Before we examine the risk factors and consequences of stress affecting the college student, and ultimately the avenues for preventing and ameliorating this stress, it is important that we clarify what is meant by *stress*. As is often the case with psychological terms that are widely adopted throughout popular culture, there is no single agreed-on definition. Stress, now most often thought of in the context of psychological coping, was first described from a physical disease model perspective. Hans Selye (1950), through early animal studies, identified a universal physiological response to noxious stimuli (e.g., light, water, noise) that, regardless of stimulus type, is also found in humans. From his observations, he coined the term *general adaptation syndrome* to define the series of stages an organism undergoes when attempting to respond to a challenge or *stressor* from the environment. When a pathogen or other noxious stimulus is first introduced, the body responds with *alarm*, during which the autonomic nervous system is activated, leading to physiological arousal marked by increased heart rate, decreased body temperature, and the secretion of cortisol and adrenaline by the adrenal glands, preparing the organism to fight or flee. Following these initial hormonal and physiological changes, the parasympathetic nervous system then attempts to regain its original physiological and psychological homeostasis (*resistance* or *adaptation*). If the stressor exceeds the organism's capacity to cope, the system is overwhelmed and moves into a state of *exhaustion*. Having reached the exhaustion stage, the organism is depleted and must rest and conserve resources before facing a new challenge.

Stress was first defined by Selye in the 1950s broadly as a nonspecific response of the body to any demand to change. Stress researchers have since modified this definition to include perception by the individual that the demand (stressor) exceeds capacity (resource) to cope. It is important to highlight that by Selye's original definition, stress is not inherently bad. In fact, response to the demand to change is at the foundation of healthy growth and learning. Much like muscles are built through a series of tears and repairs by applying stress in the form of weight, psychological strength is also built by the successive facing and overcoming of challenges. The key to healthy *eustress* versus unhealthy *distress* then lies in the organism's ability to meet and ultimately overcome the challenge. As contemporary psychological researchers highlight, not only is stress at times adaptive, but the absence of challenge is actually problematic because it leads to disengagement and boredom (Csikszentmihalyi 1990; Csikszentmihalyi and Asakawa 2016). Thus, optimal engagement and performance in college require a balance between challenge and skills to meet that challenge.

Individual differences in capacity to cope and perception of coping skills are thus important for predicting college student *dis*tress. However, consideration of challenges that stretch but do not exceed capacity also becomes important at the student body level as universities consider things such as curriculum and policies around academic expectation and the concrete resources provided to students. The general adaptation process is designed to help an organism cope with an acute, short-term stressor; the process becomes problematic when stressors are severe, chronic, or multiplicative. In the context of college student stress, then, it is important that colleges and universities first understand the typical challenges faced by students as well as the resources and capacities students have to cope with and overcome these challenges and then contribute to setting the level of challenge that stretches students and helps them to develop and grow without exceeding capacity to cope.

Population-Level Risks for Stress

THE CHANGING FACE OF COLLEGES AND THE COLLEGE STUDENT

Improved access to education has resulted in a more diverse student body than ever before, leading college students to more closely mirror the general population. This advancement in access is accompanied by new challenges for colleges and universities in supporting students with the type and intensity of stressors they are facing. Data from college counseling centers suggest that historically student mental health centers were tasked with treating concerns of college adjustment such as homesickness, roommate conflict, or romantic relationship breakup. As students once excluded from college are increasingly able to access higher education, centers are now seeing students with preexisting major mental illness and developmental disability, such as schizophrenia, autism, and bipolar disorder (Center for Collegiate Mental Health 2017). In the past three decades, the college student body has also broadened in cultural diversity, with the number of women now exceeding that of men and ethnic minorities making up more than one-third of the student population (Iarovici 2014). Numbers of international students have more than doubled in the past 20 years, and sexual minorities are more likely to be open about their identity and orientation than they were in the past, with the average age of coming out having dropped from a postcollege age of 23 to a high school age of 16 (Iarovici 2014).

A survey of first-year college students (Eagan et al. 2015) indicated increasing rates of self-identification with minority sexual orientations (i.e., lesbian, gay, bisexual) and nonbinary or nonconforming gender identities (i.e., transgender, bigender, gender queer). While these statistics reflect a growing diversity in college student identities and willingness to communicate openly about gender identity, they also capture important areas for potential stress and vulnerability. Many students experience significant stress and uncertainty around how to communicate about sexual and gender identity and navigate the coming out process. Students may also experience internal conflict with other aspects of their identity (e.g., religion, family, ethnicity) or have limited awareness of or access to resources, such as psychotherapy, medical services, or hormone therapy. Findings suggest that lesbian, gay, bisexual, transgender, and queer/questioning (LGBTQ) students who identify with minority sexual orientations or gender identities report more serious mental and emotional health concerns than do heterosexual peers (Eagan et al. 2015). Additionally, sexual minority status is a risk factor for suicide (Rankin 2003). Many academic institutions and college counseling centers acknowledge limitations in their education and resources relevant to these students, and college campuses often reflect ongoing social issues and national intolerance in response to the LGBTQ community, resulting in students facing greater discrimination and harassment than other minority groups (Iarovici 2014).

Rising numbers of first-generation and socioeconomically disadvantaged students introduce another area of stress. College students now graduate with higher levels of debt than ever before. In one survey of more than 2,000 students, 67% endorsed finances as a top stressor (mtvU/Associated Press 2009).

Immigration status is another aspect of identity that uniquely contributes to the experience of student stress in higher education. Almost 30% of young adults ages 18–34 years are foreign-born or have a foreign-born parent, and 17 million children under age 18 are immigrants or children of immigrants who will be transitioning to adulthood in the next two decades (Passel 2011). These youth are increasingly pursuing higher education, with 37% of male and 46% of female immigrant children and children of recent immigrants enrolled in or completing a bachelor's degree by age 25 (Children of Immigrants Longitudinal Study; Feliciano and Rumbaut 2005). For these students, the stressors that impact their transition to adulthood differ from those of youth with United States–born parents; the groups have wide disparities in parental economic value, family and neighborhood context, cultural influences, opportunities during early education, and access to citizenship (Hofferth and Moon 2016). Additionally, social, political, and institutional factors contribute to the stress experienced by students who are immigrants. Immigration status can be a critical source of stress due to the related uncertainty, discrimination, and lack of transparency regarding impact of status on education rights and access. Although recent cohorts of children who are immigrants without documentation have access to more opportunities than their predecessors (Hofferth and Moon 2016), the policies that dictate higher education admissions and academic resources vary widely. An absence of federal or state laws that dictate admissions policies for undocumented immigrants to U.S. colleges results in students navigating an often-confusing institution-specific policy and process. Even the experience of applying to and beginning a college education can induce anxiety and fear due to incidences of discrimination and harassment, lack of resources and knowledgeable administrators and faculty, lack of family support, issues around acculturation and social exclusion, and lack of familiarity with academic settings and demands. These combined factors exacerbate students' abilities to cope effectively with and adapt to changes associated with pursuing higher levels of education.

In sum, the changing face of the college student means a wider array of stressors and greater challenges for universities seeking to address student stress at a systems level. In concert with a broader array of students attending college, there are also changes to the expectations that students as a whole are facing. The competitive landscape for admittance into a higher education institution sets the stage for increased stress from the outset. Emerging adults hoping to enter college are faced with more rigorous academic challenges, lower admission rates, and often intense familial and peer pressure to be successful (Iarovici 2014). This pressure is not alleviated on entry into college when focus shifts to achieving those milestones indicative of adulthood, such as choosing a career path, getting a diploma, or solidifying long-term intimate relationships (Hermann et al. 2014).

ROLES OF EXPECTATIONS AND PARENTING

Familial and generational patterns create a context for additional stress. Current college students are predominantly from the millennial generation, or "generation me," which has been characterized as "confident and achievement-oriented" as well as "sheltered and pressured" (Iarovici 2014), potentially further exacerbating stress response due to both self-expectation to achieve and reduced practice at facing and overcoming challenge. These traits are theorized to have developed, in part, because of parenting styles that have prioritized safety, protection, and overinvolvement. The concept of "helicopter parents" represents overly invested parents eager to give their children every opportunity possible, while inadvertently setting them up to be less equipped to cope with stress and more developmentally fragile. From the lens of stress researchers, these students have not had adequate experiences of eustress prior to facing the challenges of college and are thus ill prepared for the independence and freedom that college brings. Without their parents' continued protective buffer from environmental stressors, students face stress that exceeds their learned coping skills, and they may be at risk of unhealthy behaviors due to a lack of either skill or related cognitive maturity (Hermann et al. 2014).

It is important to acknowledge, however, that this depiction of millennial generation students as overparented has also been criticized for failing to take into consideration the growing cultural diversity of this population (Iarovici 2014). Students representative of a broader range of socioeconomic and racial backgrounds often experience a different set of risk factors for stress that are equally worthy of the attention of university administration and mental health professionals. Students who have grown up in economically unstable conditions where there may be less parental oversight and perhaps more familial responsibility placed on them face their own pressures to succeed in college that can also exacerbate stress. These students may be balancing the demands of continued familial responsibilities while pursuing independent educational goals. They may also perceive that to succeed, they need to assimilate in the dominant culture, for example, by downplaying aspects of their racial identity (Iarovici 2014). Further, the American Psychological Association's 2017 report on stress suggests that in the previous year, media attention on police violence toward minorities resulted in increased concern with environmental safety by emerging adults, who appear to be most attuned to these stressors than any other surveyed age group.

DEVELOPMENTAL PERIOD OF EMERGING ADULTHOOD

The typical college ages of 18–25 years fall within a distinct developmental stage referred to as *emerging adulthood*, marked by a period of transition from adolescence to young adulthood (Arnett 2012) that comes with its own set of stressors. During this time, youth not only are tackling the demands of college, but they are also doing so while navigating a set of developmental tasks that include developing identity, gaining self-sufficiency, solidifying intimate relationships, pursuing personal responsibility, and achieving a specific skill. Most students have not yet accomplished the traditional developmental tasks that signify entry into adulthood, such as establishing a stable profession or becoming a parent. Yet, expectations and messages about successfully completing this transition are often palpable to students during the college experience, intensifying their experience of stress. Moreover, emerging adulthood and the college years are an extended period of exploration in which students are gaining exposure to a wide range of cultures, opportunities, and identities, which come with inherent opportunity for change. There is some evidence that sensation-seeking and risky behaviors increase in part as a result of this exploration process (Arnett 2012), making students vulnerable to both stress and negative outcomes that may result from these riskier behaviors. Well-being often changes dramatically over this period, and stability during transition to college is not necessarily associated with overall life satisfaction. This evidence suggests that some stress in navigating the college transition may be normative and even characteristic of emerging adulthood (Hermann et al. 2014). Several theories of college student development shed further light on the complexities of navigating emerging adulthood and the contribution of development to stress. Hermann et al. (2014) provide a concise review of three primary theories: 1) Erik Erikson's life span development theory, 2) Urie Bronfenbrenner's ecological model, and 3) William Perry's intellectual schema.

Erikson highlighted the importance of psychosocial conflict across eight stages of development. In his sixth stage, young adulthood, individuals are seeking intimate and meaningful connections with peers in the face of possible interpersonal isolation. Students may experiment with romantic commitment and partnership during this period and begin to identify their feelings about forming a family of their own in the future (Hermann et al. 2014). Reconciling the conflict between intimacy and isolation can be particularly challenging for students in the later years of college. As students approach graduation, they must balance possible competing desires, from meaningful intimate relationships to career opportunities and obligations. Erikson's model illustrates how stress can naturally arise in this negotiation between intimacy, isolation, and identity.

In Bronfenbrenner's ecological model, emerging adulthood is conceptualized within the context of transition from a familiar adolescent environment to a new college environment. Bronfenbrenner examined identity development within the individual's current environment vis-à-vis the person's environmental history and defined *microsystems* as the person-environment relationships related to a specific setting—its place, time, and activity—and the role of the individual. He examined how microsystems, such as student-student interactions, are influenced by *mesosystems* (interactions with other influences, including family, other peers, and school organizations), *exosystems* (interactions with greater social influences, including school policies, media, and geographic location), and *macrosystems* (broader cultural and social influences that interact with each of the previous systems) (Hermann et al. 2014). Students may grapple with isolation and disengagement if they do not connect with their educational communities at any one of these levels. Research demonstrates that this connection or sense of engagement can support student retention, specifically if established in the first year (Tinto 2006). Students are entering university with increasingly diverse personal experiences and perspectives, which add to the challenges faced by educational institutions to effectively support its students at this life transition.

Finally, Perry's intellectual schema or theory of intellectual and ethical development offers a four-stage developmental pathway that can illustrate how college students make meaning of their academic and personal collegiate experiences. Students progress through stages of intellectual and moral development, beginning with dualistic thinking, in which they perceive answers to questions and challenges as "right or wrong" and believe there is a clear path to success. The second stage, multiplicity, reflects a transition to perceiving knowledge as subjective and consisting of multiple truths. As students continue to search for answers in the third stage, relativism, they may become more tolerant of ambiguity or experience disorientation due to uncertainty in answers. Perry's final stage, commitment, is signified by a student's ability to hold conflicting information while moving toward a personal career or specific set of beliefs or ideals (Hermann et al. 2014). Ideally, students progress linearly through these stages from their first year of college to graduation; however, research suggests conflicting evidence about the consistency of stage development at time of graduation (Hermann et al. 2014). Additionally, students can respond to environmental stressors and uncertainty by regressing to earlier developmental stages for security or comfort. For those students who struggle to advance beyond dualistic reasoning, whether as a result of environmental stressors or life circumstances, it can be particularly challenging to navigate the complexities of the later college years and after graduation.

Clearly, college students as a population face a considerable array of stressors from the environment, including the challenges of their specific phase of life development, cultural and political climate changes, the increasingly high standards for admittance at top universities, the financial pressures of paying for college and navigating a changing postcollege job environment, and the balancing of school demands with preexisting vulnerabilities such as greater mental health concerns. In addition to these cohort-level concerns, there is also variability, of course, in the resources brought by the individual student to cope with the stressors of college. In general, college students report high levels of effort to cope with stress in concert with the sense that they are not doing as much coping as they would like (American Psychological Association 2017). Interestingly, Center for Collegiate Mental Health (2017) data indicate that over the past 6 years, mental health diagnoses and a mental health treatment history at the time of admittance to college did not increase. However, rates of suicidal ideation and nonsuicidal self-injury in the college population have increased, suggesting that a subset of today's students may not have access to sufficient tools to effectively handle stress and its common consequences, anxiety and depression.

Internal Resources to Manage Stress

Depending on a student's prior experiences and coping style, the ability to adapt to the stressors of the college period can vary greatly. As noted by stress researchers after Selye (1950), individuals' perception of their capacity to cope and their resources to do so is an essential determinant of whether facing a stressor is ultimately an adaptive or maladaptive life event. In fact, the experience of transition to college itself is predicted by both a student's belief regarding how stressful the transition will be and the self-perception of having resources to respond to the stress (Kerr et al. 2004). Precollege perceptions may be particularly important in first-year adjustment and have been found to be predictive of academic success, as well as social and emotional adjustment and ultimately college graduation.

With regard to internal resources to cope, studies suggest that the ability to identify, name, and process emotions related to stress are key elements to stress management (Kerr et al. 2004). Cognitive elements such as flexibility of thinking and ability to tolerate and rebound from setbacks are also important, as are an internal locus of control and adaptive problem-solving skills. In addition, behavioral skill sets such as time management and the ability to offset stress with self-care play a central role. One psychological construct that captures the cognitive challenges of stress management is perfectionism. A cross-culturally relevant construct, perfectionism is valued and instilled across environments through messaging about the pursuit of achievement and excellence. Current conceptualizations of perfectionism reflect a multidimensional construct with adaptive and maladaptive components. Aspects such as high standards, motivation to work toward goals, and conscientiousness have been associated with adaptive perfectionism and are often encouraged in higher education. However, university mental health settings are increasingly aware of the potential for maladaptive perfectionism to result in distress and ineffective coping (Iarovici 2014). Perfectionism becomes problematic when it involves unrealistic and rigid standards, intolerance of mistakes, fear of failure, or pursuit of socially prescribed expectations. These aspects of perfectionism have been associated with psychological distress, depression, and increased suicidal risk (Iarovici 2014). The dualistic model of perfectionism, with both adaptive and maladaptive aspects that are influenced by biological, environmental, and interpersonal factors, mirrors the distinction between eustress and distress.

Increasing Stress Management Skills for College Students

Students' internal resources for managing stress may be enhanced through a variety of avenues, including teaching skills of meditation, cognitive flexibility, emotion regulation, adaptive problem solving, clarification of personal values and priorities, interpersonal relationship navigation, and time management, among others. Sleep, nutrition, exercise, and social support are thought to be core areas for self-care that can reduce overall vulnerability to stress (American Psychological Association 2017). Several factors, however, make college students particularly vulnerable in these domains. For instance, poor sleep is ubiquitous in college. In the American College Health Association's (2016) survey, only

15% of male and 10% of female college students reported getting enough sleep for 6 or more nights per week. Poor sleep is often precipitated by a late-night college lifestyle that is not conducive to good sleep. Also, during adolescence, changes in biorhythms occur such that young adults naturally go to sleep later, wake later, and need more hours of sleep than their older and younger counterparts. The combination of these factors can accentuate normal adolescent circadian rhythms such that reverse sleep-wake cycles can occur. In the area of exercise, college students are doing only somewhat better, with only half meeting guidelines for recommended physical exercise (American College Health Association 2016).

Interestingly, the stress management strategies endorsed by all adults, as reflected in the findings of the American Psychological Association's (2017) study on stress, suggest lifelong room for improvement in coping.

Of these strategies, exercising, seeking social support, and praying are frequently recommended skills in stress management approaches, whereas pursuing screen-based activities and eating tend to promote avoidance and numbing. The apparent reliance among many adults on relatively less adaptive coping skills (e.g., television, eating, screens) and the absence of data on the use of high-impact coping skills such as meditation further highlight the potential benefits of teaching a wide array of adaptive stress management skills during the vulnerable college years to set strong life-long coping in place. Clearly, there is room for improving coping skills use at the population level. Colleges and universities may be well positioned to contribute to improved stress management by emphasizing population-wide prevention efforts in emerging adulthood, making stress management a higher-education curriculum goal. Many universities offer stress management tools through the auspices of college mental health services. Although such an approach yields an important service, it may inadvertently send the message that stress management is only necessary for those with established mental health concerns. To destigmatize and further enhance knowledge about stress and coping, more universities might introduce stress management concepts to students during first-year orientation; offer or even require a stress and coping course; or set a more general requirement of stress reduction practice that could be met via different avenues either in the classroom or in applied experiences.

Case Example

Sara is a Mexican American college sophomore majoring in premed at a small, private university. The daughter of undocumented immigrants and the first of her family to attend college, Sara received a scholarship for her first 2 years of school and has a part-time job to help pay her living expenses. A strong student, Sara excelled academically during her first year. She has high standards for herself and is prone toward perfectionism that is exacerbated by her awareness of how much her success in college means to her family, both in terms of the family's pride in her and the financial support she may help provide with a strong job and career path after college. Sara drives herself hard in her studies and spends long hours at the lab perfecting her work in her required science courses. As a result, Sara often gets limited sleep and frequently misses out on unstructured socializing in her dorm. Although well liked by peers, she rarely has time that she feels she can allocate outside of her studies and so has not created the depth of sharing in her friendships that makes her feel she can talk openly about her stressors.

This semester Sara is enrolled in organic chemistry and is maintaining a strong grade, but her chemistry professor has noticed that Sara frequently looks worn down, is quiet in class, and recently appeared tearful after receiving a B on an exam. When she stopped Sara after class to inquire, Sara initially denied any concerns, but ultimately, she shared her disappointment with herself in her grade, mentioning that her scholarship ends after this year and that recent political events have her concerned about risks of deportation of her parents. She wonders what would happen to her two younger siblings then and whether she should leave school to help her family. Her professor suggests she make an appointment at the campus counseling center for further support.

An analysis of Sara's case illustrates the concepts of both eustress and distress. Sara's commitment to medicine, a rigorous academic path, likely has already presented significant academic challenges (or *stressors*). In her first year, her resources to meet those academic demands were sufficient such that she excelled (*adaptation*). This year, however, she is facing more challenging course work (organic chemistry, which is challenging for most students) as well as additional stressors in the form of financial, familial, and sociopolitical pressures. As she attempts to drive herself forward academically at the same pace despite competing stressors, the impact of her overworking is beginning to take a toll, and if it continues, she risks exhaustion. Currently, Sara is getting insufficient sleep and is receiving limited social support, which are both major risk factors for additional physical and mental health effects. These stressors are resulting in the *distress* observed by her professor—the demands are exceeding Sara's capacity to cope.

Sara herself reflects the changing face of the college student in that she is female (once in the minority, women now exceed men in college numbers), is from an ethnic minority, and is from an immigrant family of which she is the first to attend college. She is facing substantial financial pressures with her scholarship ending after this year and may feel overwhelmed by the idea of pursuing alternatives such as financial aid, given the uncertainties of navigating the university system as well as the typical requirement of parental information on financial aid applications; this may feel risky to Sara, given her parents' undocumented status. Sara is also dealing with significant sociopolitical stressors in terms of the more general worries about her parents' immigration status.

INTERNAL COPING

As noted, Sara is getting poor sleep and is socially isolated due to overfocus on her schoolwork. Sara is additionally prone to perfectionism; her distress about her B grade suggests potentially unrealistic and rigid standards and intolerance of mistakes. These aspects of perfectionism have been associated with psychological distress, depression, and increased suicidal risk. She would likely benefit from skills to help her recognize the value of social support and the need to make more space for prioritizing this and the value of recalibrating her perfectionistic self-standards.

DEVELOPMENTAL TASKS

Sara is navigating issues of autonomy and individuation in balancing the needs of her family for financial support and values around her achieving success in medicine with her own needs for individuation and identity development. Additionally, from the perspective of Erikson, Sara's work is not leaving much time or space for a focus on the developmental task of intimacy (dating and a romantic relationship) at this stage in her life. Utilizing Bronfenbrenner's ecological model, one might also note the ways in which Sara is experiencing stress within multiple levels of the system, including balancing her family and her own needs within the mesosystem, the school scholarship and financial assistance needs within the exosystem, and the sociopolitical stressors around immigration status within the macrosystem (Hermann et al. 2014).

COLLEGE COUNSELING

Sara's professor does a great job of attuning to Sara, noticing that something is off, and taking the time to check in after class. The suggestion to seek college counseling services is a great one but may not be sufficient in itself. Less than 20% of college students said they would seek out this resource (mtvU/Associated Press 2009), and there are greater barriers to access for ethnic minorities, who seek these services even less, in part because of stigma (Iarovici 2014). Additionally, referring Sara for services may inadvertently send the message that there is something wrong with her or that she is not coping well enough. Additional avenues for intervention might include advocating for mandatory stress management classes for all premed students or indeed for all students, requesting that the college reexamine its financial assistance policies, and initiating broader discussions about how to address immigration challenges.

Conclusion

The growing trend of increasing levels of stress for college-age populations is cause for concern for higher education administrators and mental health professionals. The capacity to adapt to the college environment and to cope effectively with normative stress and prevent psychological harm is a paramount developmental task for emerging adults. Complicating this process are the numerous internal and external risk factors to stress facing emerging adults. Stress research indicates that many emerging adults either feel ill prepared to cope effectively or they engage in problematic coping strategies. Subsequently, stress continues to be a primary contributor to negative physical and mental health outcomes, decline in well-being, and poor academic performance. Universities have an opportunity to enhance student coping and access to resources and to ultimately optimize engagement, academic performance, and ability to navigate life challenges. With this understanding of the complex relationship between stress and adaptation, universities can mitigate negative outcomes through education and prevention programs. Whether stress management is being discussed across core curricula or incorporated into mandatory orientation programs, the university has a captive college audience primed and receptive to helpful interventions at this developmentally critical juncture.

KEY CONCEPTS

- General adaptation syndrome, first identified by Hans Selye in the 1950s, describes the three-stage process by which an organism attempts to respond to a *stressor* or demand from the environment to change. These stages include alarm, resistance or adaptation, and exhaustion. Although originally described in the physical health system, today the concept is most often applied to psychological health.

- Popular notion would suggest that stress is inherently negative; however, this is not the case. Stress describes the attempt by an organism to adapt to a challenge, and therefore is inherent in the process of growth. The difference between healthy *eustress* and unhealthy *distress* lies in a person's self-perception of having the resources and capacity to cope with and ultimately adapt to the stressor or challenge.

- The traditional college student is in a distinct developmental phase of life marked by specific changes in cognitive, social, emotional, and psychological development. During this period, students are tasked with developing identity, autonomy, and intimacy, and thereby defining themselves alone and in connection to others. These developmental tasks are often simultaneously exciting, challenging, and confusing, adding to the stress of college. This period extends from ages 18 to 25, the border between adolescence and full adulthood, and thus it is labeled emerging adulthood.

- *Adaptive coping* refers to the ability of the student to meet successfully the demands and challenges of college and of life beyond. Rather than attempting to eliminate stress, a goal both unrealistic and counterproductive, learning adaptive coping strategies helps students manage stress by strengthening their capacities and promoting resilience. Interventions include optimizing self-care (e.g., sleep, nutrition, exercise, relaxation); practicing mindfulness and balance or modulation; enhancing cognitive flexibility, emotion regulation, and problem solving; clarifying personal values and priorities; improving interpersonal relationships; and teaching time management skills.

Recommendations for Psychiatrists, Psychologists, and Counselors

1. The universality of college student stress and the widespread struggles with stress of American adults should not be taken to mean that stress is inevitable, harmless, or a badge of honor. It is important to keep in mind that unmitigated stress causes physical illness and disease; is a precursor to mental health conditions such as anxiety, depression, and suicide; and interferes with the academic mission more than any other barrier. Every educator, administrator, and college health professional should consider, "How am I modeling healthy coping, self-care, and work-life balance in my own life every day?"

2. The aspirational solution need not be the elimination of student stress. Stress is a natural and even adaptive part of development and growth, provided that demand does not exceed resource. Rather, universities would do well to play an active role in reducing excessive, unnecessary, or maladaptive stress where possible and simultaneously to strive to enhance students' internal resources and capacities to cope.

3. Reducing maladaptive stress as an educator, administrator, or college mental health professional means being well educated regarding the changing face of the college student and well versed in the unique stressors of the current generation. This includes being sensitive to the unique stressors experienced by minority students and committed to promoting social justice causes on campus—espousing zero tolerance for prejudice, discrimination, and acts of hate; providing platforms for empowering students; and recognizing these struggles and their ultimate resolutions as belonging to the university system as a whole and not to the individual alone.

4. Building resilience and adaptive coping in college students begins with the message that stress is universal, problematic, and treatable for all human beings. Colleges and universities can help to empower all students with stress management and adaptive coping skills by building these offerings into the core academic curriculum or campus-wide residential life experiences such that learning adaptive coping is a value woven into the day-to-day fabric of the university. Also, this strategy enables all students to learn adaptive coping by default rather than having to seek out services or be identified as needing mental health treatment in order to be exposed to these offerings.

Discussion Questions

1. Are challenges with stress management and adaptive coping best considered vulnerability factors for some students, which might interfere with learning, or as normative developmental tasks typical of the period of emerging adulthood?

2. Given the educational mission of a college or university as well as its in loco parentis role, to what extent should the development of students' social-emotional well-being, stress management skills, and adaptive coping skills be an explicit university objective?

3. If universities are tasked with this role, how might enhancement of coping and stress management be best integrated into educational curriculum, student life, or other facets of the college experience?

Suggested Readings

American Psychological Association: Stress in America: Coping With Change, 10th Edition. Washington, DC, American Psychological Association, February 15, 2017. Available at: http://www.apa.org/news/press/releases/stress/2016/coping-with-change.pdf. Accessed February 15, 2017.

Arnett JJ: New horizons in research on emerging and young adulthood, in Early Adulthood in a Family Context, Vol 2. Edited by Booth A, Brown SL, Landale NS, et al. New York, Springer, 2012, pp 231–244

Lythcott-Haims J: How to Raise an Adult: Break Free of the Overparenting Trap and Prepare Your Kid for Success. New York, Henry Holt, 2016

References

American College Health Association: American College Health Association–National College Health Assessment II: Spring 2016 Reference Group Executive Summary. Hanover, MD, American College Health Association, 2016. Available at: http://www.acha-ncha.org/docs/NCHA-II%20Spring%202016%20US%20Reference%20Group%20Executive%20Summary.pdf. Accessed January 19, 2017

American Psychological Association: Stress in America: Coping With Change, 10th Edition. Washington, DC, American Psychological Association, February 15, 2017. Available at: http://www.apa.org/news/press/releases/stress/2016/coping-with-change.pdf. Accessed February 15, 2017.

Arnett JJ: New horizons in research on emerging and young adulthood, in Early Adulthood in a Family Context, Vol 2. Edited by Booth A, Brown SL, Landale NS, et al. New York, Springer, 2012, pp 231–244

Center for Collegiate Mental Health: 2016 Annual Report. Publ No STA-17-74. University Park, PA, Center for Collegiate Mental Health, Penn State University, January 2017. Available at: https://sites.psu.edu/ccmh/files/2017/01/2016-Annual-Report-FINAL_2016_01_09-1gc2hj6.pdf. Accessed January 19, 2017.

Csikszentmihalyi M: Flow: The Psychology of Optimal Experience. New York, HarperCollins, 1990

Csikszentmihalyi M, Asakawa K: Universal and cultural dimensions of optimal experience Jpn Psychol Res 58(1):4–13 2016

Eagan K, Stolzenberg EB, Bates AK, et al: The American Freshman: National Norms, Fall 2015. Los Angeles, CA, Higher Education Research Institute, UCLA, 2015

Feliciano C, Rumbaut R: Gendered paths: educational and occupational expectations and outcomes among adult children of immigrants. Ethn Racial Stud 28(6): 1087–1118, 2005

Hermann KM, Benoit ES, Zavadil A, Kooyman L: The myriad faces of college student development, in College Student Mental Health Counseling: A Developmental Approach. Edited by Degges-White S, Borzumato-Gainey C. New York, Springer, 2014, pp 1–12

Hofferth SL, Moon UJ: How do they do it? The immigrant paradox in the transition to adulthood. Soc Sci Res 57:177–194, 2016 26973039

Iarovici D: Mental Health Issues and the University Student. Baltimore, MD, Johns Hopkins University Press, 2014

Kerr S, Johnson VK, Gans SE, Krumrine J: Predicting adjustment during the transition to college: Alexithymia, perceived stress, and psychological symptoms. Journal of College Student Development 45:593–611, 2004

Mattlin JA, Wethington E, Kessler RC: Situational determinants of coping and coping effectiveness. J Health Soc Behav 31(1):103-122, 1990 2313073

mtvU/Associated Press: mtvU AP 2009 Economy, College Stress and Mental Health Poll. Available at: http://cdn.halfofus.com/wp-content/uploads/2013/10/mtvU-AP-2009-Economy-College-Stress-and-Mental-Health-Poll-Executive-Summary-May-2009.pdf. Accessed February 16, 2017.

Passel JS: Demography of immigrant youth: past, present, and future. Future Child 21(1):19–41, 2011 21465854

Rankin SR: Campus Climate for Gay, Lesbian, Bisexual, and Transgender People: A National Perspective. New York, The National Gay and Lesbian Task Force Policy Institute, 2003

Selye H: Stress and the general adaptation syndrome. BMJ 1(4667):1383–1392, 1950 15426759

Tinto V: Research and practice of student retention. What next? Journal of College Student Retention 8(1):1–19, 2006

A Developmental Perspective on Risk Taking Among College Students

Michael Kelly, M.D.
Anne McBride, M.D.
Whitney Daniels, M.D.

FOR many individuals, the college years are a time of burgeoning opportunities for self-expression, creativity, collaboration, exploration, and experimentation. Depending on one's perspective, these terms may be considered euphemisms for a more blunt characterization: risk taking. Numerous researchers have suggested that risk taking is a developmentally appropriate and necessary aspect of adolescence despite the fact that it can at times lead to negative consequences. In this chapter, we review factors that make the college years a unique time of development and important concepts associated with experimentation and risk taking among adolescents and emerging adults. We provide an overview of the types of higher-risk behaviors that are frequently associated with college campuses, including supporting evidence from the literature, and review strategies for mitigating the risk of serious or long-lasting harm befalling students on college campuses.

Emerging Adulthood

Jeffrey Arnett (2000) coined the phrase *emerging adulthood* to describe the period of typical development for many young adults ages 18–25 in Western countries. In his 2016 article, Arnett describes how American college students, particularly those who live on campus, are immersed in an environment that encourages them to seek challenges and expand their worldviews (Arnett 2016). College also provides the opportunity to explore a variety of potential career paths. For many students, these exciting opportunities occur in settings with relatively large amounts of unstructured time, diverse groups of peers, and the potential for a variety of romantic partners and/or sexual exploration. Arnett summarizes as follows:

> The social experiences, the intellectual experiences and the experience of being on their own and learning to take responsibility for the day to day tasks of life combine to transform the green emerging adults who entered as freshmen into graduating seniors who have taken great steps toward becoming an adult. (p. 1)

As described in *Childhood and Society*, Erik Erikson (1950/1993) labels the period of adolescence as "identity versus role confusion," incorporating the notion that the time period between childhood and adulthood *typically* includes the exploration and discovery of one's own identity in the world. Erikson describes the next stage of psychosocial development, the period of time associated with young adulthood, as "intimacy versus isolation," which is characterized by the individual's exploration of intimate relationships with others, both friendships and sexual relationships.

The college years may be the first opportunity for young adults to establish their independence and expand their sense of responsibility. Most of these individuals have freedom for the first time in their educational experience to pursue a variety of academic opportunities and explore future professional interests. Young adults may establish peer friendships and romantic interests that sometimes lead to lifelong relationships. College may be a period of time during which individuals learn to navigate the challenges of living with virtual strangers in small dormitory settings or transition to living independently for the first time. Emerging adults inevitably find themselves navigating various developmental hurdles along their journeys through college. Some of the most salient hurdles include those discussed further in this text.

Experimentation Versus Risk Taking

For many individuals, the college years are a time of life associated with the greatest amounts of substance use and sexual activity; however, some researchers maintain that the risk taking that leads to potentially negative consequences is simply part of typical and necessary development. In a small study, Dworkin (2005) examined the ways in which 32 college students viewed their own risk-taking behaviors. She found that the students tended to see themselves as "experimenters" rather than "risk takers." The students also generally saw their experimentation as successful, even when it led to negative consequences, because it served as a learning experience. In our view, this study highlights the importance of avoiding judgment and pejorative labels when talking about "risky" behaviors (e.g., unprotected sex, binge drinking) that many young adults may view as "experiments" or learning opportunities. Conversely, individuals may be at risk of underestimating potential harm from so-called experimental behaviors when these behaviors are normalized among same-age peers. Finding a balance between experimental behaviors that represent typical development and potentially harmful behaviors that could lead to significant repercussions is essential.

Dual Systems Model

Steinberg's (2010) article "A Dual Systems Model of Adolescent Risk-Taking" examined the hypothesis that reward seeking and impulse control have distinct neural underpinnings. This dual systems model regarding adolescent risk-taking behavior theorizes that risky behavior is the product of distinct developmental trajectories involving two neurobiological systems. The model suggests that what Steinberg called the "social-emotional" system, involving the limbic and paralimbic areas of the brain, develops at a different rate from the "cognitive control" system, involving mostly the lateral prefrontal and parietal cortices of the brain, interconnected by the anterior cingulate cortex. In this model, adolescent risk taking increases following a surge in dopaminergic activity within the social-emotional system during puberty, leading to increased reward-seeking behaviors. However, the cognitive control system, leading to improved impulse control and self-regulation, continues to mature and develop throughout adolescence and early adulthood. A gap develops between these evolving systems of brain maturation, leading to heightened risk taking during adolescence.

In the study, Steinberg and colleagues included 935 youth and adults between ages 10 and 30 years (Steinberg 2010). Patterns of impulsivity and reward seeking were examined using both self-report and behavioral measures. Consistent with the dual systems model, Steinberg and colleagues found that reward seeking tends to rise significantly from the preteen years through mid adolescence and then subsides. However, impulsivity drops steadily after age 10, and individuals continue to make gains in impulse control throughout adolescence and into young adulthood. Thus, from a neurodevelopmental perspective, the high degree of risk taking associated with mid adolescence could be a direct result of a peaking tendency to engage in reward-seeking behavior mixed with a relatively immature capacity to limit impulses.

Steinberg's (2010) results indicate that self-reported tendencies toward reward seeking and impulsivity drop significantly between ages 18–21 and ages 26–30, a time period that is relevant when examining college-age students. Thus, it stands to reason that from a developmental perspective, students' incomplete neurodevelopment combined with the relatively unrestricted opportunities that campuses offer can lead these young adults to engage in a variety of potentially risky behaviors (e.g., substance use, sexual exploration). The dual systems model of adolescent risk taking offers some explanation for the risk taking that is often seen as an integral part of the college experience. In our view, such a perspective lends itself toward incorporating a harm reduction model when designing interventions to address risk taking among adolescents and college students alike.

Types of Risk

At first pass, one might presume that the types of risky behaviors associated with college life have been known to include substance use, sexual risk taking (e.g., unprotected sex), campus violence, reckless driving, and poor diet and self-care. The American College Health Association–National College Health Assessment (ACHA-NCHA) survey conducted in 2008 included responses from over 80,000 students that attended 106 institutions (American College Health Association 2009). The ACHA-NCHA report provided valuable information regarding a variety of factors influencing the overall health and academic success of college students, supporting the presupposition stated in the first sentence of this paragraph, with only slight synonymous changes, such as weight, nutrition, and mental health versus poor diet and self-care.

SEXUAL BEHAVIORS

Nearly 4% of women responding to the survey reported receiving verbal threats for sex against their will in the previous year. Just over 10% of women surveyed reported being touched in a sexual manner against their will, and nearly 4% reported being victims of attempted sexual assault. Approximately 2% of the surveyed women reported being victims of nonconsenting sexual penetration within the past year. Men surveyed reported similar incidents, only in much smaller percentages.

VIOLENCE

In regard to physical fights and assaults over the past year, 6% of students responding to the survey indicated that they had been in a physical fight over the past year, and 3.5% reported having been physically assaulted. Of note, this figure did not include sexual assaults.

SUBSTANCE USE

Over one-third of the students who drank alcohol reported consuming five or more alcoholic beverages the last time they attended a party. Of the surveyed men and women who reported drinking alcohol, nearly 31% reported symptoms of blacking out (i.e., "Forgot where you were or what you did"), 18.6% reported alcohol-related injuries, and 14.5% reported having unprotected sex in the context of drinking within the past year. Over 30% reported drinking on 3 or more days within the past month. Also, of the surveyed men and women who drank, 34.1% reported driving after drinking alcohol within the previous 30 days.

Pathways to Risk Taking

Luo and colleagues (2015) conducted an online survey with 996 college students at Indiana University that led to the identification of four different "classes" of students based on seven different risk factors. These factors included binge drinking, sleep habits, smoking, and diet. Luo and colleagues found that students tended to fall into one of four categories with regard to risk-taking behaviors: a "healthy" group; a group that did not engage in high levels of substance use but had poor overall health behaviors; a group that engaged in a high degree of alcohol and/or other substance use; and a group whose responses indicated higher levels across the board with respect to the survey questions. The young men and women in this study tended to have different risk-taking patterns based on differing determinants. For example, male students in general tended to report more risky behaviors, including increased substance use and poorer diet, than female counterparts. Also, the researchers found that young women from ethnic minorities and those with lower parental education may have preventive health and treatment–related needs, especially related to diet and physical activity, that are distinct from other young women in college. In another example, students who were age 21 years or older or who were taking more advanced undergraduate coursework tended to engage in the highest degree of substance use. This study's findings carry important implications for identifying high-risk groups within the college environment based on sociodemographic variables alone.

Additional considerations are whether gender, race, culture, and ethnicity are related to pathways to risk taking and whether these factors have any impact on types and levels of risk taking. Although much has been written about the presence of risk perception differences based on race, gender, and culture, there is minimal literature directly addressing these differences among college students. Several attempts have been made to describe ethnic identity development, expanding on the Erikson (1950/1993) theories discussed above (see section "Emerging Adulthood"). There is agreement that an ethnic identity formation is a process that occurs during adolescence and emerging adulthood, and yet, many questions remain. How does gender identity, ethnic identity, cultural identity, or race affect one's degree of risk taking and for the emerging adult, does continuing the developmental task of further refining identity, specifically with regard to gender, culture, and ethnicity, encourage or discourage risk-taking behaviors? Using the cultural and ethnic contextual lens may provide additional clues to finding successful risk reduction strategies. This topic deserves closer study with regard to risk taking among college students. Until such work is conducted, it is critical to be aware that ethnic identity formation may play an important role in risk taking and that research is needed to better inform practices for risk reduction.

Ravert and colleagues (2009) looked at how students' tendencies toward sensation seeking and perceived invulnerability impacted behaviors with potentially negative health consequences (e.g., sexual behaviors, substance use, driving while intoxicated) within the past 30 days. The study's sample consisted of 1,690 students across nine colleges and universities within the United States. Ravert and colleagues found that higher levels of sensation seeking were associated with the greatest likelihood of engaging in risky behaviors in general. However, students who tended to perceive of themselves as invulnerable despite engaging in risk-taking behavior tended to engage in less common and more severe forms of risk taking, such as driving while intoxicated, more frequent casual sex, and use of "hard drugs (such as ecstasy, cocaine, speed, meth and ice)." This study showed that students' levels of sensation seeking and self-perceived invulnerability were both relevant in gauging their degree of health-compromising behaviors but tended to confer different types of risk. Ravert and colleagues' findings carry important implications for care professionals and college or university staff when attempting to get a sense of the vulnerabilities a concerning student may possess.

A literature review by Cooper (2002) showed that alcohol use is strongly associated with engaging in sexual activity in general and engaging in riskier forms of sexual activity (e.g., multiple casual partners) specifically among college students, although it did not appear to increase the likelihood of unprotected sex. A recent study by Moore and colleagues (2017) looked at the relationship between personality, potentially traumatic events (e.g., exposure to actual or threatened death, serious injury, sexual violence), and risky sexual behaviors (e.g., sexual behaviors increasing the likelihood of unplanned pregnancy and/or sexually transmitted disease) in 970 college students. Results indicated that risky sexual behavior was highly associated with impulsivity and extraverted personality characteristics. Physical and sexual potentially traumatic events were also highly associated with engaging in risky sexual behaviors. In our view, this study underscores the importance of obtaining a thorough psychosocial history when working with college students, especially when there are concerns about said students engaging in patterns of risky sexual behavior.

Finding Hard-to-Reach Students

It is important to note that not all college students actively take part in campus life and/or feel comfortable accessing their school's health services. For example, in 2011, Eisenberg and colleagues reported that among college students with mental health issues, only around 30% of men and 39% of women received treatment. What can institutions do to mitigate risk among students who are wary of, or simply not interested in, college health services? Addressing such a broad and important question is beyond the scope of this chapter; however, we briefly review some literature to add clarity and identify potentially helpful strategies.

Eisenberg and colleagues (2012) identify that barriers to college students' seeking help may include stigma associated with mental health treatment; the absence of perceived need and/or time for help; limited previous exposure to mental health professionals (i.e., knowing friends or family who have received treatment); and the lack, and/or perceived lack, of cultural competence among college mental health staff. On the basis of what we know about barriers to help seeking among students, campus-wide psychoeducational programs focused on reducing stigma are one potential avenue for promoting harm reduction. "Gatekeeper" programs that involve training faculty, student life personnel, and student leaders how to recognize warning signs and provide referrals have become more popular on college campuses. In addition, Web-based health screenings are becoming more common throughout college campuses around the country. Data on the effectiveness of programs designed to reach students who are less likely to seek services have been mixed, and more studies addressing this issue are needed. From our perspective, efforts to reach students may still be helpful and worth pursuing while research expands in this field. The following section describes some specific programs that have been developed to address different types of risk.

Programs for Reducing Risk

SEXUAL VIOLENCE

In 1990, the passage of the Jeanne Clery Act, named after a Lehigh University student who was tragically raped and murdered by a fellow student in 1986, required all colleges and universities that offer federal financial aid to track and disclose crime statistics from events that occurred on and near campus. In 2013, the Campus Sexual Violence Elimination (SaVE)

Act, an amendment to the Clery Act, mandated that college campuses implement "primary prevention and awareness programs" related to sexual violence. The need for a mandate like the Campus SaVE Act becomes clear in light of the fact that nearly a quarter of young women attending college report having been the victim of rape or attempted rape (see Chapter 21, "Response to Survivors of Campus Sexual Assault").

RISKY SEXUAL BEHAVIORS

According to Satterwhite and colleagues (2013), approximately 50% of the 20 million sexually transmitted diseases diagnosed in the United States each year occur in young people ages 15–24. In 2002, Yale University began having formal "sex weeks" designed to promote discussion about sex, safe sexual practices, and sexuality in general. A number of universities around the country have since followed suit. Although common sense would dictate that psychoeducation on safe sex practices for college students is a good thing, we personally do not know of any recent studies showing evidence for the effectiveness of formal "sex weeks" on college campuses.

SUBSTANCE USE

Screening for substance use disorders is an important preventive measure to mitigate risk. The Rutgers Alcohol Problem Index (RAPI) is a well-validated measure that can be used to assess for problem drinking patterns among adolescents and college-age adults (White and Labouvie 2000). This measure assesses only problems associated with drinking (e.g., whether the respondent has ever gone to work or school drunk, experienced withdrawal symptoms, noticed personality changes associated with drinking) and is insufficient to make a diagnosis of an alcohol use disorder. That said, the RAPI is a quick and efficient means of getting a lot of information about a student's drinking habits (see Chapter 14, "Alcohol and Substance Use and Co-occurring Behaviors").

The Brief Alcohol Screening and Intervention for College Students (BASICS; Dimeff 1999) is a program designed to limit problem drinking patterns and their associated negative effects among college students through cognitive behavioral, motivational enhancement, and harm reduction techniques. A number of studies attest to the benefits of the BASICS program in reducing risky behaviors and negative consequences related to alcohol consumption. Additional information about the BASICS program can be found at the Web site for the Addictive Be-

haviors Research Center at the University of Washington (https://
depts.washington.edu/abrc/).

POLICY LEVEL CHANGES

Another method for reducing risky behaviors in college-age students
focuses on overarching policy changes to reduce exposure to potentially
harmful environments. This model draws on the idea that as young
adults' brains continue to mature and develop, the most effective
change may come from the environment rather than trying to change
risky behaviors. For example, in his article "How to Improve the Health
of American Adolescents," Steinberg (2015) suggests changing public
health policies to prevent harm rather than trying to change adolescents
themselves. He provides examples of potential policy changes for adolescents, such as delaying high school start time to accommodate for adolescent sleep deprivation, raising the minimum age of legal tobacco
purchase to 21 to prevent smoking among adolescents, and prohibiting
retail sales of alcohol within a certain distance from schools to limit minors' use of false identification to purchase alcohol. For college-age students, policy changes could include limiting access to alcohol on or near
campus and reducing access to less healthy dietary options in dormitory settings (Table 7–1).

Case Example

Daniel is an 18-year-old first-year college student with no formal psychiatric history. Daniel blacked out at keg parties twice because of severe alcohol intoxication during the first 2 months of his fall semester
and was taken to the emergency room following the most recent incident. Daniel's resident assistant (RA) heard some of Daniel's neighbors
discussing his recent "wild night," contacted Daniel, and scheduled a
time to meet. The RA and Daniel had an open conversation about his alcohol use and the negative impact that "partying" was having on his academic performance. Daniel's RA referred him to the school's student
mental health services.

Daniel underwent two sessions within his school's BASICS program.
Daniel completed a questionnaire during the first session that identified
multiple concerns related to his alcohol use. Daniel spoke with a mental
health counselor at his next session and obtained feedback on information obtained from his intake questionnaire. A thorough psychosocial
history revealed that Daniel first began experimenting with drugs and

TABLE 7–1. Using policy changes to deter risky behavior on college campuses

Examples of risky behaviors	Examples of campus-wide policy
Alcohol-related behaviors	Limiting access to alcohol on or near campus
Ignoring crime on campus (e.g., physical assault, sexual assault)	Increasing educational efforts to foster awareness and safety
Poor dietary choices	Reducing access to less healthy dietary options in dormitory settings and/or around campus
Driving while under the influence of alcohol or drugs	Expanding campus transportation options

alcohol on the weekends during high school. There was a strong history of addiction in both his mother's and father's families. Daniel's driver's license was suspended during high school after he was pulled over for speeding in a residential area. Daniel revealed that he had been smoking marijuana prior to the driving incident; however, this went undetected because he passed a field sobriety test. Daniel's parents attributed his behavior to the youthful exuberance of a new driver. Daniel endorsed experiencing multiple blackouts and was told that he had sex with a classmate during his most recent episode. Daniel was unsure whether he used protection during intercourse. Daniel related that both he and his parents have become concerned that his behavior is getting "out of hand," and he was considering taking a leave of absence from school.

Daniel and his counselor talked about a variety of treatment options that ranged from individual counseling with motivational interviewing to participation in 12-step programs. Daniel enrolled in substance use counseling at his school and signed a release of information that enabled his parents to participate in his treatment plan. He was ultimately diagnosed with a severe anxiety disorder and benefited from a combination of psychotherapy and medication. Despite having several more concerning experiences with alcohol over the course of the next year, Daniel was never hospitalized. Daniel stopped drinking entirely midway through his junior year and went on to graduate from college.

Conclusion

The college years are a time of transition with a host of associated developmental challenges. In recent years there has been a growing recognition of a distinct developmental stage often referred to as "emerging adulthood." The idea of an emerging adulthood stage fits nicely within a developmental framework, given the increasing knowledge about brain maturation combined with the unique challenges associated with transitioning to college life. A conglomeration of factors, including personality characteristics, neurodevelopmental maturity, trauma exposure, and substance use, all seem to have a significant impact on college students' levels of risk taking. Furthermore, evidence suggests that college students may not see their risk-taking behaviors as "risky"; instead, they see their behaviors as experimental. An understanding of this perspective may be helpful for college mental health professionals and staff who wish to connect with students and promote safe practices. More research in this area is clearly necessary; however, it is encouraging that a number of promising interventions and psychoeducational programs have already been designed to address risky behaviors on college campuses. These programs and interventions will likely serve as the building blocks to establish protocols for mitigating risk among college students.

KEY CONCEPTS

- Risk taking is a normal part of human development that tends to peak around late adolescence.
- According to the dual systems model, increased reward seeking during puberty, coupled with an immature cognitive control system, makes late adolescence a particularly risky time of development.
- Most college students do not seek out mental health services on their own.

Recommendations for Psychiatrists, Psychologists, and Counselors

1. Given that increased risk taking during late adolescence and the early college years is a normal part of human development, clini-

cians should avoid judgmental statements when expressing concerns to students.

2. Clinicians should keep in mind that students frequently perceive their risky behavior as experimentation rather than overt risk taking.

3. A thorough psychosocial history focusing on personal beliefs, cultural attitudes, sexual practices, violence and/or trauma history, and substance use is invaluable when determining a student's level of risk and treatment needs.

4. Programs seeking to make contact with hard-to-reach students should understand the most common barriers to help seeking (e.g., stigma, lack of cultural competence, perceived time constraints, lack of previous exposure to mental health professionals).

Discussion Questions

1. What impact, positive or negative, might limiting and or eliminating alcohol use on college campuses have on campus violence and/ or sexual violence?

2. How do harm reduction models differ from abstinence-based or "zero tolerance"–based approaches for reducing problematic behaviors on campus?

3. How can gender identity, ethnic identity, cultural identity, or race affect one's degree of risk taking?

Suggested Readings

Arnett, J: Emerging Adulthood: The Winding Road From the Late Teens Through the Twenties. New York, Oxford University Press, 2004
Erikson EH: Childhood and Society (1950). New York, WW Norton, 1993
Steinberg, L: Age of Opportunity: Lessons From the New Science of Adolescence. New York, Houghton Mifflin Harcourt, 2014

References

American College Health Association: American College Health Association-National College Health Assessment Spring 2008 Reference Group Data Report (abridged): the American College Health Association. J Am Coll Health 57(5):477–488, 2009 19254888
Arnett JJ: Emerging adulthood: a theory of development from the late teens through the twenties. Am Psychol 55(5):469–480, 2000 10842426

Arnett JJ: College students as emerging adults: the developmental implications of the college context. Emerg Adulthood 4(3):219–222, 2016

Cooper ML: Alcohol use and risky sexual behavior among college students and youth: evaluating the evidence. J Stud Alcohol Suppl 14(14):101–117, 2002 12022716

Dimeff LA (ed): Brief Alcohol Screening and Intervention for College Students (BASICS): A Harm Reduction Approach. New York, Guilford, 1999

Dworkin J: Risk taking as developmentally appropriate experimentation for college students. J Adolesc Res 20(2):219–241, 2005

Eisenberg D, Hunt J, Speer N, Zivin K: Mental health service utilization among college students in the United States. J Nerv Ment Dis 199(5):301–308, 2011 21543948

Eisenberg D, Hunt J, Speer N: Help seeking for mental health on college campuses: review of evidence and next steps for research and practice. Harv Rev Psychiatry 20(4):222–232, 2012 22894731

Erikson EH: Childhood and Society (1950). New York, WW Norton, 1993

Luo J, Agley J, Hendryx M, et al: Risk patterns among college youth: identification and implications for prevention and treatment. Health Promot Pract 16(1):132–141, 2015 24514018

Moore AA, Overstreet C, Kendler KS, et al: Potentially traumatic events, personality, and risky sexual behavior in undergraduate college students. Psychol Trauma 9(1):105–112, 2017 27348066

Ravert RD, Schwartz SJ, Zamboanga BL, et al: Sensation seeking and danger invulnerability: paths to college student risk-taking. Pers Individ Dif 47(7):763–768, 2009

Satterwhite CL, Torrone E, Meites E, et al: Sexually transmitted infections among US women and men: prevalence and incidence estimates, 2008. Sex Transm Dis 40(3):187–193, 2013 23403598

Steinberg L: A dual systems model of adolescent risk-taking. Dev Psychobiol 52(3):216–224, 2010 20213754

Steinberg L: How to improve the health of American adolescents. Perspect Psychol Sci 10(6):711–715, 2015 26581723

White HR, Labouvie EW: Longitudinal trends in problem drinking as measured by the Rutgers Alcohol Problem Index. Alcohol Clin Exp Res 24(5, suppl 1), 2000

Friendships and Romantic Relationships of College Students

Douglas S. Rait, Ph.D.

NO aspect of college life is more defining of the college experience than the nature, characteristics, and quality of the relationships that students form. As they loosen their ties to high school friends and family, college students begin the critical developmental task of forming new attachments in an academic and social community of peers that will temporarily become their new home. The relationships they develop span all types: roommates, close friendships, classmates, casual acquaintances, Facebook and other social media friends, dating relationships, committed romantic relationships, long-distance relationships, hookups, and "friends with benefits." If college provides a crucial transition between an extended adolescence and young adulthood, how student relationships form, are maintained, and end may become an important determinant of how individuals' lives will unfold throughout the college years and afterward. These relationships may be steady and comforting, exciting and confusing, or brittle and volatile. What is certain is that this diverse array of relationships occupies a central place in most students' minds and lives.

On campus, students regularly display how their dynamic, changing social lives feel vitally important to them. Small clusters of undergraduate or graduate students might chat together as they leave the classroom, but what they do next is as predictable as the rising and the setting of the sun: they reflexively turn to their phones and check to see who has contacted them through whatever social media or communication applications they use (e.g., SMS [Short Message Service], Facebook Messenger, Snapchat, WhatsApp, Instagram). It is not surprising that the social networks were conceived, were built, and caught fire on university campuses. For most students, college has been, and will likely continue to be, an intensely social experience.

Generalizations about college relationships are, of course, difficult to make, because relationships in college assume many forms and follow unpredictable courses. Roommates can form fast friendships or might avoid each other entirely. Many students acquire their closest, most lasting lifelong friendships with those they meet in college. Some students who enter into relationships are lifted by elation and confidence, not realizing that their friends may feel left behind and lonely. Most, if not all, students experience the sharp sting of occasional jealousy, envy, and even rejection. On most campuses, students encounter peers from different cultural, racial, religious, and socioeconomic backgrounds, an experience that can be both exciting and unsettling. Finally, striking the right balance between friends, roommates, and sexual or romantic interests can become preoccupying as students manage the competing demands of class, papers, problem sets, extracurricular activities, eating, exercise, sleep, and socializing.

Having taught a course called "Understanding Relationships" at Stanford University for a decade, I have developed a helpful perch from which to observe and make sense of relationships on campus. Both undergraduates and graduate students read and review work from psychology, psychiatry, sociology, anthropology, family-systems theory, and neurobiology, disciplines that together form the developing and rapidly burgeoning field of "relationship science." In entering into the serious study of relationships, they are also exposed to a new vocabulary. Students come to appreciate how complementarity functions as a defining principle in every relationship.

As Minuchin and Nichols (1984) observed, "In any couple, one person's behavior is yoked to the other's. This simple statement…means that a couple's actions are not independent but codetermined, reciprocal forces" (p. 63). As students begin to see patterns of complementarity in their own relationships, they observe how one young woman's fearful, passive role in her relationship is maintained by her partner's belittling, self-centered behavior (and vice versa). In another instance, a male student begins to notice that when he intentionally avoids his friend's anxious, clingy pursuit, she redoubles her effort to seek him out. By beginning with a microscopic focus on the individual, the students gradually add a wide-angle lens that enables them to better perceive the powerful social factors that influence, and are affected by, their own behavior. This helpful lens enables students to begin to see how their own roles and behaviors in relationships—be they with roommates, friends, romantic partners, or even their own family members—function as parts of a larger system.

Roommates

Among the first relationships that new students encounter as they arrive on campus are those with roommates. Whether students live in campus residence halls, fraternity or sorority houses, or off-campus housing, college roommate relationships are unique among students' interpersonal relationships because the individuals share the same physical space and live together. There are basic tasks that roommates typically must address because of their high level of contact, such as negotiating the structure and management of their living environment. The selection of decor, the use of space, agreement about noise level, boundaries around sleep and waking hours, and norms about visitors and guests may evolve organically or be discussed explicitly. For many students, roommates may be the first non–family members with whom they live, and they may become trusted, lifelong friends.

Because first-year students generally do not choose their roommates, it is normal to experience occasional tensions during the first year at school. However, selecting one's roommate in later years by no means ensures a friction-free relationship. In their review of the research on college roommates, Erb and colleagues (2014) describe a study based on 31,500 college students in a nationwide survey in which roughly half of both male and female college students reported "frequent" or "occasional" conflict with roommates or housemates. These difficulties can also affect undergraduates' academic performance, such as receiving a lower grade on an exam, receiving an incomplete, or dropping a course. Normalizing the notion that roommate discord and its resolution are expected, frequent experiences among college students is important. Empirical evidence suggests that roommate relationships can affect mental health and adjustment to college in enhancing, protective, and diminishing ways (Erb et al. 2014; McCabe 2016a, 2016b).

Friendships

While roommate relationships develop into important, close ties for many students, their friendship networks often extend beyond their dorm room. Relationships with friends, as with roommates, can enhance and discourage adjustment, well-being, and academic performance. Friendships can provide the social support that helps students navigate difficult experiences, yet the patterns of relationships that students construct during their college years can differ dramatically. In her study of the friendship groups of 67 students at a Midwestern university, McCabe (2016a, 2016b) asked students to identify their friends and then mapped out the webs of connections that comprised each person's social network at school. She characterized these friendship networks as grouping into three distinctive types: tight-knitters, compartmentalizers, and samplers. These friendship networks are helpful to understand because they shed light on how students' normative relational worlds can differ in distinct ways.

Tight-knitters had a single cluster of friends who all knew each other and did seemingly everything together, and they often described those friends as like "home" or like "family." Tight-knitters' networks might be described as a ball of yarn (McCabe 2016b) (Figure 8–1). In McCabe's sample, the tight-knitters named an average of 13 friends.

In contrast, *compartmentalizers* identified two to four unrelated groups or clusters of friends (Figure 8–2). For example, one friend group might comprise fellow engineering majors, while another friend group might consist of teammates from a sports team. With two clusters, a compartmentalizer pattern looks like a bow tie (McCabe 2016b). Compartmentalizers typically reported having at least one group of friends that was more academically oriented as well as a group that was identified as more social. Some students reported feeling spread thin socially

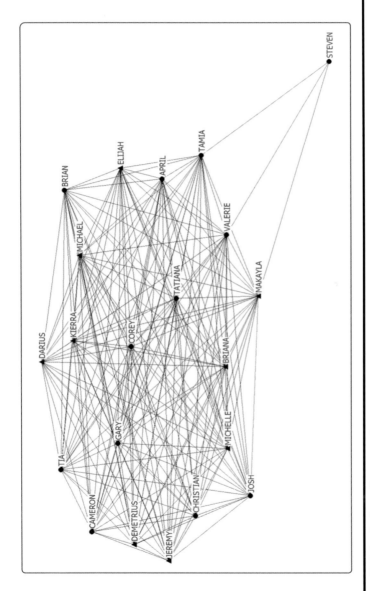

FIGURE 8–1.   "Tight-knitter" network.

Reprinted with permission of Sage Publications from McCabe J: "Friends With Academic Benefits: Valerie's Friendship Network: A Tight-Knitter." *Contexts* 15:22–29, 2016; permission conveyed through Copyright Clearance Center, Inc.

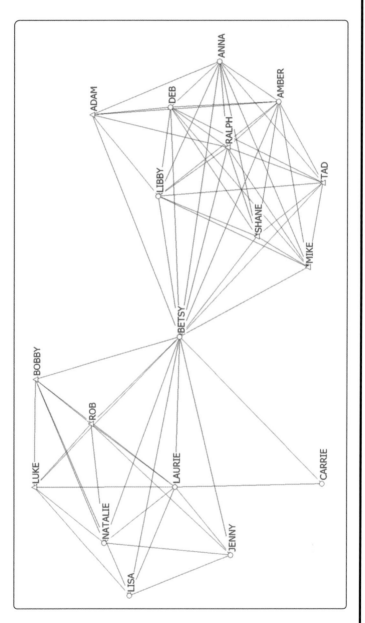

FIGURE 8–2. "Compartmentalizer" pattern.

Reprinted with permission of Sage Publications from McCabe J: "Friends With Academic Benefits: Betsy's Friendship Network: A Compartmentalizer." *Contexts* 15:22–29, 2016; permission conveyed through Copyright Clearance Center, Inc.

when juggling between more than two clusters, a common experience described by many college students.

Finally, *samplers* were characterized by one-on-one friendships with individuals who did not necessarily know one another. Their networks resembled a hub-and-spoke system or a daisy (McCabe 2016b) (Figure 8–3). Samplers reported having about the same number of friends as compartmentalizers (roughly 20), but their relationships largely composed a series of one-on-one ties. Samplers were often successful academically, but they were more likely to report being "very lonely" and socially isolated.

McCabe (2016a, 2016b) points out that although having strong friendships may be associated with academic as well as social benefits, the type of network that a student forms is also important. Most students strive to find a good balance between their academic and social lives. For example, they may meet with one group of friends when working on a problem set or preparing for an exam, whereas with other friends, they are able to relax, unwind, and "be social." Sometimes, the same groups of friends provide these functions, whereas at other times, different groups of friends or individuals offer these opportunities. Finally, the degree of emotional closeness that men and women develop in their friendships can vary by gender. Women traditionally consult each other about their internal worries, relationship questions, and vulnerabilities. For men to form close friendships, they also benefit from acknowledging insecurities, asking for help, and engaging in helping behaviors.

Not every college or university student finds navigating the social sphere on campus to be easy or gratifying. In fact, many students find their college years to be a painfully lonely, isolating time in their lives. In comparing themselves with roommates and friends who are comfortably juggling a range of friendships, romantic adventures, and academic challenges, they may feel inhibited, envious, and sad. Students who begin to withdraw socially inevitably miss out on opportunities to expand their social lives. This decision to retreat, in turn, only reinforces their social disconnection.

Romantic and Sexual Relationships

College is often a time for romantic and sexual exploration as well. Students engage in many different types of romantic relationships: dating relationships, long-distance dating relationships, hookups, and friends with benefits. In addition, these variations in romantic and sexual relationships may unfold in a way that parallels students' developmental pathways.

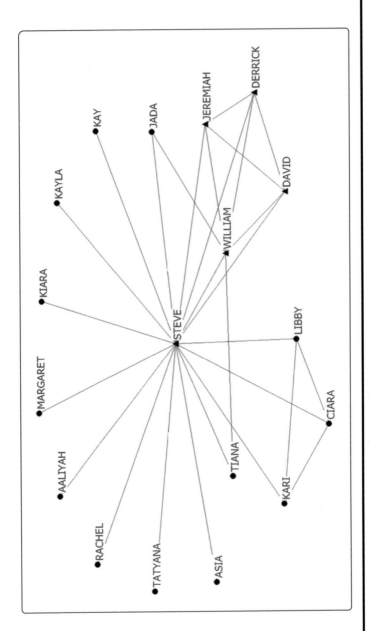

FIGURE 8–3.   One-on-one relations of "samplers."

For example, early in students' college experiences, as students step away from parental supervision, there may be more experimentation with casual sexual relationships. Romantic or sexual relationships may form and rapidly disintegrate as students encounter one another in residence halls, in classes, at parties, through common friends, or through Internet-based dating.

By the end of their sophomore or the beginning of their junior year, many students find themselves less interested in the party scene and more intent on dating and finding a steady, monogamous relationship. Graduate students often have already committed to long-term relationships and marriages, as have students returning to school after the military or time spent in the workforce. Therefore, the variations in developmental trajectories for students ranging in age roughly from 17 to 35 make it difficult to describe the modal college student's romantic relationship opportunities.

Although the majority of students engage in heterosexual forms of emotional, romantic, and sexual relationships, sexual-minority (lesbian, gay, bisexual, transgender, and queer/questioning [LGBTQ]) students in college describe specific challenges in terms of how they are perceived and treated as a result of their sexual orientation, gender identity, or gender expression. LGBTQ college students report higher levels of stigma, hostility, discrimination, shame, guilt, disapproval, and social rejection than heterosexual peers (Tetreault et al. 2013). Intersectionality represents a powerful heuristic for understanding how individuals may identify with more than one social group, whether it is cultural, ethnic, religious, gender, or sexual. As a result, not only is identity experienced as more dynamic, fluid, and complex, but student relationships bear many of the same social and emotional burdens that students experience individually.

HOOKUPS

Probably no topic regarding college relationships has been more controversial than what is widely described as the "hookup culture" on college campuses. In the literature, *hookup culture* is defined as casual sexual contact, which may or may not include sexual intercourse, between nondating partners without an expressed or acknowledged expectation of forming a committed relationship (Garcia et al. 2012; Heldman and Wade 2010). The typical hookup occurs at a nighttime party and involves an exchange of verbal and nonverbal communication signaling mutual attraction, followed by sexual contact either at the party, in a dorm room, or at some other location. After hooking up, participants generally do not spend the night with each other. Much has been written about problems with the hookup culture, in that the sex is often experienced as risky, coercive, guilt-inducing, and unpleasurable (especially for women), and hookups are frequently associated with alcohol use, depression and emotional distress, problems with attachment, and family stress (Garcia et al. 2012; Heldman and Wade 2010; Wade 2017).

In her analysis of 101 student journals from undergraduates at two liberal arts colleges, Wade (2017) found that 91% of college students agreed that their lives were dominated by the hookup culture, that the median number of hookups for a graduating senior was seven, and that only about 40% of those hookups included sexual intercourse. Students also varied widely in the extent to which they participated in the hookup scene. Only 14% of students hooked up more than 10 times in 4 years, and these students were more likely than others to be white, higher socioeconomic status, heterosexual, and attractive. Students who did not fall into these categories hooked up significantly less often and were more likely to disapprove of or be uninterested in the whole hookup culture. Still, over three-quarters of students report that they participated in at least one hookup while in college (Garcia et al. 2012; Heldman and Wade 2010; Wade 2017).

FRIENDS WITH BENEFITS

Hookups appear to differ from more protracted mutual arrangements that are sexual yet not romantic. These relationships, termed "friends with benefits," are typically initiated and maintained by two good friends who have casual sex without any kind of emotional or romantic commitment (Owen and Fincham 2011). These relationships offer the security of a sexual opportunity without some of the perceived disincentives of a committed, monogamous relationship. Avoiding the risk of emotional entanglement is typically viewed as a primary motivation for these relationships. Men are more likely than women to cite sex as an impetus; however, women do cite emotional connection as a motivation more than men (Owen and Fincham 2011).

ON-CAMPUS DATING RELATIONSHIPS

Although on many campuses hooking up has replaced dating as the primary form of sexual interaction among many heterosexual college students, dating continues as a familiar form of romantic commitment. Typically, the man follows a traditional script that includes asking a woman out, and the quality of the encounter dictates whether the couple will continue to see each other. Many young adults begin serious dating relationships during the developmental stage of emerging adulthood, and researchers have found that individuals who have committed relationships during their college years experienced fewer mental health problems than those who do not (Braithwaite et al. 2010). Students on campus often refer to their friends who are in committed relationships as "married." Not surprisingly, the protective nature of these relationships may offer comfort and security during what many see as a turbulent, emotionally challenging stage of development.

LONG-DISTANCE DATING RELATIONSHIPS

As a subset of committed relationships, long-distance dating relationships are fairly common, with some researchers reporting that they constitute 25%–50% of college student dating relationships on residential campuses (Dargie et al. 2015). Although geographic separation can pose a challenge for relationship partners as they try to maintain their dating relationships, these long-distance relationships are often very functional. Facilitated by the various forms of digital communication, students can maintain emotional contact as if they were in closer proximity.

For example, students may hang out together on Facetime or Google Hangouts, do their homework together, venture into difficult conversations about their relationship, and even engage in "phone sex." In a large study comparing college undergraduates in geographically close versus long-distance dating relationships, Dargie and colleagues (2015) found that individuals in long-distance relationships did not report lower levels of relationship or sexual satisfaction than those in geographically close relationships. These results indicate that individuals in long-distance dating relationships are not necessarily at a disadvantage and that these relationships represent a manageable alternative to on-campus relationships.

Case Example

Marie quietly recounted how the weekend had gone. On Saturday night, she and some of her friends had "pregamed" in their suite before heading to one of the notorious all-campus parties. They had a shared ritual: each of them would drink shots as they counted down the last 5 minutes before heading out. At the party, the music was deafening. Marie met up with her boyfriend, Alex. He had partied with his friends. After dancing a little bit, he headed to refill their drinks. Soon after, Marie noticed that he was flirting with Karen, his girlfriend from the year before. After a few interminable minutes, the old girlfriend reached over and gave him a long kiss. Marie's heart dropped. She broke into tears and found her friends, some of whom were dancing together. "It's the third time this has happened at a party; I can't trust him at all." Her friends tried to console her, and she angrily pushed them away. After a couple of guys tried to hit on her, she wandered back to her house, fell asleep, and woke up alone well after noon. She felt despairing, lonesome, and concluded that her roommate would be of no help because she had boy problems of her own. Marie texted some friends to go to brunch, but they had already eaten and were now heading for the library. With no one to turn to, she went to the store, bought a box of cookies and a quart of ice cream, went back to her room, and, full of self-loathing, ate everything she had just purchased. Late that evening she called the student health crisis number and began by saying, "I just don't know why this happens...."

Conclusion

Friendships and romantic relationships during the college years take many forms, often flow seamlessly into one another, and represent one of the greatest determinants of students' health and well-being during this important developmental transition. During this period of intellectual, emotional, and social exploration, college students are testing their own limits, finding new ways to experiment and express their desires for connection and sexuality, and taking interpersonal risks. How they manage the inevitable, sometimes dramatic fluctuations with their roommates, friends, sexual partners, and romantic relationships will establish models for them in how they deal with subsequent people and significant relationships in their lives.

College has become, for many young people, the laboratory in which they learn to show caring, experience comfort, deal with conflict, show responsibility, display respect, and manage asymmetries in relational power. Administrators, faculty, staff, and health care professionals on college and university campuses can increase their own sensitivity by expanding their perspectives on students to include a wide-angle lens that will assist in better perceiving the powerful social factors that influence, and are affected by, students' roles and behaviors. In addition, we would all be well advised to remember that "it is easy to forget that life is lived in relationships, and the quality of those relationships has much to do with how life turns out" (Lewis 1998). There is little question that for young adults attending colleges and universities, their relational world is precisely where their lives are lived.

KEY CONCEPTS

- Relationships are a critical contributor to students' college experiences and should be considered in any assessment of students' experiences.

- The types of relationships in which college students engage include roommates, friendships, and a range of different kinds of romantic and sexual relationships. Some students, however, have few ties and are quite lonely.

- The types of student relationships can also vary with students' normal developmental changes as they move through their college years.

Recommendations for Psychiatrists, Psychologists, and Counselors

1. It is important to think contextually about the students' experiences, because relationships have a continuing, changing, and significant influence on students' psychosocial well-being and adjustment.
2. Relationships can be a source of pride, anxiety, pleasure, or shame, so a sensitive, nonjudgmental inquiry to understand the full range of students' experiences is essential.
3. Relationships on campus can feel exciting and validating, confusing and volatile, and confining and intimidating. Students spend considerable time thinking about and discussing their relationship worries, problems, and wishes. Considering and honoring the full range of a student's relationship concerns will facilitate rapport, the development of the therapeutic alliance, and the therapeutic process.

Discussion Questions

1. In what ways do relationships play a critical role in college students' experiences?
2. What types of college student relationships are important, and how do they differ?
3. If college students' experiences are primarily rooted in their relational world, how does this perspective change the views of administrators and health care professionals about psychopathology and mental health intervention?

4. How does thinking systemically and relationally about student relationships influence programming on the part of administrators and health care professionals in the college or university context?

Suggested Readings

Garcia JR, Reiber C, Massey SG, Merriwether AM: Sexual hookup culture: a review. Rev Gen Psychol 16(2):161–176, 2012
McCabe J: Connecting in College: How Friendship Networks Matter for Academic and Social Success. Chicago, IL, University of Chicago Press, 2016
Wade L: American Hookup: The New Culture of Sex on Campus. New York, WW Norton, 2017

References

Braithwaite S, Delevi R, Fincham F: Romantic relationships and the physical and mental health of college students. Pers Relatsh 17:1–12, 2010
Dargie E, Blair KL, Goldfinger C, Pukall CF: Go long! Predictors of positive relationship outcomes in long-distance dating relationships. J Sex Marital Ther 41(2):181–202, 2015 24274061
Erb S, Renshaw K, Short J, Pollard J: The importance of college roommate relationships: a review and systemic conceptualization. Journal of Student Affairs Research and Practice 51:43–55, 2014
Garcia JR, Reiber C, Massey SG, Merriwether AM: Sexual hookup culture: a review. Rev Gen Psychol 16(2):161–176, 2012 23559846
Heldman C, Wade L: Hook-up culture: setting a new research agenda. Sex Research and Social Policy 7:323–333, 2010
Lewis JM: For better or worse: interpersonal relationships and individual outcome. Am J Psychiatry 155(5):582–589, 1998 9585706
McCabe J: Connecting in College: How Friendship Networks Matter for Academic and Social Success. Chicago, IL, University of Chicago Press, 2016a
McCabe J: Friends with academic benefits. Contexts 15:22–29, 2016b
Minuchin S, Nichols M: Family Healing: Strategies for Hope and Understanding. New York, Simon & Schuster, 1984
Owen J, Fincham FD: Effects of gender and psychosocial factors on "friends with benefits" relationships among young adults. Arch Sex Behav 40(2):311–320, 2011 20349207
Tetreault PA, Fette R, Meidlinger PC, Hope D: Perceptions of campus climate by sexual minorities. J Homosex 60(7):947–964, 2013 23808345
Wade L: American Hookup: The New Culture of Sex on Campus. New York, WW Norton, 2017

Family Relationships During the College Years

Sujata Patel, M.D.

Bina Patel, M.D.

THE college years are a time of incredible growth for students who enter college straight from high school. They often arrive at school with little to no experience managing life on their own. If all goes well, they graduate as mature, functional adults. Although the college years are often seen as a time of increased independence and separation from parents, many students today remain strongly connected to their families, and parents often expect continued involvement in their children's lives. With this change in parental and student expectations, mental health clinicians and student life staff (e.g., student resident associates in campus housing, faculty fellows in student dormitories, and student life deans who are available to support a range of student needs) need to develop a thorough and nuanced understanding of students' family relationships to foster productive collaboration with students and their families.

Transition to College

When a student leaves home to attend college, everyone in the family must adapt to the change in circumstances. It can take time for family members to settle into a new equilibrium; they must learn to adapt to their new roles while giving up old ones.

THE STUDENT'S PERSPECTIVE: FROM ADOLESCENT TO ADULT

For many of today's college students, moving into a college dorm for the first time marks the most abrupt transformation they have yet experienced. They change overnight from adolescents under parental care to adults responsible for making their own decisions. In our work as child and adolescent psychiatrists in college counseling centers, we have witnessed firsthand the challenges posed by this transition and its impact on family relationships.

First-year college students must adjust to new academic and social expectations while also learning how to take care of routine tasks that were previously handled by parents. These tasks can include arranging for medical and mental health care, filling prescriptions, and communicating with clinicians about past treatment. Students who are living on their own for the first time are also responsible for making choices about time management, drug and alcohol use, sexual activity, romantic and social relationships, and academic engagement.

THE PARENT'S PERSPECTIVE: FROM CAREGIVER TO CONSULTANT

As students adjust to being on their own, parents often struggle with the change in their own role. Parents who are used to being intimately involved in the lives of their children are now caught between wanting to foster their children's independence and worrying about their children's ability to manage new challenges. Recent articles in the popular press have characterized parents of today's college students as "helicopter" parents who hover over their children or as "snowplow" parents who are intent on removing all obstacles in their children's path (English 2013). One study found that "helicopter behaviors were associated with lower levels of perceived autonomy, competence, and relatedness" in college students (Schiffrin et al. 2014, p. 554). In our experience, these hovering parents are a small minority of those who have children in college. Most parents welcome their children's growing independence.

Factors Affecting the Student-Parent Relationship

Families from different backgrounds experience and react to students' transition to college in different ways. Socioeconomic status, ethnicity, cultural background, and community and family norms all affect this process.

RELATIONSHIP COMPLEXITIES

Although the move to college happens suddenly, students and parents must negotiate family relationships and roles over time, in a back-and-forth exchange. There may be different expectations between and within families for how much autonomy a student can handle at a particular stage or how much separation from a family is desirable. Some students will keep some aspects of their lives private but involve their families in other domains. For example, students might not share details of their dating life or their romantic relationships, but they might consult their parents about their academic courses or their choice of major. Each family has a unique way of approaching and resolving these issues, and students and parents need to work together to shape the roles that parents will play in students' lives.

For students, autonomy and closeness with their families are not always correlated. A recent study grouped students into four categories based on high or low "separateness" (independent functioning) and high or low "connectedness" (emotional closeness with parents). Students who were highly separate and also highly connected were categorized as "individuated"; those with low levels of both "separateness" and "connectedness" were categorized as "ambiguous." According to the study, individuated students tend to report more positive affect and lower depressive symptoms than ambiguous students (Kenyon and Koerner

2009). Students in the latter group, who are dependent but also emotionally disconnected, tend to express frustration and resentment toward their parents.

CHILDREN OF COLLEGE GRADUATES

Many middle-class and upper-middle-class students remain financially dependent on their parents during the college years. Students may take this support for granted, but it can undermine their efforts to assert themselves as independent adults. When parents are footing the bills, they can exert leverage over students' choices and behaviors.

Parents who are college graduates generally feel qualified to offer guidance to their students and to advocate for their students in the university setting. Many are able to sympathize with the challenges that students face because they recall their own college experiences. At the same time, students whose parents have attained a high degree of career success may feel pressure to live up to their parents' expectations for academic, social, and career achievement (Grigsby 2009).

FIRST-GENERATION COLLEGE STUDENTS

Students who are the first people in their family to attend college—a category that may include individuals from all socioeconomic backgrounds and diverse ethnic and cultural backgrounds—typically find themselves navigating cultural milieus with behavioral norms that are unfamiliar to them. For these students, transitions to and from home and school can feel jarring. Many feel pressure to obtain a lucrative job after college so they can improve their family's financial circumstances. Some send scholarship money home. These students sometimes also express concern that they will grow apart from family members as they pursue career trajectories that lead them into the middle or upper-middle class.

First-generation college students often report feeling close to their home communities but also describe how difficult it is to explain the challenges they face to family members (Grigsby 2009). Many of them feel guilty that they have access to opportunities and resources that some of their family members and peers lack. They also feel distant from more affluent students, who have access to resources and connections that are out of reach for them.

Students from less affluent backgrounds are more likely than their more affluent peers to have assumed some household responsibilities in high school, and thus they often arrive at school with a higher level of independence and self-sufficiency than those peers. Many students in this category worry about how their absence may affect family members who have depended on them, because they see themselves as contributing to—as well as receiving support from—their families (Grigsby 2009).

In addition to managing financial challenges on their own, first-generation college students must navigate the bureaucracy at their university and make decisions about their academic path without the guidance of parents who understand how the system works. At the same time, the parents of first-generation students still often want to be engaged in their children's lives. Indeed, many of these parents are deeply invested in their students having opportunities that they themselves did not have. However, they may lack confidence in their ability to guide students through educational challenges. A culturally sensitive clinician can serve as a valuable bridge between these parents and the university and can help parents appreciate the crucial role that they continue to play in their children's lives.

Changes in Patterns of Communication Between Parents and Students

Technology can be a blessing for college students and their family members; it allows families to stay connected regardless of the physical distances between them. Technology can also be a curse; it can interfere with the separation process that college students have traditionally experienced when they leave for college.

ROLE OF TECHNOLOGY

College students today have grown up with laptops and mobile phones. Many have had a mobile phone since middle school. As a result, many parents are used to having instant access to their children and to knowing their children's whereabouts at all times. Many parents, moreover, can track their children's activities on social media. In short, for millennial adolescents, a physical separation from home no longer leads automatically to a psychological separation from parents.

PARENTAL EXPECTATIONS

When students today leave for college, parents often anticipate staying in close communication with them. It is not unusual for parents and students to text, e-mail, or call each other multiple times per day (Stein et al.

2016). This practice is a far cry from the once-weekly phone call to parents that was typical for earlier generations of college students. As a result, parents are often aware of their students' shifting moods. Because students tend to call home more often when they are unhappy, parents may form an inaccurate impression of their mood patterns. Student life staff and clinicians in college counseling centers describe receiving calls from parents who are frantic because they have gone just a few hours without hearing from their student.

SETTING BOUNDARIES

Students today are so accustomed to constant communication that they can struggle to set boundaries with parents. Clinicians can help them with this process by exploring how much contact with parents they actually want and by discussing the times and methods of communication that would work best. The content of student-parent interaction and the meaning attached to it are as important as the frequency. Students often feel that their parents' calls, texts, and e-mails indicate a lack of confidence in them. It can be helpful to reframe such attempts to communicate as an expression of parental anxiety rather than a statement about a student's competence. In these cases, clinicians can advise students that initiating an occasional update will keep their parents happy while allowing the students some privacy and separation. The goal is to foster independence without sacrificing emotional support. Students may consult parents when making major decisions but will ideally begin to develop their own judgment.

Relationships With Siblings and Other Family Members

Although much attention is focused on the parent-student relationship, other family connections are also important to consider.

SHIFTS IN SIBLING RELATIONSHIPS

As college students separate from their families, their relationships with siblings also shift. Sometimes, distance from each other allows siblings to see each other as people and reduces rivalry and conflict. A student who had been accustomed to being dismissed may start to be consulted, confided in, and taken seriously by older siblings. Conversely, students who had little time for younger siblings may find themselves missing little brothers and sisters when away at school and looking forward to time at home together during breaks.

On the other hand, some sibling relationships can become more conflicted during the college years, as students and their siblings take different paths in life and set different goals and priorities. Some students may feel that they have little in common with their siblings once they no longer live at home together. Others may feel an increased sense of competition with siblings. In some cases, changes in values or beliefs can lead to rejection or a cooling of sibling relationships.

SIBLINGS AS A SOURCE OF CONNECTION AND SUPPORT

Particularly when student-parent relationships are fraught with tension, siblings can offer a less stressful way to maintain family connections. Older siblings with college experience can be a valuable source of advice for students. Many students object to their parents having full access to their social media but are more likely to be connected to siblings on Facebook and other sites. One recent study suggests that "synchronous communication" between college students and their siblings—including texts, phone calls, and in-person conversations—may be correlated with more positive sibling relationships (Lindell et al. 2015).

EXTENDED FAMILY TIES

Students with close connections to grandparents, aunts and uncles, or cousins can rely on them for different perspectives as they figure out their own identities and roles within their nuclear family and their extended family. These relatives can often mediate conflicts with parents or provide a different point of view. Asking a student about these relationships can be useful in treatment planning, particularly when communication with parents proves to be challenging. For some first-generation students, an extended family member who is a college student or college graduate can provide mentoring and guidance that parents cannot provide. Similarly, students from immigrant families can sometimes draw on the support of a relative who has greater familiarity with the dominant culture or language than the students' parents have.

Family-of-Origin Issues

For some college students, the family of origin is a source of stress rather than comfort and support. This can be due to abuse or neglect, family conflict or estrangement, or situations that develop at home while a student is at school. Support on campus can help students cope with these challenges.

ABUSE AND NEGLECT

Students who have suffered abuse or neglect by their parents or other family members do not leave these issues behind when they arrive at college. This transition may provide their first opportunity to address their trauma in a clinical setting. Clinicians working with these students are mandated to report incidents of abuse to Child Protective Services if any minor children remain at risk of maltreatment. Because disclosures of this kind can greatly affect the therapeutic alliance, clinicians should be sure to discuss such disclosures with affected students.

Students with a documented history of abuse or neglect may be eligible for financial aid through what is known as a "dependency override" (Federal Student Aid 2017). In these situations, the parents' financial status is no longer taken into account in determining a student's eligibility for aid.

ESTRANGEMENT FROM FAMILY OF ORIGIN

Some students, when they arrive at college, are estranged from one or both parents. Others may become estranged from their parents during their college years. The reasons for estrangement include differences in religious belief, parental rejection of a student's sexual orientation or gender identity, and disagreements regarding lifestyle choices. Although parental threats of abandonment do occur, permanent estrangement from a family of origin is rare. Parents may initially refuse to accept a student's identity or choices but usually move toward acceptance when they realize that their connection to their child is at stake. Clinicians can help students and parents see each other's point of view and suggest ways to reopen channels of communication.

DIFFICULT SITUATIONS AT HOME

Students who no longer live at home are still deeply affected by what happens there. Parental separation or divorce, parental illness or death, financial difficulties, or problems experienced by a sibling can lead to student distress. It can be jarring for students to speak with family members about challenges that happen at home and then return to their on-campus lives. Some students decide to take time off from school and return home during times of crisis. Changes at home can also lead to sudden shifts in the family roles that students are asked to play.

Students who feel that family members are withholding stressful information from them during times of crisis can experience a heightened sense of worry. Direct and transparent discussions between students and families about how and when to share distressing information can go a long way toward fostering trust and connection. Ongoing work with a mental health clinician can help students cope with all of these changes.

Parents and the University

Changes in university culture and parental expectations are transforming the relationship between parents and universities. Gone are the days when parents dropped their children off and disappeared, never to be heard from again. Clinicians and campus officials working with college students should keep abreast of these changes.

THE UNIVERSITY'S ATTITUDE TOWARD PARENTS

Colleges and universities send parents mixed signals. Parents are responsible for paying tuition to the extent that they are able. They are welcomed on campus when students are deciding which college to attend. However, once a student is enrolled, parents are largely left out of the college experience—unless a student is in trouble. For a generation of parents who are used to being highly involved in their children's lives, this shift can be difficult to handle.

Institutions of higher education must make a special effort to engage parents who did not attend college, who are not comfortable communicating in English, or who belong to minority groups that are underrepresented on college campuses. Making these parents feel welcome on campus is the first step toward helping their children feel welcome as well (Kiyama et al. 2015).

PARENTS AND STUDENTS AS CONSUMERS

Across the United States, colleges and universities have been beautifying their campuses, building fancy gyms, and improving food services (Martin 2012). Meanwhile, the price tag of a college education has climbed much faster than the rate of inflation. Added to this are concerns about increased selectivity at the nation's top schools, increased numbers of international applicants, and widening economic inequality. It is no wonder, then, that many parents today see a college education as an expensive investment on which they expect a return. As the percentage of Americans with a college degree has climbed, a bachelor's degree is no longer seen as a guarantee of financial security. Parents may have preconceived ideas about what academic path their students should follow, and students, in turn, may feel pressure to conform to parental expectations.

PARENTAL CONTACT WITH CLINICIANS AND STUDENT LIFE STAFF

In the past, college counseling centers prioritized student privacy and the fostering of independence. As a result, clinicians typically contacted parents only in urgent or critical situations. Today, however, clinicians should keep in mind the developmental stage of a student as they decide whether and when to involve parents. In the case of a first-year student who experiences a difficult transition to college, for example, a phone conversation between a clinician and a parent can help to allay parental worries, to obtain key information about student and family histories, and to increase the odds that a student will remain in treatment. Parents who have spoken with a clinician are much more likely to call the clinician if a concern arises in the future.

Parents often call college counseling centers to share or obtain information about students. When parents seek confidential information, clinicians can discuss clinic policies and services but should also point out that a release-of-information authorization is required to share any clinical information about a student. Clinicians should keep in mind that parents' perspectives are valuable and that even without a release-of-information authorization, they can listen to parents' concerns.

Obtaining a release-of-information authorization also means that a clinician can involve parents if a student stops attending appointments or experiences a change in functioning or mood. In our experience, students are most likely to grant permission to speak with parents when the clinician frames such communication as a way to help parents understand a student's experience, to reassure parents, or to obtain medical or family history that the student may not be aware of. By interacting with parents in a thoughtful manner, clinicians can model a way for students to communicate collaboratively with their families.

HIPAA AND FERPA

The Health Insurance Portability and Accountability Act (HIPAA) and the Family Educational Rights and Privacy Act (FERPA) govern the disclosure of students' medical and educational records, respectively. FERPA allows disclosure of educational records to those on campus "whom the school has determined to have legitimate educational interests" or to "appropriate officials in connection with a health or safety emergency" (Family Policy Compliance Office 2017). This means that a student life official who is concerned about a student can inform residence life staff or contact the counseling center if a situation is deemed urgent. Counseling centers receive these calls frequently.

Disclosure of information without student permission can also occur "[t]o parents of an eligible student if the student is a dependent for IRS tax purposes" (https://www2.ed.gov/policy/gen/guid/fpco/faq.html). This applies to most full-time college students under age 24, unless they earn a majority of the income to support themselves through college. Parents can also be informed when a student under age 21 violates the law or school policies related to alcohol or other substances. Because FERPA guidelines are generally less strict than HIPAA guidelines, campus life or student affairs staff can often share information with parents about a student when clinicians do not have permission from the student to do so.

ROLE OF CLINICIANS AND STUDENT LIFE STAFF

Clinicians and student life staff working with college students need to understand the dynamics of each student's family when communicating with parents. This is especially important when a student is struggling with academic, medical, or mental health challenges that can affect the timeline on which a student moves toward independence. Partnering with parents can help to ensure that they are aligned with—and not in opposition to—campus support staff and clinicians. Parents can be valuable allies when appropriately engaged. They know their child's history and can also arrange for services at home or off-campus when needed. If a student would benefit from taking time off from school, involving parents can smooth the exit from and return to school. Parents can also help to persuade a reluctant student to pursue treatment.

When students and their parents agree on how quickly and how much to separate, there is usually little conflict. However, problems can arise when students and parents expect a level of parental involvement that is not congruent with current campus norms. For example, parents who expect to communicate directly with a professor regarding a student's grade will usually encounter resistance. In that kind of situation, a clinician who has earned the trust of both the parents and the student can encourage them to take small steps toward independence over time. Cutting out the parents entirely tends to backfire. Highly involved parents, we have found, are eager to receive information and guidance from university staff and clinicians.

Case Example

Robert is an 18-year-old first-year undergraduate student who presented to his university counseling center early in his second semester to seek treatment for anxiety and depressed mood. He described a difficult transition to college. He was an only child and was extremely close to his parents, particularly his mother. Robert called or texted his parents several times per day during the week. They lived a few hours from his college and drove to pick Robert up and take him home most weekends during his first semester. Robert avoided socializing with his peers in his dorm and felt anxious around his roommate. After spending winter break at home, he dreaded the return to school and became increasingly anxious and sad when the second semester started. After calling home in tears a few times, he decided to seek help at the counseling center.

Over the course of several therapy sessions, he discussed his loneliness and his lack of confidence in navigating college on his own. He was used to seeking parental advice for major and minor decisions. He had not developed a supportive network of peers on campus and had not yet connected to any mentors or advisors. Robert and his therapist decided to invite his parents to participate in a joint therapy session to discuss Robert's struggles to become more independent. His parents were able to acknowledge that the time had come for Robert to make more decisions on his own and to spend more time on campus during weekends so he could bond with peers.

Over the next several months, Robert joined clubs and activities and made an effort to talk to more people in his dorm. His mood improved, and he became less anxious when he learned that many of his peers were also struggling to adjust to college life. He still communicated with his parents frequently, but he sought advice less often and instead shared updates on his activities. By the end of his first year of college, Robert had connected with a friend group and developed an increased sense of confidence in his own ability to navigate the challenges of college life.

Conclusion

As they move toward increasing autonomy and independence, most college students remain closely connected to their families. Clinicians working with the college-age population must learn how and when to involve parents and other family members while keeping in mind issues of privacy. Young adults must learn to navigate the changes in family roles and relationships that occur during this stage of life.

KEY CONCEPTS

- The developmental transition from adolescence to adulthood that occurs in college also transforms students' relationships with their families.
- Many factors influence the ways in which students and families navigate the changes in roles that occur during this crucial time.
- Thoughtful engagement with parents by clinicians and student life staff can help students thrive on campus.

Recommendations for Psychiatrists, Psychologists, and Counselors

1. Mental health clinicians should consider involving parents or other family members when providing care to college students.
2. Clinicians should stay informed about the legal issues involved in disclosure of clinical information to family members of college students.
3. Clinicians should be aware of the myriad ways in which family relationships can influence the mental health of college students.

Discussion Questions

1. How are student-family relationships affected by socioeconomic status, ethnicity, race, country of origin, and other demographic variables?
2. How have communication patterns between college students and their families changed over time? What are the advantages and disadvantages of current patterns compared with those of the previous generation?
3. What strategies can clinicians and university officials use to engage parents who do not feel connected to the university?

Suggested Readings

Grigsby M: College Life Through the Eyes of Students. Albany, NY, SUNY Press, 2009

Kiyama JM, Harper CE, Ramos D, et al: Parent and family engagement in higher education. ASHE Higher Education Report 41(6):1–94, 2015

Schiffrin HH, Liss M, Miles-MacLean H, et al: Helping or hovering? The effects of helicopter parents on college students' well-being. Journal of Child and Family Studies 23:548–557, 2014

Self C: Parent involvement in higher education: a review of the literature. AHEPP Journal 4(1):1–11, 2013

References

English B: "Snow-plow" parents overly involved in college students' lives. The Boston Globe, November 9, 2013. Available at: https://www.boston-globe.com/arts/2013/11/09/parents-overly-involved-college-students-lives/mfYvA5R9IhRpJytEbFpxUP/story.html. Accessed July 21, 2017.

Family Policy Compliance Office, U.S. Department of Education: Model notifica-tions of rights under FERPA for postsecondary institutions. Available at: http://familypolicy.ed.gov/content/model-notifications-rights-under-ferpa-postsecondary-institutions. Accessed July 21, 2017.

Federal Student Aid, U.S. Department of Education: Dependency override. Available at: https://fafsa.ed.gov/fotw1718/help/fahelp26h.htm. Ac-cessed July 21, 2017.

Grigsby M: College Life Through the Eyes of Students. Albany, NY, SUNY Press, 2009, p 1552

Kenyon DYCB, Koerner SS: College student psychological well-being during the transition to college: examining individuation from parents. College Student Journal 43(4):1145–1160, 2009

Kiyama JM, Harper CE, Ramos D, et al: Parent and family engagement in higher education. ASHE Higher Education Report 41(6): 2015

Lindell AK, Campione-Barr N, Killoren SE: Technology-mediated communication with siblings during the transition to college: associations with relationship positivity and self-disclosure. Fam Relat 64:563–578, 2015

Martin A: Building a showcase campus, using an I.O.U. New York Times, Decem-ber 13, 2012. Available at: http://www.nytimes.com/2012/12/14/business/colleges-debt-falls-on-students-after-construction-binges.html. Accessed July 21, 2017.

Schiffrin HH, Liss M, Miles-MacLean H, et al: Helping or hovering? The effects of helicopter parents on college students' well-being. J Child Fam Stud 23:548–557, 2014

Stein CH, Osborn LA, Greenberg SC: Understanding young adults' reports of con-tact with their parents in a digital world: psychological and familial relation-ship factors. J Child Fam Stud 25:1802–1814, 2016

Distress and Academic Jeopardy

Bina Patel, M.D.
Sujata Patel, M.D.

EMOTIONAL well-being is central to college students' academic performance, to the development of their professional and social identities, and to their overall ability to thrive in a university setting. Students cite mental health concerns as the main obstacle to their academic functioning, and 85% report that they "felt overwhelmed by all that [they] had to do" during the previous year (American College Health Association 2016).

As large numbers of college students struggle with mental health concerns, clinicians working with these students face the challenge of distinguishing normal *stress* from more impairing forms of *distress*. To address that challenge, clinicians need to understand how common mental health issues may manifest in the college years, how to collaborate effectively with university partners to address students' needs, and how to support students who are experiencing some form of academic difficulty.

Understanding Barriers to Success

Students devote a great deal of attention to the academic preparation that is necessary to enter college. Typically, this work begins several years before a student graduates from high school. On the other hand, students may give less attention to their well-being and the emotional challenges inevitably encountered in college.

STRESS VERSUS DISTRESS

Normal *stress* responses are expected and necessary for emotional growth during the college years, as students cope with new challenges in both academic and social domains. Adaptive responses to stress in a college setting include feeling motivated to address challenges in a focused way; engaging with external sources of support, such as peers, friends, family members, advisors, and faculty members; and viewing stress as a natural response to changing circumstances and as an opportunity to learn and grow (Li and Yang 2016).

Feelings of *distress*, however, are often paralyzing rather than motivating. Students may feel overwhelmed by challenges and respond to them in a disorganized way that leads to increased frustration and a sense of hopelessness. Instead of seeking support, they may withdraw from people who can help them cope with problems and gain perspective on those problems. This kind of withdrawal often leads to increased isolation, and as a result, students experience their struggle not as a necessary process but as a reflection of an internal flaw.

Most students will experience periods of both stress and distress. If they are able to recall and draw on strengths that allowed them to navigate previous challenges, then the experience of distress can lead them to pursue more adaptive responses. For some students, however, especially those who present in clinical settings, periods of distress may become cyclical and lead to further isolation and impairment.

IMPOSTER SYNDROME

The term *impostor syndrome* describes high-achieving individuals who struggle to identify their success as being linked to stable and enduring qualities. Although this phenomenon was first studied in women (Clance and Imes 1978), it resonates with many successful individuals who face a major transition in their academic or work life and fear that they will be revealed as a "fraud" in a new setting. They attribute their success to luck or to other factors that are distinct from their abilities and efforts.

Students making the transition to college often worry that they will not measure up to their peers. This concern is particularly common among students entering highly competitive colleges and universities. In our work with students at such institutions, we have found that many express the belief that their acceptance was a "fluke" based on a random demographic variable or that the "admissions committee made a mistake." As a consequence, these students are often afraid to stretch themselves or to ask for help when they encounter academic difficulties; they fear that if they do so, someone will discover that they "don't belong here." This negative cycle has been associated with students experiencing depressive symptoms in college (McGregor et al. 2008).

SENSE OF BELONGING

Concerns about belonging in college and succeeding academically can be especially acute among first-generation college students and students from underrepresented groups. For these students, having a framework that will help them anticipate and respond to normal stressors is critical. A recent study that encompassed three large-scale randomized controlled trials examined the effects of providing 9,500 incoming college students with narratives by older students from varied backgrounds (Yeager et al. 2016). The older students described the social and academic challenges that they encountered in the transition to college and told the incoming students that these difficulties were typical and improved over time. The incoming students were then asked to reflect on their own experiences and expectations. According to the study, this kind of intervention reduced institutional achievement gaps between students from disadvantaged backgrounds and other students by up to 40%.

"FIXED" MIND-SET VERSUS "GROWTH" MIND-SET

Having a "fixed" mind-set rather than a "growth" mind-set can affect how students cope with academic challenges. Students who believe that intelligence is a fixed quality that they cannot change are more likely to perceive academic setbacks, or the need to expend extra effort in their course work, as proof of a deficiency. This view leaves them less likely to take on challenges in the first place and more likely to give up when they encounter obstacles (Dweck 1986).

In contrast, students who believe that intellectual abilities can grow through effort are more likely to seek challenges and to persist when they have setbacks. Interventions aimed at cultivating a growth mind-set have been shown to foster greater academic achievement at all stages of education, and more vulnerable students are especially likely to benefit from such interventions (Rattan et al. 2015).

By discussing the "growth mind-set" concept with students, educators and mental health clinicians can help normalize academic challenges and reinforce the message that academic struggle is a key element of intellectual growth. In this way, educators and mental health clinicians can have a significant impact on students' efforts to reduce academic stress.

MENTAL HEALTH ISSUES

Although concerns about belonging and academic competence are expected in the transition to college, staggering numbers of college students also report significant mental health concerns that affect their academic functioning. Data from the spring 2016 American College Health Association–National College Health Assessment Survey cover 95,761 students at 137 postsecondary institutions (American College Health Association 2016). When asked about their experiences over the preceding 12 months, these students reported the following experiences: "felt overwhelming anxiety" (58.4%), "felt things were hopeless" (49.8%), "felt overwhelming anger" (39.6%), "felt so depressed that it was difficult to function" (36.7%), and "seriously considered suicide" (9.8%).

These students were also asked if any of a broad range of factors (physical, behavioral, psychological, social, or financial) had adversely affected their academic performance in the previous year. The top four stressors reported (American College Health Association 2016) were the following: stress (31.8%), anxiety (23.2%), sleep difficulties (20.7%), and depression (15.4%).

As these data show, mental concerns are the primary factors affecting academic functioning. The connection between academic functioning and emotional well-being is bidirectional: academic performance can also affect students' mental health. More than 47% of undergraduate students report that academic challenges felt "traumatic or very difficult to handle" in the preceding year (American College Health Association 2016). Academic struggles can, in turn, cause students to experience crises of confidence that make them more vulnerable to impairing forms of distress and more likely to exhibit mental health concerns.

For mental health professionals, discerning whether a student may be in crisis can be challenging. Although some students explicitly describe symptoms of anxiety, depression, or overwhelming stress, others manifest symptoms through behavioral or functional changes. Students may start to miss assignments and classes, or they may start to avoid interaction with advisors and faculty members. They may also withdraw from activities and social interactions, or they may increase their use of alcohol and other substances. Physical complaints such as fatigue and sleep difficulties are also common (American College Health Association 2016). Clinicians working with students should be aware of the various ways in which symptoms can manifest. To address these issues effectively, clinicians may also need to consult with campus medical, academic, and student life professionals.

Collaboration With Campus Partners

Each college has its own structure and culture of academic and student life support, and navigating the landscape of a particular school is a bit like traveling in a foreign country. Mental health clinicians should therefore consider this question: What are the languages, customs, regulations, norms, and expectations that a student will encounter? Asking detailed questions about students' lives on campus will not only help clinicians to build a therapeutic alliance with students but will also provide information to help clinicians understand students' needs and the resources available to help them.

STUDENT LIFE STAFF

Student life staff members have a unique window into students' experiences and functioning. People in this group include student resident associates in campus housing, faculty fellows in student dormitories, and student life deans who are available to support a range of student needs. These officials are often the first point of contact both for students in distress and for family members and others who have concerns about a particular student. Faculty fellows and student life deans can also reach out to academic departments and families to help support a student of concern. As they take this step, they should follow guidelines set forth under the Family Educational Rights and Privacy Act (FERPA; Family Policy Compliance Office 2017).

For clinicians working with students who may benefit from additional frontline support, student life staff members can be a valuable resource. In addition to directing students to sources of academic support on campus, they can engage students who may be in crisis but are ambivalent about accessing mental health care. Discussions with students about connecting with student life staff can cover a spectrum of options:

- Informing students of the availability of student life staff and explaining the role that this group plays on campus
- Obtaining a release of information from a student to contact staff about a specific student need, or to let staff members know that a student they referred has connected for treatment
- Telling students the circumstances under which a clinician may consider contacting student life staff without explicit permission from a student—circumstances that include acute concern about a student's safety or the safety of other students and events (e.g., hospitalization) that require a student to leave campus abruptly (American Psychiatric Association 2016)

STUDENT DISABILITY OFFICE

In the case of students diagnosed with mental health disorders or learning needs that affect their academic functioning, it can be helpful for clinicians to obtain permission from students to communicate with a school's disability office. Clinicians who request potential accommodations or services for a student should focus on how a specific concern affects the student's ability to learn. They can make recommendations about such accommodations, but student disability advisors will usually need to meet with a student directly to determine which services are appropriate. Potential interventions may involve providing a student with extra time to take exams, extensions on assignments, note-taking or tutoring services, reduction in the student's credit requirements per term, and housing accommodations (U.S. Department of Education 2011).

FACULTY AND ACADEMIC ADVISING STAFF

Students are often directed to seek mental health care by academic advisors or faculty members who notice a change in a student's functioning or hear directly from a student about symptoms or thoughts that raise concern (Harper and Peterson 2005). Sometimes, however, students may be reluctant to tell an advisor or faculty member that they are seeking services because they are wary of the stigma that may come with appearing less than able. Stigma is a particular concern among graduate students. Their relationships with faculty members can be intense and complex, and they often fear that a faculty member's confidence in them or support for them will diminish if they disclose difficulties. For faculty members, meanwhile, a change in a student's functioning can feel bewildering, particularly if they do not understand the context for that change.

Discussions with students in treatment about whether, how, and when to involve faculty members and advisors should take into account the following questions:

- What is the likely impact of students' symptoms on their near-term and future academic functioning?
- What are realistic academic goals for students given their current symptoms?
- Do students have an accurate perception of their past and current academic functioning?

Students often have a distorted view of how well or how poorly they are doing, and without objective information from faculty members or advisors about their performance, it can be difficult to formulate realistic treatment plans.

Communication with advisors and faculty members can occur in a variety of ways. In the case of undergraduate students, a student disability office can contact faculty members regarding the need for accommodations without disclosing specific medical information. For this reason, many college mental health centers have a policy that calls for clinicians to work with the disability office instead of sending information directly to faculty members.

In the case of graduate students, faculty members may need to have more information about a student's functioning in order to address long-term issues related to the student's academic work and funding. For this reason, students often choose to talk directly with faculty members about their situation. Alternatively, they may ask clinicians to communicate with faculty members on their behalf. Although taking that step may be appropriate in some cases, clinicians should keep in mind the need to protect a student's medical privacy and should first assess whether there are other campus entities (e.g., the disability office or the student life office) that can help advocate for a student (American Psychiatric Association 2016).

Academic Review Process

Academic performance is a key measure of how well students are functioning in college. Some students who grapple with mental health concerns will continue to do well in their course work. However, students who struggle to meet minimum academic standards are very likely to experience major challenges to their well-being and self-esteem.

All colleges have standards set by faculty for expected academic progress. Students who are on the borderline of meeting those standards are considered to be in "academic jeopardy." If their term or cumulative grade point average (GPA) falls below an expected standard or they earn too few credits per term, they are placed on academic probation.

Each institution reviews students' grades at the end of each academic term. Most institutions also provide students with midterm warnings if their performance falls short of established benchmarks. These warnings encourage students to connect with faculty members and advisors for additional support while there is still time for helpful intervention. Students who do not meet minimum GPA and credit standards at the end of a term are notified that they are on academic probation and are instructed to meet with advisors who can help them develop a plan for returning to good academic standing. Students may be subject to academic dismissal or suspension if they remain on academic probation for two or more consecutive terms.

In working with students who are struggling academically, mental health clinicians should become familiar with the standards for academic progress at the students' institutions. Academic advisors will share information on standards directly with students, and such information is typically available online. However, feelings of shame may prevent students who are in jeopardy or on probation from fully acknowledging the academic difficulty that they face, and thus they may not fully use the resources available to them. Clinicians should inquire frequently about students' academic lives. If they become aware that students are in academic difficulty, they should urge these students to meet regularly with their advisors, who can provide clarifying feedback and critical support in developing appropriate educational plans (Gehrke and Wong 2007).

Mental health professionals can also help to assess a student for potential academic accommodations. Colleges can allow students to reduce the number of credits per term that they must take or to take extra terms toward degree completion if students meet criteria for disability accommodations (U.S. Department of Education 2011). These types of accommodations require clinicians to submit supporting documentation to the student disability office at a student's university. Student athletes, international students, and students who receive financial aid or scholarship funding may have to meet additional eligibility standards.

In most institutions, the decision to suspend a student for failure to make expected academic progress usually occurs only after a careful review by a committee that includes advisors, faculty members, and student life staff members. Students facing suspension typically have an opportunity to submit a personal statement and a plan for addressing the obstacles that have interfered with their academic work (R. Williams, Associate Dean for Undergraduate Advising and Research, Stanford University; L. Schlosberg, Director of Academic and Educational Support Programs, Undergraduate Advising and Research, Stanford University, personal communications, November 11, 2016).

For students facing an academic suspension ruling, clinicians may conclude that it is appropriate to share information with a review committee. Clinicians should do so only with a student's authorization and only after determining which committee representative is designated to receive confidential information. Situations in which it is suitable to share information vary. A student may be experiencing a specific stressor that is approaching resolution, for example. Or a student may be undergoing treatment for a condition that is likely to stabilize enough to allow the student to learn effectively by the next academic term. Review committees do not want or need detailed clinical information but are likely to welcome a clinician's input regarding a student's ability to succeed academically in the near future.

Most schools establish a minimum amount of time that students who are on academic suspension must be away from school before they can return. Institutions vary on the expectations and requirements for return. Although students receive detailed guidelines about such policies at the time of suspension, they may not absorb such information fully during this stressful period. School officials emphasize that the suspension process is not punitive; instead, it is meant to allow a student time to address obstacles to learning and to develop a plan for moving forward. The elements of an effective plan include an assessment of factors that led to academic difficulty, a strategy to address academic and other relevant stressors, and a commitment to communicating regularly with academic advisors and other campus resources.

Mental health professionals can support students on academic suspension in several ways: by helping them find appropriate treatment resources when they need to leave campus; by encouraging them to stay in contact with academic advisors during their time away; by working with them to explore any mental health, developmental, or psychosocial obstacles to academic success that they face; and by helping them maintain confidence in their ability to learn.

Case Example

James is a 20-year-old sophomore student at an elite private university. He had been estranged from his biological parents since middle school, and had lived with relatives and in foster homes prior to entering college. His academic talent had been recognized and nurtured in the large public high school he attended, resulting in his getting a full scholarship in college. However, during his first year, he found that his level of academic preparation was behind that of many of his peers. His sense of academic competence, which had been a source of pride and resilience for him throughout high school, began to falter. He felt sensitive about his multiracial background and his lack of a "traditional" family at home. He also found it difficult to feel fully connected to peers and faculty members whose identities, life experiences, and economic resources often differed widely from his own.

By his sophomore year James had begun to experience episodes of significant anxiety, which led to his missing classes and assignments and resulted in his becoming further isolated from his peers. He was placed on academic probation at the end of his sophomore fall term. After being placed on probation, James met with his academic advisor and disclosed the struggles he had been having with anxiety and the shame he felt about his academic difficulties. His advisor helped to decrease James's sense of shame by expressing appreciation for James's openness during their discussion, by validating James's ability to do well in college, and by conveying that the probation process was meant not to be punitive but to help students engage with key supports. James's advisor also connected him with tutoring resources on campus, set up regular check-in meetings throughout the term, and referred him to the university counseling center.

James went to the counseling center and met with a therapist for several sessions during his sophomore spring term. Initially, they worked on approaches to stabilize his anxiety, which was interfering with his daily functioning. James gave his therapist permission to provide documentation of his anxiety symptoms to the university's student disability office. After meeting with a disability advisor, James was allowed to take a reduced course load while his anxiety symptoms were being stabilized.

James and his therapist also explored factors that had affected his self-esteem in college. They examined and questioned James's assumption that his academic struggles were due to a lack of ability, instead of being an expected part of the transition to a more competitive environment. As James began to view academic challenges as reflective of growth instead of vulnerability, he was able to engage more effectively with academic life. He developed a strong connection with a faculty member in the setting of a small seminar class, where he felt comfortable expressing how his life experiences had contributed to his perspective on key topics. This faculty member remained available as a mentor who helped to foster James's academic confidence. As James became less anxious and more confident in contributing to discussions in and out of class, he began to develop friendships with peers, which added to his sense of belonging.

By the end of his junior year, James had been in good academic standing for three consecutive terms, was making expected progress toward his degree, and had made lasting connections with several peers.

Conclusion

Clinicians who work with college students must be knowledgeable about the range of expected stressors and mental health concerns that can arise during the college years and the impact that these experiences may have on everyday functioning and academic performance. When caring for students in academic difficulty, clinicians also need to learn about the specific supports and processes within each student's institution. As clinicians encourage students to engage with campus resources, they must sensitively address issues such as shame, isolation, and self-criticism, which may prevent students who are struggling academically from seeking help.

KEY CONCEPTS

- Psychological distress and mental health concerns are the primary factors that affect academic functioning of college students today.

- Educators and mental health professionals working with college students need to understand and address common barriers to students' sense of competence and belonging in college.

- Students in academic distress typically require the support of multiple campus resources.

Recommendations for Psychiatrists, Psychologists, and Counselors

1. Mental health clinicians should screen for and address common emotional challenges that students face in the transition to college.

2. Clinicians should consider collaborating with campus partners in support of students' academic and emotional needs.
3. Clinicians should support students who are struggling academically in key ways: encouraging early and frequent contact with academic advising staff; considering if students would benefit from academic accommodations because of their symptoms; and helping students to understand the standards for academic progress at their institutions.

Discussion Questions

1. What are the most common mental health concerns affecting academic functioning, as reported by college students?
2. What are some key emotional and social issues that affect how students respond to academic challenges? How can educators and mental health professionals discuss these issues with students?
3. Which campus partners offer resources that can help mental health professionals to support students in academic jeopardy?
4. What are some of the common components of an academic review process? What role can mental health professionals play in that process?

Suggested Readings

American College Health Association: American College Health Association–National College Health Assessment II: Spring 2016 Reference Group Executive Summary. Hanover, MD, American College Health Association, 2016. Available at: http://www.acha-ncha.org/docs/NCHA-II%20Spring %202016%20US%20Reference%20Group%20Executive%20Summary.pdf.
Rattan A, Savani K, Chugh D, Dweck CS: Leveraging mindsets to promote academic achievement: policy recommendations. Perspect Psychol Sci 10(6):721–726, 2015
Yeager DS, Walton GM, Brady ST, et al: Teaching a lay theory before college narrows achievement gaps at scale. Proc Natl Acad Sci USA 113(24):E3341–E3348, 2016

References

American College Health Association: American College Health Association–National College Health Assessment II: Spring 2016 Reference Group Executive Summary. Hanover, MD, American College Health Association, 2016. Available at: http://www.acha-ncha.org/docs/NCHA-II%20Spring %202016%20US%20Reference%20Group%20Executive%20Summary.pdf. Accessed January 2, 2017.

American Psychiatric Association, Council on Psychiatry and Law: Resource Document on College Mental Health and Confidentiality. Arlington, VA, American Psychiatric Association, 2016. Available at https://www.psychiatry.org/psychiatrists/search-directories-databases/library-and-archive/resource-documents. Accessed January 2018.

Clance PR, Imes SA: The impostor phenomenon in high achieving women: dynamics and therapeutic intervention. Psychotherapy 15(3):241–247, 1978

Dweck CS: Motivational processes affecting learning. Am Psychol 41(10):1040–1048, 1986

Family Policy Compliance Office, U.S. Department of Education: Model notifications of rights under FERPA for postsecondary institutions. Available at: http://familypolicy.ed.gov/content/model-notifications-rights-under-ferpa-postsecondary-institutions. Accessed July 21, 2017.

Gehrke S, Wong J: Students on academic probation, in Advising Special Student Populations. NAAA Monograph Series, No 17. Edited by Huff L, Jordan P. Manhattan, KS, National Academic Advising Association, 2007, pp 135–185

Harper R, Peterson M: Mental Health Issues and College Students: What Advisors Can Do. Manhattan, KS, NACADA Clearinghouse of Academic Advising Resources, 2005. Available at: http://www.nacada.ksu.edu/tabid/3318/articleType/ArticleView/articleId/141/article.aspx. Accessed July 21, 2017.

Li M, Yang Y: A cross-cultural study on a resilience-stress path model for college students. Journal of Counseling & Development 94(3):319–332, 2016

McGregor LN, Gee DE, Posey KE: I feel like a fraud and it depresses me: the relation between the imposter phenomenon and depression. Social Behavior and Personality 36(1):43–48, 2008

Rattan A, Savani K, Chugh D, Dweck CS: Leveraging mindsets to promote academic achievement: policy recommendations. Perspect Psychol Sci 10(6):721–726, 2015 26581725

U.S. Department of Education, Office for Civil Rights: Students With Disabilities Preparing for Postsecondary Education: Know Your Rights and Responsibilities, Washington, DC, U.S. Department of Education, 2011. Available at: http://www.ed.gov/ocr/transition.html. Accessed July 21, 2017.

Yeager DS, Walton GM, Brady ST, et al: Teaching a lay theory before college narrows achievement gaps at scale. Proc Natl Acad Sci USA 113(24):E3341–E3348, 2016 27247409

Caring for Students With Mental Health Issues

Psychiatric Evaluation of the Young Adult University Student

Matthew Pesko, M.D.

Amy Alexander, M.D.

Douglas L. Noordsy, M.D.

IN this chapter, we review the elements of a complete evaluation of the young adult university student. University students can include a broad range of undergraduate, graduate, and postdoctoral learners who are typically ages 18–30 years. These individuals are in the midst of intense social change and may have just left their childhood home for the first time. Many have traveled across the country or around the world to attend their university. They are experiencing substantial academic demands in addition to maintaining athletic training, club, or teaching responsibilities; arranging study abroad and internships; and discovering a hidden curriculum that seems to require competitive perfection. Students face critical decisions about career goals during their academic progression, and they may not yet have the experience and perspective of being unable to master challenging tasks. An astute psychiatric evaluation of university students takes this context into consideration.

Information Gathering Before the Evaluation

It is prudent for any mental health professional practicing with young adults to obtain information about each student ahead of time to more accurately guide the psychiatric evaluation in an efficient manner. Our experience is that time spent gathering information about clinical history can provide dividends in terms of time saved and accuracy during the evaluation. Additionally, it is likely that students will appreciate that the clinician has put in the work ahead of time to get to know them, thus building rapport and trust in the therapeutic relationship. First, the clinician must understand the nature of the referral, which should be straightforward and easily available: is it an urgent, walk-in appointment; consultation; or routine appointment to establish an ongoing treatment relationship?

Next, it is helpful to know who placed the referral. Many students will have online or phone access and be able to set up an appointment for themselves. Other potential referral sources include a primary care physician who is concerned about mental health symptoms observed in or reported by a student, a psychologist or case manager seeing the patient for therapy who requests a medication evaluation, or parents who wish that their child continue ongoing mental health services after moving away from home and commencing higher education. Referrals that are unique in the college or university setting could come from an academic dean, housing dean, friends, or peers who have witnessed concerning behavior from the student (Kirsch et al. 2014). Last, a student may be referred for evaluation after completing an inpatient hospitalization.

It is also likely that there will be some information available from a screening/triage mechanism. This information would ideally include a chief complaint that is the impetus for the student to seek mental health treatment. Although the chief complaint expressed during a screening appointment can be helpful in guiding the evaluation, it is often general or vague for college students because of their lack of experience with mental health treatment; frequent general complaints that could lead in many different directions include "stress," "feeling overwhelmed," "lack of sleep," and "relationship problems." Lists of medications and allergies, if available, should be reviewed and recorded in an easily accessible format for reference during the evaluation. It will be helpful to note whether a student has ever seen or is currently seeing a psychiatrist, therapist, or other mental health professional. Advance knowledge about identity-related information such as the following can help to establish rapport more quickly: the student's year in college, the name the student wishes to be called, the student's gender identification, and the student's preferred personal pronouns (these include but are not limited to he/him, she/her, they/them). Perhaps the most important screening-related item relevant to a psychiatric evaluation is whether the patient has any suicidal ideation or self-harm behaviors currently or has had them in the past. A screening protocol would likely help in directing the student to the appropriate level of care (e.g., inpatient vs. outpatient); however, caution should be taken to prevent errors or misunderstandings that could lead to a referral, for example, of an actively suicidal patient to a routine outpatient evaluation. After all this information is reviewed, the psychiatrist may pause and consider whether it makes sense that the student is being referred to a psychiatrist. Perhaps the concern is more easily addressed by a primary care physician, a neurologist, a social worker, or a student services liaison.

Next, the psychiatric professional should further review other information available in the student's medical record. This may include labs (e.g., thyroid stimulating hormone, vitamin B_{12}, complete blood count, comprehensive metabolic panel), imaging, and the nature of other medical visits (e.g., sexual health, substance use). Also, scanned records may be available within the patient's medical record that detail past psychiatric history and treatment if the patient has been seen before by mental health professionals.

All the information up to this point can be gathered solely by the clinician, likely from within the medical record. For particularly challenging or unclear referrals, a direct conversation with the referral source may be advisable. In rare cases, the clinician may need to discuss certain items with the student before the first meeting (e.g., scheduling conflicts, forms/documents needed ahead of time, problems with insurance coverage).

Setting the Stage Immediately Prior to Evaluation

At the time of the psychiatric evaluation of the young adult university student, the clinician is equipped with knowledge gleaned ahead of time regarding the new patient. A few additional steps should be pursued to maximize patient comfort and minimize distraction during the visit. The clinician will want to pay attention to the room environment, including lighting and the number and spacing of chairs in the room. Keeping in mind the comfort of the student and the importance of establishing the therapeutic alliance, the psychiatrist will need to decide whether to interview from across a desk or an open space. Having ready access to several items will also ensure efficiency during the evaluation; these may include release-of-information forms, privacy information for the clinic, standardized screening instruments such as the Patient Health Questionnaire (PHQ; Spitzer et al. 1999), and contact information or business card for the clinician.

Start of the Evaluation

First impressions are important in all areas of life, no less so for a patient's first impression of a new mental health professional. This will likely be formed within the first several minutes of the interview. The first impression is especially important at a young-adult student's first-ever mental health visit because it can influence the individual's experience of psychiatry and all mental health care for years to come. The clinician should be aware of preconceptions that the student might have of psychiatric services, based on popular culture depictions or experiences of other students at their institutions (a very prudent approach is to regularly read the student-published newspaper if existent and available). In one cross-sectional study (Downs and Eisenberg 2012), personal stigma (one's own attitudes of mental health diagnoses and treatments) was shown to be associated with lower use of treatment services.

The very first interaction is in the waiting room. The psychiatric professional will want to use the student's preferred name, provide an introduction, and invite the student back to the office or evaluation room. The student may be accompanied to the appointment by someone else—parents, partner, or friends. The clinician can ask whether the student wants the other(s) to join them; if the student does, the clinician may want to explain that the other(s) can join for most of the visit but that some information would have to be gathered from the student alone for privacy and confidentiality reasons and, although it does not need to be stated, to allow the student to be as open as possible regarding symptoms and concerns.

When present and seated in the evaluation setting, the physician will reintroduce himself or herself and explain the job of the psychiatrist in layman's terms, such as, "I am a doctor who specializes in mental health care and can help with understanding your experience, as well as treatment with medications, therapy, and lifestyle interventions." We recommend that the clinician then explain the process of the evaluation *before* launching into questioning. It is easy to forget that the format of a mental health evaluation, while familiar for clinicians, is not necessarily known to the patient. An opening line may take the following form: "I understand a little about what brings you in today, but I want to hear more about what has been concerning you in general, and then I will ask a series of questions so that I can more completely understand your mental health history. Does that sound okay?" It is helpful to explain the difference between the questioning, assessment, and treatment planning (recommendations and discussion) elements of the evaluation and the order of those items. The psychiatrist briefly discusses time available for the evaluation, explains confidentiality issues (with provision to break confidentiality if safety issues arise), and invites questions from the student throughout the intake.

The transition from start to the main body of the psychiatric evaluation can be approached in several ways. Some psychiatrists prefer to start with open-ended inquiry to let the patient tell their story without constraint; however, it is reasonable to begin with collecting some basic demographic information in closed-ended questioning format. The latter approach may be particularly helpful to gently ease in and build rapport with a seemingly reticent or nervous interviewee. This information, whether obtained at the start, middle, or end, should include the patient's gender identification and preferred pronouns (if not obtained already from screening information), sexual identification and current relationship status, race and ethnicity, year in school and choice of study, housing situation (e.g., commuting from home, living on campus or off campus), and financial issues or stressors (e.g., student loan debt, need to work many hours while taking classes to support tuition). All of this information should be asked about sensitively with allowance for the student to forgo any of these demographic questions if not comfortable answering them.

Elements of a Psychiatric Evaluation

The psychiatrist should seamlessly transition to the bulk of the information gathering in order to obtain a complete history and mental status evaluation (Table 11–1). The student's chief complaint often leads directly to a history of present illness, and open-ended questioning (e.g., "Can you tell me more about that?") can facilitate the student's expression of the story. The psychiatrist can use various strategies to clarify the student's symptoms and understand whether syndromes or diagnoses are present. One helpful tool is for the psychiatrist to use the patient's words while not anchoring them to the professional understanding of such terms (e.g., "Can you describe what 'panic' means to you in your own words so I can better understand your experience?"). The clinician must understand elements of the symptoms, including duration and severity of the symptoms currently and in the past, number and frequency of episodes, the time when the symptoms first appeared, and factors that have helped or made them worse. A chronological history may be helpful if symptoms are complex or long-standing (e.g., "Let's go back to the beginning, when you first felt that something was wrong, and tell me what then developed over time"). While perhaps going above and beyond the norm of practice, the mental health professional who develops a written or drawn time line with the student may help the student to feel engaged and to feel that the development of their symptoms is understood.

After the history of present illness is concluded, a psychiatric review of systems must be completed to assess for psychiatric comorbidities or contributions to the chief complaint not already addressed. We generally include at least mood, anxiety, psychosis, substance use, and trauma screens in our evaluations (mnemonic: MAPS-T). To assess mood symptoms, the psychiatrist screens for episodes of depression, with emphasis on understanding the student's sleep, diet, and exercise habits. Suicidal ideation must be assessed in every psychiatric evaluation, and doing so at this point is logical given its inclusion in the diagnostic criteria for major depressive disorder. We recommend a more inclusive screening for suicidal ideation at first: "Have you ever had a time in your life where you were considering ending your life?" If the answer is positive, the psychiatrist should ask about past or current plans, attempts, or nonsuicidal self-injurious behavior. Likewise, the psychiatrist should screen for homicidal ideation or past aggressive behaviors or legal issues. Additionally, screening for hypomanic or manic episodes must be included, ideally for any patient, but especially for those with whom there is a con-

---

TABLE 11–1. Selected components of a psychiatric history

Components of the evaluation

Chief complaint	Inviting patients to express their concerns in their own words.
History of present illness	Open-ended questions initially Symptoms and episodes Chronological history, if needed

Review of systems	MAPS-T
	  Mood
	  Anxiety
	  Psychosis
	  Substance use
	  Trauma
	  Attention-deficit/hyperactivity disorder
	  Eating disorders

Past psychiatric and medical histories	Diagnoses Hospitalizations Suicide attempts or other self-harm behaviors Past treatment modalities
Social history	Childhood experience Sexual and relationship history Social belongingness
Family psychiatric history	Diagnoses Hospitalizations Suicide attempts or other self-harm behaviors Past treatment modalities Responsiveness to treatment

Note.   MAPS-T=mnemonic device for mood, anxiety, psychosis, substance use, and trauma.

cern of a depressive disorder, because many individuals with bipolar disorder initially present with a major depressive episode (Goldberg et al. 2001). Although it may not be efficient to screen for every part of the criteria for bipolar disorder, a general screening question may take the following form: "Have you ever had periods in your life when, perhaps instead of feeling down and depressed, you felt an elevated mood or perhaps were more productive and energetic than usual?" The clinician may wish to use a standardized instrument to assess for mood symptoms now or at the beginning or end of the evaluation to provide quantitative data that can be followed over time.

Second, the clinician will want to screen for several different disorders that fall within the general anxiety spectrum, the "A" in the MAPS-T mnemonic. The psychiatrist should assess briefly for symptoms of generalized anxiety, social anxiety, panic, and obsessive-compulsive disorders. Again, the clinician may want to use standardized instruments to quantitatively assess for these symptoms and disorders.

Psychosis is the "P" in the MAPS-T mnemonic. Young adults may present with attenuated psychotic symptoms, in addition to full psychosis. Attenuated psychosis syndrome, defined among the "Conditions for Further Study" in Section III of DSM-5, is characterized by subthreshold hallucinations, delusions, or disorganized speech with intact reality testing (American Psychiatric Association 2013). Psychosis can be related to other disorders as well, including depression, mania, and substance use disorders. The psychiatrist should perform a general screening for history of paranoia and hallucinations, followed by further review as needed based on positive answers.

An especially important symptom and diagnosis category to review in this young adult population is substance use, the "S" in MAPS-T, because of its prevalence in college and university settings, its common comorbidity with other mental health diagnoses, its potential to trigger or mimic the symptoms of other disorders, and the tendency for young adults to minimize or reluctantly share their use with their clinicians. The psychiatrist must strike a balance between allowing the young adult to open up about substance use comfortably while not giving the sense of condoning problematic use. The clinician's guided exploration of the pattern and timing of substance use will allow the student to better understand and weigh the benefits and detriments of substance use. Necessary components of a review of alcohol use include frequency of use, number of drinks per episode, number of drinks per week, presence of binge drinking, drinking with others or alone, blackouts, drunk driving, other social or legal repercussions, ability to regulate consumption, and compulsive drinking habits (Ham and Hope 2003). Marijuana is also a frequently used substance in campus settings. Although decreasing stigma is associated with its use, especially in states where marijuana has been legalized, clinicians should review the student's perceptions of marijuana use, frequency, quantity, and delivery form. Tobacco, other recreational drugs, misused prescription medications (especially medications for attention-deficit/hyperactivity disorder [ADHD]), and substances used for bodybuilding (e.g., steroids, testosterone) round out this review section.

Trauma, the final review category in our MAPS-T mnemonic, must also be screened for because of its centrality to many areas of psychopathology, including but not limited to trauma-specific disorders such as posttraumatic stress disorder. A basic screening question may take the following form: "This may be a difficult question, but one that will help me understand you and your history more completely: Have you ever been physically, sexually, or mentally abused or traumatized by others or a situation?" Recently experienced or on-campus sexual or physical assault deserves special care and attention and should prompt an immediate set of questions in the interviewer's mind: Is this a situation where the police would ideally be involved? Should the student be referred to a campus sexual-assault response team?

ADHD, although not part of the mnemonic, is also a helpful diagnosis to screen for because of its prevalence and its potential impact on academic performance. Review of past psychiatric history is important in all cases, but especially for ADHD because symptoms must have been present before age 18 to meet diagnostic criteria. The clinician would want to understand whether the diagnosis was made in childhood, and if so, how. Additionally, past testing, history of accommodations, and past treatments would be helpful to explore. The clinician may want to advise the student of the necessity to obtain parent/guardian collateral information regarding childhood symptoms of ADHD.

Finally, eating disorders should be reviewed separately because of prevalence and impact in the college-age population.

After completing the review of systems, the clinician will question the patient about past psychiatric and medical histories. In regard to the past psychiatric history, the clinician would want to inquire about past diagnoses, past hospitalizations, past suicide attempts or nonsuicidal self-injurious behavior (if not yet discussed), past clinicians and forms of therapy or other interventions (e.g., transcranial magnetic stimulation), and past psychiatric medications. Questions about psychiatric medications include when the medication was started, how long it was used, what maximum dosage was achieved, whether the student used it as prescribed, whether it was effective, whether it had side effects, and why it may have been stopped. The clinician should ask similar questions about over-the-counter medications and supplements. A complete past medical history would include review of other medical conditions, past hospitalizations and surgeries, allergies, and nonpsychiatric medications. The clinician would also want to explore whether there was any relation between the student's mental health symptoms and other medical disorders or medications, as well as the potential for interactions with psychiatric medications under consideration. A careful sexual history, including screening for high-risk sexual behaviors or abusive relationships, should be pursued. Special emphasis must be placed on assessment of sexual activity and associated use of contraceptive method for patients in this age cohort. Engaging the patient in a discussion of the potential risks of psychiatric medications during pregnancy is always good practice and is particularly important when students identify inadequate use of contraception.

One of the richer elements of the initial evaluation is social history. It can be helpful to revert to a more open-ended question strategy when beginning to obtain this information, such as, "Tell me a little about your childhood and growing up." A helpful prompt to investigate patterns of attachment that may continue to influence current relationships is "How would you describe your relationship with your parent(s) in several words?" (C. George, N. Kaplan, and M. Main, "The Adult Attachment Interview," unpublished manuscript, University of California, Berkeley, 1985). The psychiatrist can ask further questions to obtain the student's educational history and sexual and relationship history (some of this information may have been garnered during the past medical history above) and about current peer groups, extracurricular activities, sense of social belonging, and history of being bullied or of bullying others. Identities with regard to race, ethnicity, country and location of origin, religion, and socioeconomic status should also be explored (sensitively) and prompt the clinician to consider campus connections that may allow the student to find community around their identities.

Family psychiatric history should also be explored. If the psychiatrist is considering medication treatment recommendations, it is helpful to understand whether any psychiatric medications have been tried by immediate family members and how they responded to them. Students are frequently not aware of their parents' psychiatric history, but may have knowledge about siblings or others in the family. This discussion presents a nice opportunity to explore mental illness stigma that may exist within the student's family of origin. The clinician can ask whether mental health is discussed in the family and, if so, how. Another useful question is "How comfortable would you feel asking a parent about response to psychotropic medications?"

Throughout the interview, the astute clinician will be filing away observable data from the whole interaction to compile the mental status evaluation. Components include the student's appearance (e.g., hygiene and choice of clothes), behavior (e.g., forthcoming or evasive and superficial—the latter may be related to goals of the evaluation for the patient), speech patterns, affect, mood, perceptions (e.g., responding to internal stimuli), thought process and content, insight and judgment, and cognitive capacity. A pertinent physical examination may also be useful based on the history (e.g., testing for neurological side effects if the patient is currently taking antipsychotic medication).

As the psychiatrist nears completion of data collection, it is helpful to pause to provide the student with a brief summary of the information gathered, checking for correctness along the way. This process provides validation of the student as the expert in their personal experience. It is also useful to inquire about the patient's goals for treatment and perceptions of different treatment modalities.

Conclusion of the Evaluation

When the data-gathering portion of the interview is complete, the evaluation enters the treatment-planning phase, starting with a discussion of the mental health professional's assessment and diagnostic impressions. Note that caution must be exercised regarding making a firm diagnosis at the first evaluation in order to allow for more cross-sectional evaluation and collection of collateral history. The psychiatrist should also consider the effect that a concrete diagnosis could have on the still-developing student. Nuanced delivery such as, "It sounds like you have developed some obsessive thinking patterns," rather than, "You have obsessive-compulsive disorder," may be less stigmatizing and allow for more optimistic self-assessment by the patient. It can be helpful to encourage the student to weigh in on the assessment and their perception of diagnoses under consideration. On the other hand, accessing treatment modalities and services should not be delayed, especially in clinical circumstances in which early intervention is known to lead to far improved health outcomes, for example, schizophrenia or bipolar disorder.

Education about the disorders being considered and potential treatments is a cornerstone of shared decision making (Barr et al. 2016). Because many students may be experiencing psychiatric symptoms for the first time, education about potential disorders, their prognosis and functional impact, and responsiveness to treatment is essential. An overview of viable treatment options, including pharmacologic, psychotherapeutic, and lifestyle interventions (e.g., physical exercise, diet, substance use, sleep, stress management), is also important to ensure that the student is fully aware of the choices to be made. It may be helpful to encourage the student to do some research about the disorders and treatments under consideration.

An open, interactive conversation can now be pursued with the patient regarding treatment decisions. In high-risk situations, the first priority is to determine whether a higher level of care is needed, such as an inpatient hospitalization or partial hospitalization program. Every clinician working with young adult students in an outpatient setting, for example, must understand the organization's protocol for providing in-patient hospitalization for students who are a danger to themselves or others or who are gravely disabled. Next, treatment decision making around lifestyle interventions, such as sleep, exercise, and socialization, can be discussed. The clinician may ask the student to help provide more objective data, which could include vital signs, height and weight, or results from electrocardiogram, labs, or imaging modalities.

Referrals to specialty mental health care, other medical disciplines, case management services, and other campus services can be considered (Chan et al. 2015). Depending on the situation, the clinician can discuss psychotherapy and/or medication interventions that may be indicated, stating the pros and cons of the different approaches of therapy or classes of medications. Risks and benefits of and alternatives to the potential treatments must be thoroughly communicated. In many cases, permission to speak with parents or previous clinicians may be sought to collect collateral information, which may provide a more complete clinical picture and can affect treatment planning and recommendations. The student's preferences for including parents in the decision-making process should also be considered. Whereas some students prefer to make their decisions alone or even keep them from their parents, other students will want their parents' advice and support in making decisions about their health care. Family may also be an important source of social support for some students, and their involvement may be facilitated by student or clinician contact. The student who needs more time to research treatment alternatives or consult family members who are not immediately available may prefer to briefly delay a treatment decision.

Prior to the patient leaving, a follow-up schedule, if needed, can be arranged. Any remaining forms that are needed, such as release of information, should also be filled out at this time. Prescriptions or other orders that need to go with the patient can be written. Last, the psychiatrist should consider obtaining the student's feedback, either verbal or written, about the session.

After the Evaluation

In addition to spending some time ahead of the visit to adequately prepare to evaluate the student, the clinician must follow up on loose ends after the evaluation to ensure that the assessment and treatment recommendations are accurate and helpful. When it is appropriate to seek additional information from family members, consent from the student should be obtained, and follow-up communication with the family should be initiated. The clinician will want to follow up with the results from any remaining orders or referrals to supplement the evaluation. The clinician can also communicate with the referral source regarding the assessment and plan, as needed. Finally, the evaluation should be comprehensively documented in the medical record.

Case Example

Sophia is a 19-year-old sophomore who has decided to reach out to the college counseling center. In high school, she did quite well, had good grades, and played varsity softball. She was well liked, close to her teammates, and recognized as a scholar-athlete. She was recruited to play softball at her university. However, a snowboarding accident during her first year caused an athletic career–ending injury. She lost control and crashed into a tree, fracturing her collarbone and elbow. She had surgery, missed several weeks of school, and made up the work, but her arm did not work the way it used to, and she had to quit the softball team. This was disappointing and socially difficult because she had just made friends with her new teammates. By the end of the first year, she didn't feel very close to them anymore. It was difficult to make new friends, because everyone else seemed to have "paired up" and established groups of friends already. She found college to be more challenging academically, and slowly her grades worsened. She was starting to feel out of place and found that she was not enjoying school very much anymore. She also was unsure about what she wanted to major in or what career path to take.

The summer after her first year, she continued to slowly heal from her injuries while at home and was no longer in much pain. She spent time resting and socializing with her high school friends. However, she felt that they were all doing better than she was: some were playing college softball, some had joined sororities, and everyone seemed happy with their college experiences. It was difficult for her to relate to them. During her sophomore year, her grades continued to worsen, and she was eventually missing half of her classes. She would mostly stay in her room, isolated, and would often lie awake in bed during the day. Many thoughts went through her head, including fears of not passing her classes or graduating. "Why is it so hard to get to class and to concentrate on schoolwork? What if I switch schools and move closer to home? Why can't I seem to succeed in making friends, dating, and doing well in school, like everyone else?"

During the winter break, the subject of her grades was broached with her parents. Her mother was concerned that Sophia's grades were lower than they had ever been. Her mother also noticed that Sophia was sleeping more than usual, seemed to have lost weight, and was not socializing with her high school friends like she usually would. She confronted Sophia about these concerns and asked whether Sophia was depressed. Sophia agreed to contact the college counseling center when she returned to school.

However, after the spring semester started, Sophia thought she would wait and see if she felt better with the new course schedule rather than make an appointment right away. When her mother asked her about the appointment, Sophia would brush it off and say, "Don't worry, I'm on it," and would not elaborate further.

Following her first set of exams, Sophia realized the semester was not going to be any better, because she kept missing classes and her grades continued to be poor. She called the counseling center and requested an appointment. The person she spoke with took down her information and told her that the triage nurse would call her back that day. When the nurse returned the call, Sophia described her situation and answered the screening questions. It was determined that a routine appointment with a psychiatrist would be most appropriate. She made an appointment to see one the following week.

On the day of Sophia's appointment, the psychiatrist saw that a new student was on the schedule. The psychiatrist took 10 minutes before the intake appointment to review Sophia's chart. Sophia was self-referred and had called the counseling center to make the appointment. She told the triage nurse that her grades were poor and "I feel terrible all the time." She had passive thoughts of death: "I would never do anything, but if something happened to me, it wouldn't be the worst thing." Because she had no psychiatric history, active suicidality, prior history of suicide attempts or self-harm, or psychiatric hospitalizations and was deemed to be at low risk for self-harm, she was given a routine appointment by the nurse. While reviewing the rest of Sophia's medical chart, the psychiatrist saw that Sophia had been in treatment and had follow-up appointments for her snowboarding injuries. The labs that had been done were all normal, although no thyroid tests had been ordered. Sophia had also been seen for strep throat once but otherwise had no other contact with the health care system at the school.

There was also a note in the chart about Sophia's mother, and then the psychiatrist recalled a conversation with the nurse a few days ago. The nurse said that a student's mother had called the counseling center three times since the semester started, asking if her daughter had been seen by the counseling center. Each time, she was told by the receptionist that students have to sign a consent form before they can release any information. She was advised to talk with her daughter directly. The third time she called, Sophia's mother was extremely frustrated. She wanted her concerns to be escalated "to a manager," and ended up talking with the nurse for 20 minutes. Sophia's mother explained her concerns, including that depression "runs in our family and it gets very bad." Her sister, Sophia's aunt, dealt with severe depression all her life as an adult. She was worried that Sophia "is in a bad place" and "she isn't herself at all." Although she did try to talk with Sophia, as suggested, Sophia wouldn't give her any details about what was happening with the counseling center. Although the nurse empathized with Sophia's mother about how frustrating the situation was, she again explained the limitations. The nurse relayed this conversation to the psychiatrist, and there was also a reminder in the chart for the psychiatrist to ask Sophia if she would be willing to sign a consent form for her mother.

Sophia had been asked to arrive 20 minutes early to the appointment, and at that time, she filled out a questionnaire on a computer tablet in the waiting room. In responding to the survey, Sophia reported that she identifies as a woman (female), and uses she/her pronouns. In responding to the survey, Sophia reported a history of binge drinking in high school. She also indicated less often drinking to excess in college. She currently smokes marijuana and has occasionally used caffeine pills and energy drinks to stay awake to study.

The psychiatrist noted all the above and then went to the waiting room to meet Sophia. Sophia appeared a bit nervous and self-conscious of the students around her, so the psychiatrist spoke in a low tone of voice and was conscious of ensuring privacy for her. As Sophia sat down in the office, she said she had "never been to a place like this before." The psychiatrist made a point to orient Sophia to the appointment and clinic, telling her that her chart and questionnaire had been reviewed; that this was an intake appointment focused on understanding her situation and history; that Sophia could decline to answer any questions she didn't feel comfortable discussing; that her confidentiality is important and will be protected, but there are also some exceptions; and that at the end of the appointment, the psychiatrist would give an assessment of her situation, review the potential diagnoses, and then discuss treatment options together. The psychiatrist encouraged Sophia to ask any questions as they went through the interview.

The psychiatrist said, "Although I have some background information, I'd like to hear from you about what brings you in today." Sophia stated, "I don't know, I just feel terrible all the time. I don't know what's wrong, I used to be a good student, but I can't seem to 'do school' anymore. I made a promise to my mother to come in, because she thinks I'm depressed and she's really worried." They proceeded to review her current symptoms, as well as her history. The psychiatrist noted that Sophia was neatly groomed and thin. She appeared anxious, although she became more comfortable as the interview progressed. Sophia was able to answer the questions in a straightforward way.

At the end of the interview, the psychiatrist went on to discuss the assessment, impressions, and provisional diagnoses of major depressive episode, unspecified anxiety disorder, and marijuana use disorder. They reviewed potential options, and Sophia chose to try medications, as well as short-term therapy with a psychologist. The psychiatrist reviewed her mother's request for information, and they discussed whether Sophia would feel comfortable signing a release. Sophia said, "Of course, my mom is one of the people I'm closest to." She said she knew her mother was worried, but Sophia had felt conflicted about making an appointment and did not want her mother to know she was procrastinating about coming in. She also asked that they not discuss her daily marijuana use with her mother, saying, "It would just upset her." Sophia said that she used to smoke marijuana only socially with her teammates in high school. She remembered how it seemed to make her feel less anxious, and this year, she tried smoking marijuana alone in her dorm room. It reduced her anxiety in the moment, but she noticed that changed when she began smoking every day. The psychiatrist discussed the recommendation to consider cutting back her marijuana use, and Sophia agreed, saying she had been thinking for a while about whether it could help her situation to smoke less. She said she would try not to smoke daily, as a first step. The psychiatrist explained that the psychologist would likely continue to work with her on this issue in therapy.

After the appointment, the psychiatrist contacted Sophia's mother, who was relieved to hear that Sophia had connected with clinicians at the counseling center. Sophia's mother responded, "That is all I really wanted to hear, that she was in good hands. Sorry that I lost it talking with the nurse. I'm sure you can understand how worried I have been about Sophia." The psychiatrist validated the mother's concerns for Sophia. Her mother also offered further family history that her own sister, Sophia's aunt, has severe depression, and had to have many trials of medications before finally improving with nortriptyline. The psychiatrist thanked her for this information, explained the treatment plan, and reviewed information about the clinic, including contact information, after-hours procedures, and recommendations for emergencies.

Sophia was able to engage in treatment after this initial appointment. She began to see the psychologist weekly for therapy, and continued to see the psychiatrist monthly for medication management.

Conclusion

In this chapter, we have reviewed aspects of the complete psychiatric assessment tailored to the context and needs of university students. Clinicians have an opportunity to help these individuals to develop a positive experience with mental health care that may enable them to remain in school and maintain their academic progress, while setting them up for a lifetime of comfort with accessing psychiatric care as needed to manage their mental health. Comprehensive, sensitive psychiatric evaluation is the cornerstone of a strong therapeutic alliance and effective treatment. We hope that this chapter provides the university student mental health professional and administrator with appreciation for the vital importance of this role, validates their mission, and motivates them for excellence.

KEY CONCEPTS

- Young adults are at significant risk for the onset of psychiatric disorders.

- University students may be seeking mental health care for the first time in their lives.

- University students vary widely in their preferences for parental involvement in their care and treatment decisions.

- Clinicians caring for students should engage in a shared decision-making process when considering treatment options with their patients, recognizing that exploring health care options may be a new experience for many students.

- Clinicians should encourage the use of a comprehensive, holistic treatment approach that includes consideration of lifestyle and social interventions, psychotherapy, and pharmacotherapy.

Recommendations for Psychiatrists, Psychologists, and Counselors

1. There is a flow to a psychiatric evaluation of the young adult university student that includes components before, during, and after meeting with the student in person.

2. First impressions are important because for many students, the evaluation may be the first significant contact with the entire field of mental health care.

3. The clinician will profit from employing warmth and open-ended questions to help the student feel comfortable with the value of providing complete and accurate information.

Discussion Questions

1. What script would be useful to start an interview (including explaining the process and flow of the interview) with a young adult university student?

2. What areas of the evaluation are *more* important to obtain in this population than in the general adult psychiatric population?

3. What areas of the evaluation are *less* important to obtain in this population than in the general adult psychiatric population?

4. What strategies might be used to engage a young adult university student in shared decision making regarding treatment?

Suggested Readings

Barnhill JW (ed): DSM-5 Clinical Cases. Arlington, VA, American Psychiatric Publishing, 2014

McIntyre KM, Norton JR, McIntyre JS: Psychiatric interview, history, and mental status examination, in Kaplan and Sadock's Comprehensive Textbook of Psychiatry, 9th Edition. Edited by Sadock BJ, Sadock VA, Ruiz P. Philadelphia, PA, Wolters Kluwer Health/Lippincott Williams & Wilkins, 2009, pp 886–907

References

American Psychiatric Association: Diagnostic and Statistical Manual of Mental Disorders, 5th Edition. Arlington, VA, American Psychiatric Association, 2013

Barr PJ, Forcino RC, Mishra M, et al: Competing priorities in treatment decision-making: a U.S. national survey of individuals with depression and clinicians who treat depression. BMJ Open 6(1):e009585, 2016 26747036

Chan V, Rasminsky S, Viesselman JO: A primer for working in campus mental health: a system of care. Acad Psychiatry 39(5):533–540, 2015 25854453

Downs MF, Eisenberg D: Help seeking and treatment use among suicidal college students. J Am Coll Health 60(2):104–114, 2012 22316407

Goldberg JF, Harrow M, Whiteside JE: Risk for bipolar illness in patients initially hospitalized for unipolar depression. Am J Psychiatry 158(8):1265–1270, 2001 11481161

Ham LS, Hope DA: College students and problematic drinking: a review of the literature. Clin Psychol Rev 23(5):719–759, 2003 12971907

Kirsch DJ, Pinder-Amaker SL, Morse C, et al: Population-based initiatives in college mental health: students helping students to overcome obstacles. Curr Psychiatry Rep 16(12):525, 2014 25308393

Spitzer RL, Kroenke K, Williams JB: Validation and utility of a self-report version of PRIME-MD: the PHQ primary care study. Primary Care Evaluation of Mental Disorders. Patient Health Questionnaire. JAMA 282(18):1737–1744, 1999 10568646

CHAPTER 12

Mood and Anxiety Disorders

Allison L. Thompson, Ph.D.

Daniel Ryu, M.S.

IN recent years, an increasing number of college students have arrived on campus with a variety of mental health concerns. A survey by the American College Health Association (2015) of more than 93,000 students at 108 colleges and universities found that 34.5% reported feeling so depressed in the previous 12 months that it was difficult to function, and nearly 57% felt overwhelming anxiety in the same time period. Interestingly, in that 1-year period, only 15.8% and 13.1% of respondents had been diagnosed or treated for anxiety and depression, respectively. Given the prevalence of anxiety and depression on college campuses, it

is imperative that administrators, faculty, staff, and practitioners understand the various ways in which these disorders may manifest and be
familiar with appropriate treatment options for students.

Anna, a 19-year-old single Mexican American heterosexual cisgender female sophomore, self-referred to the college counseling center of a private university on the East Coast. Anna appeared withdrawn and made
minimal eye contact. She had never previously sought mental health
treatment and stated that her resident assistant encouraged her to go to
the counseling center after she had shared some of the difficulties she
was having since returning from winter break.

Although she was excited when she was accepted into the university she
currently attends, Anna reported that she no longer wishes to be at school.
She reported that she had historically been a straight-A student, but lately
she has been having difficulty concentrating on schoolwork and is often on
the verge of tears. She reported having trouble sleeping, but she said that
she spends much of her time in bed watching videos on her smartphone.
She added that she has begun to skip classes and has been avoiding her
friends. She denied any suicidal ideation but stated that she does not feel as
if she belongs at the university and simply wants to go home.

At intake, Anna shared that she was raised in a small Midwestern
town by a single mother, who immigrated to the United States from
Mexico before her three older siblings and Anna were born. Anna described having close relationships with her mother, sisters, and brother,
all of whom still live in their hometown and stated that it is difficult for
her to be away from them.

Despite her close relationships with her relatives, Anna described
having had a difficult upbringing. She reported often having to serve as
an interpreter for her mother, who is a monolingual Spanish speaker.
Given that she does not speak English, her mother had trouble finding
steady employment and the family often struggled to make ends meet.
Anna shared that she and her siblings were bullied throughout middle
school and high school because of their socioeconomic status and Mexican heritage. Although she was upset and saddened by the bullying,
Anna said that having the support of her siblings and her teachers
helped her cope. In addition, she reported that she put much of her energy into her schoolwork, which helped her succeed in secondary school
and ultimately get a scholarship to her university.

The family's situation worsened when Anna's mother was diagnosed with bipolar I disorder when Anna was in middle school. For several years, Anna occasionally skipped school and stayed home to help
care for her mother, who initially refused to take medication or go to
therapy. With the encouragement of her children and pastor, Anna's
mother ultimately agreed to seek services and was taking medication
and was stable at the time of Anna's intake. Despite her mother's improvement, Anna reported worrying about her and calling her daily.
Anna denied any mania but acknowledged that she worries that she or
one of her siblings will develop bipolar disorder, stating that these
thoughts often contribute to her depression.

Prevalence and Symptomatology of Mood and Anxiety Disorders

College students present with a variety of stressors, some of which are general and some of which are unique to their environment and stage of life. Concerns that are common among college students and other adult populations include sleep disturbance, relationships, health, and self-esteem. According to Beiter and colleagues (2015), the most common concerns cited by college students are college specific, including academic performance, pressure to succeed, postgraduation plans, and financial concerns.

The stressors commonly cited by students may be associated with a variety of symptom presentations, including depression and anxiety. Although Anna's sleep difficulties and academic concerns may have led to her depressive clinical presentation, other students with similar stressors might instead report feeling anxious or stressed out. Extant research indicates that anxiety is the most common issue for which students seek services. Mistler and colleagues (2012) reported that 41.6% of students who presented to college counseling centers sought services for anxiety, whereas 36.4% of students presented for treatment of depression. In 2016, Reetz et al. reported that a mean of 50.61% of students present with anxiety and a mean of 41.23% present with depression.

Although anxiety is the more common reason that students seek treatment, they are more often diagnosed with depressive disorders. In an anonymous, Web-based survey of students from more than 1,500 colleges and universities, Tupler and colleagues (2015) found that approximately 74% of respondents met criteria for major depression and approximately 30% met criteria for social phobia. Additionally, 24% met criteria for panic disorder or agoraphobia (Tupler et al. 2015).

In a sample of students from a large public institution, Eisenberg and colleagues (2007) found that nearly 14% of undergraduates and approximately 11% of graduate students screened positive for depression, whereas about 4% of both undergraduate and graduate students were diagnosed with panic disorder or generalized anxiety disorder. Interestingly, although there were no gender differences for depression, women were almost twice as likely to be diagnosed with anxiety (Eisenberg et al. 2007).

In addition to anxiety and depression, other mood disorders are seen in college populations, but at lower frequencies. For instance, according to Auerbach and colleagues (2016), less than 2% of college students are diagnosed with bipolar disorder.

It is not surprising that students seek services for and are diagnosed with mood and anxiety disorders, given that the average age at onset of many of these disorders falls within the age range for undergraduate and graduate populations. For example, for individuals with bipolar I disorder, the mean age at onset for a first manic, hypomanic, or major depressive episode is about 18 years. Additionally, the average age at onset for bipolar II disorder is in the mid-20s (American Psychiatric Association 2013).

Anxiety disorders often initially appear during adolescence or early adulthood. For example, in the United States, the median age at onset for social anxiety disorder is 13 years; this disorder is of particular concern because those diagnosed with it are more likely to drop out of school. Although panic disorder and generalized anxiety disorder have later median ages at onset, individuals diagnosed with each disorder could experience symptoms that would interfere with their education. Panic disorder, for instance, is associated with high levels of functional impairment; students diagnosed with this disorder are frequently absent from school or work. In comparison, students diagnosed with generalized anxiety disorder tend to worry about their academic and sports performance (American Psychiatric Association 2013).

Although many disorders first manifest in college, Auerbach and colleagues (2016) found that the majority of mental disorders in an international sample of college students predated the students' enrollment in college. These disorders were associated with negative outcomes for individuals, including being less likely to enter college and more likely to drop out. Jonsson and colleagues (2010) found that depression in particular seems to interfere with higher education such that adolescents diagnosed with the disorder were significantly less likely to have graduated from college by the time they turn 30. The same study showed that women with depression were less likely to enter college than women who were not depressed and that men with depression were less likely to graduate. Given how disruptive preexisting disorders can be to a student's academic career, it is imperative that college mental health professionals routinely assess for and treat these disorders to increase the student's chances of succeeding in and completing college.

Screening for mood disorders in the student population presents some unique concerns, including the fact that many symptoms that are characteristic of mood disorders are extremely common within the general student population. For instance, sleep disturbance is a hallmark symptom of depression; however, the general student population often has irregular and insufficient sleep schedules. Similarly, changes in weight and/or appetite can be signs of a mood disorder but may be difficult to differentiate from weight changes that are typical for young adults transitioning into college and adjusting to living and eating on a college campus. Last, the college years are often a time of great stress and anxiety, and individuals are under considerable social and academic pressure; although many students report feeling stressed and anxious, that does not necessarily indicate that they have a diagnosable anxiety disorder. Consequently, it is important that mental health professionals use their clinical judgment to assess premorbid functioning and symptomatology to differentiate between psychiatric concerns and shifts that are normative in this population.

Barriers to Seeking Treatment

As her intake session drew to a close, Anna thanked the clinician for her time but said she didn't think she would return for subsequent sessions. When the clinician expressed curiosity about Anna's reluctance to return, Anna listed a number of reasons, including her various commitments, finances, and embarrassment about not being able to solve her problems on her own.

Unfortunately, Anna's hesitancy to engage in treatment is not uncommon. Although a high number of college students endorse symptoms of mood and anxiety disorders, many are reluctant to seek treatment at college counseling centers or elsewhere. Researchers have identified several common barriers to help seeking among college students.

LACK OF TIME

College students have countless demands on their time. Students frequently express that they do not have enough time and are often inundated with attending classes, participating in extracurricular activities, and forming and maintaining new relationships. Not surprisingly, students, especially those who are struggling, often cite lack of time as a reason for not seeking treatment. In a study of college students at an elevated risk for suicide, nearly 27% reported that they did not have enough time to seek help (Czyz et al. 2013).

STIGMA

Although mental health treatment is more accepted than it has been historically, there still is stigma related to receiving mental health treatment. Potential patients often express concern that others will think they are "crazy" if they disclose that they are in treatment. This may be a particularly strong concern among students raised in cultures in which mental illness and psychological treatment are viewed negatively. Czyz and colleagues (2013) found that 12% of students at an elevated risk of suicide cited stigma as a reason for not seeking treatment. Furthermore, in a sample of more than 100 undergraduate students, D'Amico and colleagues (2016) found that those who perceived that their family or friends had a discriminatory attitude about or associated stigma with depression were less likely to seek treatment.

UNDERESTIMATION OF SEVERITY

Many students who endorse symptoms of anxiety, depression, or both believe that their symptoms will improve with time. Although some patients will experience a significant reduction in symptoms without any intervention, many would benefit from treatment. In Czyz and colleagues' (2013) sample of students with an elevated risk of suicide, 66% believed they did not need treatment and consequently did not seek services. Relatedly, 18% of the students in the sample preferred to manage their problems on their own and therefore did not seek help.

ACCESS

Despite the fact that students can receive low-cost or free mental health treatment on most college campuses, access remains a barrier to treatment. In a convenience sample of students from a large university in Northern California, Bohon and colleagues (2016) found that cost of treatment was the greatest barrier to seeking treatment. The study also found that students who had difficulty scheduling appointments and obtaining transportation were less likely to express intention to seek mental health treatment.

CULTURAL FACTORS

Many cultures and marginalized populations have negative views of mental illness and mental health treatment. For instance, in part due to historical medical abuses such as the Tuskegee syphilis experiment, African Americans may be skeptical of health care professionals and might look for other ways to address a mental illness, such as turning to faith. Similarly, other populations of color, such as Latinos and Asians, may be less likely to enter treatment and more likely to drop out. Other population groups, including sexual and gender minorities, have historically been pathologized by the psychiatric community; consequently, members of these communities may be less likely to seek and to remain in treatment (Reicherter et al. 2016).

Although these barriers may prevent students from seeking services at a college counseling center, clinicians can use other means to reach students in need. For instance, outreach programming is an effective way to educate students about common mental disorders and to introduce them to the services offered on campus. In addition, mental health professionals can train resident assistants, professors, administrators, and student organizers to identify students who may be struggling and to direct them to the appropriate resources.

Treatment

Anna's clinician initiated a conversation about the advantages of treatment. After this discussion, Anna agreed to a brief course of therapy and accepted a referral to a psychiatrist. She ultimately saw a psychiatrist, who prescribed Zoloft 100 mg/day. Through working with her individual therapist using cognitive-behavioral therapy (CBT), Anna learned about behavioral activation and ways to identify and challenge unhelpful thought patterns. Through the former, she began to reengage with her friends on campus and started exercising and singing in a musical group. The latter helped Anna question long-standing automatic thoughts about her abilities and her place on campus as a woman of color. After 12 sessions of individual therapy, Anna reported a significant reduction in her symptoms. Although she still missed her family, she reported feeling happier and was once again excited about being in college. At her final session, Anna expressed confidence that she could use the skills she learned in therapy to address any future depressive episodes.

Given the multiple constraints on their time, students often are not interested in long-term treatment. In addition, many college counseling centers limit the number of sessions students can receive in a given year. As a result, it is important to provide time-limited, evidence-based treatment that can give students the relief they seek in the shortest time possible (see Chapter 22, "Brief and Medium-Term Psychosocial Therapies at Student Health Centers).

CBT remains the gold standard for treating a variety of concerns, including depression, anxiety, panic disorder, bipolar disorder, and social phobia. As in Anna's case, CBT often provides rapid relief by helping patients change the distorted thoughts and unhelpful behaviors that are contributing to their mood difficulties.

In addition to CBT, researchers have pointed to the efficacy of other evidence-based treatments, such as acceptance and commitment therapy (ACT), and found innovative ways in which they can deliver these treatments. For instance, Levin and colleagues (2016) found that an online ACT intervention led to improvements in college students' anxiety and depression. Delivering an evidence-based treatment online could potentially allow clinicians to reach more students and to deliver interventions using a method that is more convenient and comfortable for students.

Other brief interventions can be effective with college students. For instance, time-limited dynamic psychotherapy can be useful when working with students with interpersonal difficulties. In addition, motivational interviewing can help explore a student's ambivalence about changing problematic behavior.

Psychotropic medication also has been shown to be effective in the treatment of college students with anxiety and depression. In fact, Kirsch and colleagues (2015) found that depression and anxiety are two of the most common problems for which students are referred for psychiatric medication evaluations and that antidepressants were the most commonly prescribed psychotropic medications. Many patients, like Anna, find that the combination of medication and psychotherapy is helpful and can lead to more rapid results.

Conclusion

An increasing number of college students are coping with mood and anxiety disorders; despite the prevalence of these conditions, many students are reluctant to seek treatment for a variety of reasons, including lack of time and stigma. For students who do present to college counseling centers for treatment, short-term, evidence-based therapies such as cognitive-behavioral therapy, acceptance and commitment therapy, and time-limited dynamic psychotherapy have been shown to be effective and appropriate for students with limited time or in centers that can only provide time-limited services. In addition, psychotropic medications may be indicated. Clinicians should also strive to reach the many students who are struggling with mood and anxiety disorders but do not seek help, by providing outreach to often overlooked segments of the university community and by enlisting allies, such as resident assistants and faculty members, who might recognize when students are struggling and can encourage students to seek treatment.

KEY CONCEPTS

- Mood and anxiety disorders are increasingly common on college campuses, with more than 34% of students reporting feeling so depressed in the past 12 months that they had difficulty functioning, and nearly 57% reporting feeling overwhelming anxiety in the same time period (American College Health Association 2015).

- Despite the high prevalence rates of mood and anxiety disorders, several significant barriers often prevent students from seeking treatment. These barriers include lack of time, stigma, and access.

- Time-limited, evidence-based treatments such as cognitive-behavioral therapy, acceptance and commitment therapy, and time-limited dynamic psychotherapy have proven effective at treating college students and addressing the barriers, such as lack of time, that might keep students from seeking help.

Recommendations for Psychiatrists, Psychologists, and Counselors

1. When assessing for mood and anxiety disorders, the clinician should consider stressors that might be seen in other adult populations as well as stressors that are specific to college, such as academic performance and postgraduation plans.
2. Because many students have disorders that predate their enrollment in college, it is important to get a comprehensive history of mental health concerns when evaluating and treating students.
3. Many symptoms that are characteristic of mood disorders, such as sleep disturbance and weight change, are common in the general college student population. Therefore, it is imperative to differentiate between psychiatric symptoms and shifts that are normative for students.
4. To address common barriers to treatment, such as lack of time and stigma, the clinician should consider using outreach programming to engage students who might be hesitant to go to the counseling center. Also, enlisting allies such as resident assistants and faculty members may aid in the identification of potential at-risk students.
5. Given students' time constraints as well as the short-term nature of the services offered by many college counseling centers, brief evidence-based treatments are often recommended. Cognitive-behavioral therapy, acceptance and commitment therapy, time-limited dynamic psychotherapy, and motivational interviewing have proven particularly useful with college students who present with mood and anxiety disorders.

Discussion Questions

1. What are ways in which counseling centers could improve outreach in order to reach and treat more students with anxiety and/or mood disorders?

2. What stressors might you see in college students that you might not see in other adult populations? What strategies might you use to address them?

3. What can college counseling centers do to raise awareness of and screen for mood and anxiety disorders on campus?

4. What barriers on your campus are likely preventing students from seeking services? How might you address them?

Suggested Readings

Borzumato-Gainey C, Degges-White S: College Student Mental Health Counseling: A Developmental Approach. New York, Springer, 2014

Kitzrow MA: The mental health needs of today's college students: challenges and recommendations. NASPA J 41(1):167–181, 2003

Zawadzki MJ, Graham JE, Gerin W: Rumination and anxiety mediate the effect of loneliness on depressed mood and sleep quality in college students. Health Psychol 32(2):212–222, 2013

References

American College Health Association: American College Health Association–National College Health Assessment II: Spring 2015 Reference Group Executive Summary. Hanover, MD, American College Health Association, 2015. Available at: http://www.acha-ncha.org/docs/NCHA-II_Web_Spring _2015_Reference_Group_Executive_Summary.pdf. Accessed January 15, 2017.

American Psychiatric Association: Diagnostic and Statistical Manual of Mental Disorders, 5th Edition. Arlington, VA, American Psychiatric Association, 2013

Auerbach RP, Alonso J, Axinn WG, et al: Mental disorders among college students in the World Health Organization World Mental Health Surveys. Psychol Med 46(14):2955–2970, 2016 27484622

Beiter R, Nash R, McCrady M, et al: The prevalence and correlates of depression, anxiety, and stress in a sample of college students. J Affect Disord 173:90–96, 2015 25462401

Bohon LM, Cotter KA, Kravitz RL, et al: The Theory of Planned Behavior as it predicts potential intention to seek mental health services for depression among college students. J Am Coll Health 64(8):593–603, 2016 27386898

Czyz EK, Horwitz AG, Eisenberg D, et al: Self-reported barriers to professional help seeking among college students at elevated risk for suicide. J Am Coll Health 61(7):398–406, 2013 24010494

D'Amico N, Mechling B, Kemppainen J, et al: American college students' views of depression and utilization of on-campus counseling services. J Am Psychiatr Nurses Assoc 22(4):302–311, 2016 27220991

Eisenberg D, Gollust SE, Golberstein E, Hefner JL: Prevalence and correlates of depression, anxiety, and suicidality among university students. Am J Orthopsychiatry 77(4):534–542, 2007 18194033

Jonsson U, Bohman H, Hjern A, et al: Subsequent higher education after adolescent depression: a 15-year follow-up register study. Eur Psychiatry 25(7):396–401, 2010 20541372

Kirsch DJ, Doerfler LA, Truong D: Mental health issues among college students: who gets referred for psychopharmacology evaluation? J Am Coll Health 63(1):50–56, 2015 25222760

Levin ME, Haeger JA, Pierce BG, Twohig MP: Web-based acceptance and commitment therapy for mental health problems in college students. Behav Modif 41(1):141–162, 2016 27440189

Mistler BJ, Reetz DR, Krylowicz B, Barr V: The Association for University and College Counseling Center Directors Annual Survey. Indianapolis, IN, Association for University and College Counseling Center Directors, 2012

Reetz D, Bershad C, LeViness P, Whitlock M: The Association for University and College Counseling Center Directors Annual Survey. Indianapolis, IN, Association for University and College Counseling Center Directors, 2016

Reicherter D, Liu EY, Roberts LW: People from culturally distinct populations, in A Clinical Guide to Psychiatric Ethics. Edited by Roberts LW. Arlington, VA, American Psychiatric Association Publishing, 2016, pp 133–145

Tupler LA, Hong JY, Gibori R, et al: Suicidal ideation and sex differences in relation to 18 major psychiatric disorders in college and university students: anonymous web-based assessment. J Nerv Ment Dis 203(4):269–278, 2015 25784307

Attention-Deficit/ Hyperactivity Disorder and Learning Disorders

Lindsay C. Chromik, M.S.
David S. Hong, M.D.

LEARNING occupies a prominent role in the lives of youth. By corollary, difficulties in this domain have significant impact on adaptive functioning. Unfortunately, challenges in this domain are common. Attention-deficit/hyperactivity disorder (ADHD) now has the distinction of being the most common behavioral disorder in children, affecting approximately 7% of the population (Thomas et al. 2015); specific learning disorders (SLDs) are similarly estimated to affect up to approximately

10% of youth (Altarac and Saroha 2007). Frequently, individuals have comorbid ADHD and SLD. There is evidence that a large proportion of youth will continue to be affected as they enter adulthood, presenting these transition-age youth with specific and unique challenges. This age group is faced with managing difficulties caused by these disorders in a college setting, but also these disorders occur in a context of global developmental challenges, including individuation, increased self-reliance, navigating work and social/romantic relationships, and the emergence of other psychiatric conditions that peak at this time of life. Specific to the college environment, ADHD and SLDs may potentially impact myriad skills that students need to successfully navigate a college program's curriculum, such as acquisition of academic knowledge, self-monitoring, and organization.

Without appropriate management, the presence of either or both disorders can result in substantial personal burden and often requires a different approach than management of symptoms during earlier stages of an individual's development. The relatively unstructured and independent nature of postsecondary education can cause students who previously were successful to seek additional support, including students needing a first-time clinical diagnosis. Additionally, students with previously well-managed symptoms may experience new difficulties due to more challenging course work or disruption in academic supports and accommodations. Much of the clinical work in these domains requires mental health professionals and students to identify and advocate for support and accommodations within the constraints of what the educational institution can and will provide. In this chapter, we explore the impact of ADHD and SLDs on functioning in college-age individuals, as well as the unique challenges of diagnosing and treating these conditions in the dynamic and complex context of college life.

Diagnosis

ATTENTION-DEFICIT/HYPERACTIVITY DISORDER

The core symptomatology of ADHD in the college-age population does not differ substantially from the childhood diagnosis. Indeed, beyond the criteria of age at onset and the number of symptoms required, DSM-5 (American Psychiatric Association 2013) does not distinguish an adult versus a childhood phenotype for ADHD (Table 13–1). Therefore, establishing a diagnosis of the condition warrants a similar approach, includ-

TABLE 13–1. Diagnostic features of attention-deficit/hyperactivity disorder and specific learning disorder

Attention-deficit/hyperactivity disorder

Diagnostic features	An overall pattern of problems related to inattention, hyperactivity, and/or impulsivity. The difficulties must cause problems in functioning in multiple settings. The pattern of behavior must have started before age 12 and should not be attributable to another mental health condition.
	Of potential relevance to college students is the "in partial remission" specifier, which is indicated when a full diagnosis was previously warranted but current symptoms would not meet diagnostic criteria, although the remaining symptoms still cause functional impairment.
Predominantly inattentive presentation	Impairment in at least six aspects of attention (five aspects in adults). Examples include making frequent careless mistakes, avoiding activities that require prolonged periods of attention, being forgetful, and being easily distracted.
Predominantly hyperactive-impulsive presentation	Impairment in at least six aspects of impulse control and hyperactivity (five aspects in adults). Examples include fidgeting, extreme restlessness, and intruding on others.
Combined presentation	Guidelines for both inattentive and hyperactive-impulsive types are met.

Specific learning disorder

Diagnostic features	Problems with learning and academics for at least 6 months that cause interference with performance, even after attempts to improve functioning in impacted areas. The problems should not be better explained by factors such as intellectual disability, educational quality, or sensory deficits. Of potential relevance to college students, the problems begin during earlier school-age years, but the extent may not be fully realized until the individual experiences increased academic demands.
	The impaired domain should be specified and may be reading, written expression, or mathematics.

ing assessment for behaviors consistent with inattention, hyperactivity, and/or impulsivity, which is often accomplished through a comprehensive clinical interview and standardized assessments. However, a specific challenge in diagnosing college-age individuals is that the ability to obtain historical data is often limited. Currently, ADHD is conceptualized as a *developmental* disorder, and evidence of symptoms consistent with ADHD is required to have been present since childhood, defined in DSM-5 as "prior to age 12 years." The burden of proof for meeting this criterion is accomplished easily for students who have a well-documented clinical history of ADHD that includes prior medical records and student and parent interviews. A more substantial challenge lies in diagnosing college students seeking a first-time diagnosis of ADHD, because a majority of individuals in this cohort self-refer for evaluations as opposed to having been identified within the educational system or by family members (as commonly occurs with childhood ADHD diagnoses). For previously undiagnosed students, obtaining historical data supporting the presence of symptoms of ADHD during childhood can present a challenge. This challenge can be further complicated when parents are no longer involved in care or when students want to pursue diagnosis and treatment independently without parental input. In these cases, the following can assist in the diagnostic process and supplement the standard clinical interview: prior school and/or medical records, adult self-report scales, and observational reports from peers, resident fellows, counselors, and parents. Some commonly used symptom scales for adults are the Structured Clinical Interview for DSM-5 (First et al. 2016), the Conners' Adult ADHD Rating Scales (available at www.mhs.com/MHS-Assessment?prodname=caars), and the Adult ADHD Self-Report Scale (Adler et al. 2003).

SPECIFIC LEARNING DISORDERS

SLDs (see Table 13–1) represent a substantial burden on affected students in the college environment and often go undiagnosed. One of the core issues regarding SLDs is the distribution of these conditions across domains of psychiatry, neuropsychology, and education, which represent different points of entry for affected individuals into systems of care. Unfortunately, consensus diagnostic criteria across these fields are lacking, resulting in a significant clinical gap that causes substantial underdiagnosis for affected students. There are several different methods of determining whether an individual has a learning disorder (Hale et al. 2010), the most commonly accepted being the ability-achievement discrepancy and response-to-intervention models (Table 13–2), both of which have been incorporated into the DSM-5 categorization of SLDs.

TABLE 13–2. Models of diagnosing learning disorders

Ability-achievement discrepancy models

Grade-level discrepancy: Presence of discrepancy between grade placement and achievement as measured by grade-equivalent scores

Simple discrepancy: Presence of discrepancy between measured ability (typically IQ) and achievement

Intraindividual discrepancy: Presence of a discrepancy between an individual's average overall cognitive ability and achievement and the individual's area-specific cognitive ability and achievement

Underachievement: Scores below average range on achievement testing

Response-to-intervention model

Diagnosis by treatment failure (treatment in this case being standard educational interventions within the classroom over a reasonable period of time)

Persistent underachievement or difficulty with learning (no requirement for formal neuropsychological testing or "failure" in academic achievement)

Unfortunately, these methods do not have a high level of agreement, and the same student may or may not receive a diagnosis of an SLD depending on the selected method. Similarly, the implementation of these diagnostic models often varies across educational and clinical settings, resulting in a poorly defined cohort of individuals who have learning challenges. Additionally, these diagnostic challenges frequently persist across childhood into college settings, where accurate evaluation of the presence of a learning disorder is often difficult and requires careful consideration of the diagnostic model that best addresses the concerns with which the student presents. In these instances, further academic histories or prior neuropsychological testing is useful, as well as an up-to-date comprehensive neuropsychological assessment. College students with a previously undiagnosed learning disorder typically need to assume responsibility for obtaining an outside evaluation.

EVALUATION IN THE COLLEGE SETTING

A standard clinical assessment for ADHD and SLD in a young adult student presenting for treatment is typically initiated with a comprehensive clinical interview. The primary components of the interview include assessment of the manifesting issues and establishment of both current and past contexts in which these problems are occurring or have occurred. The interview is focused primarily on subjective report of inattention, symptoms of hyperactivity and/or impulsivity, and learning challenges, and the impact that these potential issues have on adaptive function. Careful attention should also be given in the interview to comorbid psychiatric symptoms, substance use, academic and social histories, developmental trajectories, sleep patterns, and appetite. The extended assessment entails broader information gathering, including collateral input from any of the following: parents, roommates, friends, coworkers, resident advisors/fellows, professors, and academic advisors. Ideally, collateral information will be collected in person or by phone, although observer-reported standardized rating scales may also suffice. Access to current or historical academic reports and neuropsychological testing when indicated also provides substantive support in establishing a new diagnosis.

Treatment Options

A number of effective treatment options are available for ADHD once students struggling with this condition are appropriately identified. Broadly available therapies include medications, behavioral and psychosocial therapies, and educational resources and interventions. Learning disorders are not typically treated by mental health clinicians, and the evidence base for interventions for SLDs in the clinical literature is sparse; the vast majority of interventions for SLDs fall within the educational realm, as briefly overviewed in the last part of this section.

PHARMACOTHERAPY

Available evidence indicates that medication management of ADHD symptoms in college-age individuals can be highly effective, as it can be in childhood ADHD, although age-specific effects may emerge in later adulthood (Schrantee et al. 2016). Therefore, treatment strategies recommended for college-age students are similar to those used for children. For example, the Texas Children's Medication Treatment Algorithm includes prioritization of first-line therapies such as stimulants, within the methylphenidate or amphetamine classes, or treatment initiation with atomoxetine, especially for patients with comorbidities that may benefit from norepinephrine (and possibly serotonin) reuptake inhibition (Pliszka et al. 2006). Longer-acting formulations are generally preferred because of reduced abuse potential and duration of effect in college settings with increased cognitive load throughout the day. Side effects associated with these treatments should be expected and monitored on a regular basis, consistent with standard clinical practice. In clinical situations where stimulants or atomoxetine are ineffective or not appropriate first-line treatments, bupropion, tricyclic antidepressants, or α-agonists may also be considered.

Specific issues pertinent to college-age individuals being treated with medications for ADHD include comorbid conditions and concerns for medication abuse or misuse. Comorbidities should be carefully considered during selection of treatment medications as well as for treatment planning purposes. More complex clinical scenarios likely require closer monitoring in college settings than can be provided by occasional visits with a long-distance mental health professional, such as visiting a hometown clinician during school breaks. Mood and anxiety problems are frequent comorbidities; for students with these problems and ADHD, standard treatment protocols are generally followed. Prominent symptoms associated with ADHD are impulsivity and sensation seeking, which have particular salience within the college environment and lead to a host of complex adaptive functioning issues for affected individuals. Substance abuse is one of the most prominent sensory-seeking activities in students. Although the rate of substance abuse is increased in students as a whole, individuals with ADHD have consistently been found to have approximately a two to three times greater risk for substance use disorders (Harstad et al. 2014). Diagnosis and treatment of ADHD in the context of active and significant substance abuse is challenging, given the substantial overlap in symptoms associated with chronic substance use and the ADHD phenotype, as well as potential concerns for initiating treatment in students who are either unwilling or unable to limit use of substances. The clinical utility of making an ADHD diagnosis for symptoms occurring during active and regular substance abuse is debatable and requires substantial collateral information to support the diagnosis; if ADHD is diagnosed, treatment decisions are complicated by the substance-related management. In these instances, careful consideration of a number of factors should be taken into account for an individualized treatment plan. Sustained-release formulations, nonstimulant medications, or cognitive training interventions will likely be the therapies of choice when ADHD is diagnosed in the context of other substance use.

A related concern for the college-age population is prescription medication abuse or misuse. Estimates indicate that between 5% and 35% of college-age students have used stimulants in a nonmedical context, largely as a study enhancement aid (Wilens et al. 2008). Also, 16%–29% of students with stimulant prescriptions have received requests from peers to give, sell, or trade their medications, underscoring the pervasive nonclinical aspects associated with stimulant medications as "study drugs" (Wilens et al. 2008). Decisions to prescribe stimulants when there is concern for misuse should be made with great caution from both clinical and medicolegal perspectives. Patients given prescriptions should receive psychoeducation regarding appropriate and legal use of medications, be informed about clear guidelines regarding how early refills or "lost" prescriptions will be handled, and be told about statewide electronic databases or other prescription medication monitoring programs that ensure responsible management of prescriptions.

PSYCHOSOCIAL THERAPIES

For many students with ADHD who are transitioning from secondary school, the decreased structure of the college environment and increased emphasis on independence are challenges. These young adults will often be transitioning away from reliance on parental scaffolding for management of the complex issues associated with ADHD and therefore will require additional psychosocial support and behavioral strategies. Psychosocial therapies that directly or indirectly address core symptoms of ADHD and SLDs have been investigated. Although a number of studies suggest that behavioral therapies improve adaptive functioning for individuals with ADHD, closer analysis suggests that empirical data are limited regarding efficacy of these treatments for core ADHD symptoms (Chan et al. 2016). Nevertheless, cognitive-behavioral therapy, dialectical behavior therapy, neurofeedback, and cognitive training are all deployed in clinical practice (Daley et al. 2014) and may be included in treatment planning for college-age individuals, particularly for those with comorbid psychiatric diagnoses or sensory-seeking behaviors associated with impulsivity. Although the overlap between executive function deficits and core ADHD symptomatology has yet to be clearly defined, it is clear that cognitive processes such as planning, sequencing, and organization are often impaired in individuals with ADHD. Interventions specifically focused on these domains include ADHD coaching and organizational skills therapies, both of which have received increased attention from the research community in recent years (Gallagher et al. 2014; Solanto 2013). These interventions have focused on issues such as time management; assistance with organization in living environments and academics; and improving general health, nutrition, and sleep routines. The available evidence is sparse but seems to suggest that these interventions may positively impact adaptive functioning even if core ADHD symptoms do not improve, indicating that further research for these types of interventions is warranted.

Psychosocial therapies have similarly been implemented to help students with SLDs, although this evidence base is also limited. Notably, like ADHD, SLDs are often comorbid with mood and anxiety disorders that may benefit from validated psychosocial therapies.

EDUCATIONAL INTERVENTIONS

Both ADHD and SLD symptoms are prominently manifest in academic environments. Therefore, treatments frequently focus on assessing the student's cognitive strengths and weaknesses. Treatment then uses identified strengths to develop compensatory strategies for domains of weakness and targets areas of weakness using skill development. Additionally, appropriate educational accommodations can be requested and are facilitated in many college campuses through resources available to students with disabilities (including both ADHD and SLDs). Common accommodation examples are adjusted seating arrangements, extended time on exams, having a peer note-taker, taking exams in a separate room, and individual tutoring. Informal resources such as study groups and student organizations may also be of assistance.

In K–12 education, students' access to appropriate educational services is protected broadly by federal legislation, including the Americans With Disabilities Act (ADA), Individuals With Disabilities Education Act (IDEA), and Section 504 of the Rehabilitation Act. Although these legal protections apply only to postsecondary institutions receiving federal funding and they have limited implementation in college environments given that IDEA and most parts of Section 504 are specific to primary and secondary education, ADA and Section 504 Subpart E do apply to post-secondary students and require that colleges make reasonable accommodations. The scope of these accommodations is generally more limited. Given these differences, students who enter college with previously diagnosed ADHD or SLDs may need assistance navigating the differences between the accommodations they were guaranteed in secondary school and the protections and resources available in college. Furthermore, ADA guidelines require that qualified disabilities are current, meaning that students with past diagnoses may need new documentation indicating that their functioning continues to be impacted by their diagnoses.

School policies and available resources can vary significantly by institution and can encompass a broad range of accommodations that are considered "reasonable." For instance, accommodations at specific universities may include advisors, resource and tutoring centers, and career guidance, among others. Requests for accommodation require specific steps that are outlined in each educational institution's academic policies, which should be thoroughly reviewed by students with prior or newly established diagnoses. Guidelines for testing and evaluation are often specific to each institution, as are thresholds for documenting evidence of psychiatric or learning disabilities. The burden for notifying college administration of the need for educational accommodations falls on the student, who may benefit from receiving guidance in this area from clinicians, particularly because review and implementation of accommodation requests may take some time and should be initiated well before the accommodations are needed or adaptive function is impacted. When accommodations for disabilities are granted, the financial costs are covered by the educational institution.

Postcollege Transition

Central to the discussion on treatment for ADHD and SLDs in college-age individuals is successful transition into postcollege life, where access to medical care may be more challenging. Also pertinent to this discussion is the natural course of ADHD symptoms. Although childhood ADHD is identified in about 7% of the population (Thomas et al. 2015), approximately one-third of patients with childhood ADHD will demonstrate a remission in symptoms by adulthood, where the rate of ADHD is estimated to be closer to approximately 3% of the total population (Simon et al. 2009). Predictors for which individuals will be remitters versus persisters remain scarce. However, identifying and scaffolding those individuals whose symptoms persist into postcollege adulthood are important goals for clinicians working with this age group, particularly when considering the substantial personal and societal burden from lost work hours and disability associated with ADHD. College attendance in and of itself appears to help stabilize impairment level in young adults with ADHD, whereas equally impaired peers with ADHD who do not attend college see an increase in impairment (Howard et al. 2016). College students with ADHD, however, are likely to have lower grade point averages and graduation rates compared with peers, making appropriate treatment a significant priority for this cohort. Providing adequate support for a successful college experience may be an effective method of improving outcomes during the transition to adulthood. SLDs also often persist into adulthood, necessitating postgraduation treatment, including ongoing strategies for strengthening areas of vulnerability, which can help minimize the extent to which a student will continue to be impacted by symptoms. Having documentation of current impairment will enable the individual to advocate for necessary accommodations at postgraduate schooling or in work environments. Students may also benefit from psychoeducation around ADA guidelines and guidance in self-advocacy as they leave educational settings. Furthermore, career counseling may be useful in helping students identify a career path that best utilizes their strengths; however, learning disorders generally do not prevent an individual from succeeding in a chosen career and should not be used as a reason to discourage students from careers they wish to pursue.

Case Examples

CASE EXAMPLE 1

Sandra is a 19-year-old female student with no prior psychiatric diagnosis who presents to her college mental health center reporting struggles with academics. She states that since elementary school she has always had difficulty paying attention, has often used her phone or doodled during class, has made careless mistakes on problem sets, and has forgotten to turn in assignments. She notes that she gets easily distracted by other students in class and is completely disorganized in her study habits and management of school materials. She often finds herself avoiding term papers or procrastinating on studying for exams and instead ends up socializing with friends or going to parties. When she does study, she is often distracted, pulling all-nighters without much productive work. She is seeking help at student health services because she is currently at risk of failing the majority of her classes. She also observes that her most difficult classes tend to be ones with an intensive load of reading and writing. She feels that it takes much longer for her to get through the same amount of reading material as her peers and that she needs to constantly reread assignments to understand their meaning—a pattern that has been consistent since much earlier in her life.

CASE EXAMPLE 2

Jaime is a 21-year-old male student with a prior history of ADHD, diagnosed by his pediatrician during elementary school. He has a long history of symptoms including inattention, hyperactivity, and impulsivity, which is confirmed in his medical records. He also has a history of dyslexia for which he had an Individualized Education Program throughout his primary and secondary education. Jaime has clearly benefited from stimulant medications in the past but has only been taking his medications intermittently since starting college, because of the logistical challenges of obtaining prescriptions from his out-of-state pediatrician, who no longer feels comfortable continuing to prescribe given the

infrequent nature of their visits. Since starting stimulant treatment prescribed through campus health services, Jaime reports significant improvement in concentration and organization, although he continues to
skip classes and miss assignments. Jaime reports that he is rushing a fraternity this semester and endorses binge drinking (more than 5 drinks/
occasion) 3–4 days a week and smoking marijuana 4–5 days a week. In
the past 4 months since he began receiving medication through campus
health services, he has reported "misplacing" his prescription once and
"accidentally" dropping his pills down the sink once, resulting in two requests for additional refills.

Conclusion

ADHD and SLDs are among the most common disorders affecting children; however, access and engagement with care for these conditions decline significantly during the transition to adulthood. Indeed, there is
substantial symptom burden for many college-age individuals. While
diagnosis and treatment of individuals in this developmental period
presents some additional challenges, comprehensive clinical assessment,
neuropsychological testing, and use of rating scales allow objective diagnoses to be established. Furthermore, medications, psychosocial therapies, and educational accommodations continue to be effective in this
age group. While additional attention is needed to adapt assessment and
intervention approaches to factors associated with college, appropriate
care may significantly benefit the majority of students affected by ADHD
or SLD.

KEY CONCEPTS

- Attention-deficit/hyperactivity disorder (ADHD) and specific
  learning disorders (SLDs) both can persist into college and
  beyond. New challenges may arise during college due to
  the different environment and demands of this developmental stage.

- New diagnosis of these conditions during college often
  presents specific challenges and may require alternative
  strategies for obtaining historical data or observer report in
  establishing a diagnosis.

- The Americans With Disabilities Act requires that reasonable
  accommodation be made for students with ADHD or SLDs,
  which is a lesser requirement than that for primary and sec-

ondary school students in the Individuals With Disabilities Education Act. Students may need assistance navigating the changes in accommodations and academic support in the college environment.

- Both pharmacotherapy and psychosocial therapies can be effective in the college-age cohort. Additional attention is often needed in managing comorbid conditions and ensuring appropriate treatment compliance.

- With appropriate support, students with SLDs or ADHD can often have a successful college experience. Psychoeducation and guidance during the transition to postcollege pursuits is equally important in treatment planning.

Recommendations for Psychiatrists, Psychologists, and Counselors

1. Evaluation
   - Conduct a comprehensive clinical interview evaluation.
   - Obtain collateral input through interviews and/or rating scales.
   - Ascertain historical evidence of ADHD and/or SLD symptoms.
   - Screen for comorbid psychiatric diagnoses.
   - Obtain academic records if available.
   - Request additional neuropsychological testing as indicated.

2. Treatment for attention-deficit/hyperactivity disorder
   - Keep in mind that although medications are often effective for treatment of ADHD, they may have age-specific effects.
   - Remember that long-acting stimulants and nonstimulants may be preferred.
   - Initially, assess a student's risk for misuse or abuse of stimulants and provide ongoing oversight during treatment.
   - Consider psychosocial interventions, which may benefit adaptive functioning.
   - Treat comorbid diagnoses.

3. Treatment for specific learning disorders
   - Consider educational strategies specific to affected domains.
   - Consider academic accommodations.
   - Consider technology-assisted interventions
   - Consider psychosocial therapies when SLDs impact broader adaptive function.

4. Educational interventions

- Provide psychoeducation and guidance to help patients understand the process for notifying and requesting accommodations.
- Provide documentation as necessary when requested by college administration.
- Assist in navigating appropriateness of provided educational interventions.

5. Postcollege transition

- Reevaluate for ongoing presence of symptoms and their impact on adaptive functioning.
- Assist in transitioning care to new mental health professionals and provide clinical documentation as needed.
- Provide guidance in establishing accommodations for disability in postcollege setting as appropriate.

Discussion Questions

1. What is the natural prognosis of attention-deficit/hyperactivity disorder (ADHD) in college, and how does this map onto general developmental changes during this period?

2. How do ADHD and learning disorders coexist? How might evaluations efficiently assess issues in both of these domains?

3. What are the best ways to provide resources for young adults with ADHD and/or learning disorders?

4. Are there ways to minimize medication abuse with typical ADHD treatments?

5. What are the best ways to transition treatment of young adults with ADHD and/or learning disorders as they leave the learning environment?

Suggested Readings

Association on Higher Education and Disability (AHEAD) (Web site). Available at: https://www.ahead.org/. Accessed July 21, 2017.

U.S. Department of Education, Office for Civil Rights: Transition of Students With Disabilities to Postsecondary Education: A Guide for High School Educators, March 2007 (Reprinted March 2011). Available at: https://www2.ed.gov/about/offices/list/ocr/transitionguide.html. Accessed July 21, 2017.

References

Adler LA, Kessler RC, Spencer T: Adult ADHD Self-Report Scale Symptom Checklist. Geneva, Switzerland, World Health Organization, 2003. Available at https://med.nyu.edu/psych/sites/default/files/psych/psych_adhd_checklist_0.pdf. Accessed January 2018.

Altarac M, Saroha E: Lifetime prevalence of learning disability among U.S. children. Pediatrics 119(suppl 1):S77–S83, 2007 17272589

American Psychiatric Association: Diagnostic and Statistical Manual of Mental Disorders, 5th Edition. Arlington, VA, American Psychiatric Association, 2013

Chan E, Fogler JM, Hammerness PG: Treatment of attention-deficit/hyperactivity disorder in adolescents: a systematic review. JAMA 315(18):1997–2008, 2016 27163988

Conners CK, Erhardt D, Sparrow E: Conners' Adult ADHD Rating Scales. Available at https://www.mhs.com/MHS-Assessment?prodname=caars. Accessed January 2018.

Daley D, van der Oord S, Ferrin M, et al; European ADHD Guidelines Group: Behavioral interventions in attention-deficit/hyperactivity disorder: a meta-analysis of randomized controlled trials across multiple outcome domains. J Am Acad Child Adolesc Psychiatry 53(8):835–847, 2014 25062591

First M; Williams JBW, Karg RS, Spitzer RL: Structured Clinical Interview for DSM-5—Clinician Version (SCID-5-CV). Arlington, VA, American Psychiatric Association, 2016

Gallagher R, Abikoff HB, Spira EG: Organizational Skills Training for Children With ADHD: An Empirically Supported Treatment, New York, NY, Guilford, 2014

Hale J, Alfonso V, Berninger V, et al: Critical issues in response-to-intervention, comprehensive evaluation, and specific learning disabilities identification and intervention: an expert white paper consensus. Learn Disabil Q 33(3):223–236, 2010

Harstad E, Levy S; Committee on Substance Abuse: Attention-deficit/hyperactivity disorder and substance abuse. Pediatrics 134(1):e293–e301, 2014 24982106

Howard AL, Strickland NJ, Murray DW, et al: Progression of impairment in adolescents with attention-deficit/hyperactivity disorder through the transition out of high school: contributions of parent involvement and college attendance. J Abnorm Psychol 125(2):233–247, 2016 26854508

Pliszka SR, Crimson ML, Hughes CW, et al: The Texas Children's Medication Algorithm Project: revision of the algorithm for pharmocotherapy of attention-deficity/hyperactivity disorder. J Am Acad Child Adolesc Psychiatry 45(6) 642-657, 2006 16721314 45(6):642–657 2006 16721314

Schrantee A, Tamminga HG, Bouziane C, et al: Age-dependent effects of methylphenidate on the human dopaminergic system in young vs. adult patients with attention-deficit/hyperactivity disorder: a randomized clinical trial. JAMA Psychiatry 73(9):955–962, 2016 27487479

Simon V, Czobor P, Bálint S, et al: Prevalence and correlates of adult attention-deficit hyperactivity disorder: meta-analysis. Br J Psychiatry 194(3):204–211, 2009 19252145

Solanto MV: Cognitive-Behavioral Therapy for Adult ADHD: Targeting Executive Dysfunction, New York, NY, Guilford, 2013

Thomas R, Sanders S, Doust J, et al: Prevalence of attention-deficit/hyperactivity disorder: a systematic review and meta-analysis. Pediatrics 135(4):e994–e1001, 2015 25733754

Wilens TE, Adler LA, Adams J, et al: Misuse and diversion of stimulants prescribed for ADHD: a systematic review of the literature. J Am Acad Child Adolesc Psychiatry 47(1):21–31, 2008 18174822

Alcohol and Substance Use and Co-occurring Behaviors

Chinyere I. Ogbonna, M.D., M.P.H.

Anna Lembke, M.D.

THE increase in risky substance use on college campuses has been matched by increases in serious consequences to students, the college campus, and surrounding communities, with alcohol-related consequences being the most destructive. Consequences of substance use include academic problems, risky sexual behaviors, illness, unintentional injuries, accidental death, crime, and other disturbances on campus and in the surrounding communities. Although there is a common public perception that substance use among college students is a "normal rite of passage," the harmful consequences of risky substance use on campus can have lasting effects on student academic, mental, physical, and social well-being that often extend to life off-campus. A greater focus on prevention and reduction of student substance use via comprehensive, environmental management approaches is needed to change the prevailing culture of use. Routinely screening students for high-risk substance use behaviors is an important first step in identifying students who would benefit from more targeted, evidence-based prevention, intervention, and treatment services (National Center on Addiction and Substance Abuse 2007).

Trends in Substance Use Among College Students

The National Center on Addiction and Substance Abuse (CASA) released two landmark reports in 1993 and 1994 highlighting the growing public health concern of increased alcohol binge drinking and other substance misuse among American college and university students. In 2007, CASA published "Wasting the Best and the Brightest: Substance Abuse at America's Colleges and Universities" (National Center on Addiction and Substance Abuse 2007), providing a detailed analysis of the factors that contribute to the culture of student substance use and addiction (Table 14–1), the harmful consequences of this culture, and concrete recommendations for implementing comprehensive evidence-based practices and policies to prevent student alcohol and substance misuse on campus (National Center on Addiction and Substance Abuse 2007).

According to the 2007 CASA report, college students drink more than same-age peers not enrolled in college, a finding that has been consistent since 1993. The rates of alcohol use and binge drinking among college students have shown no sign of significant reduction from 1993 to 2005. Meanwhile, the rates of risky alcohol use (i.e., increased frequency of binge drinking, being intoxicated, and drinking to get drunk) have been on the rise, indicating increasingly dangerous patterns of alcohol misuse among college students. Because college students tend to underestimate their alcohol consumption, either by underreporting the amount consumed or by overpouring drinks, the extent of alcohol use among students may be greater than that captured by national surveys. In a sample of 10,424 first-year college students from 14 schools across the United States, 41% of male students and 34% of female students admitted to drinking more than the threshold for binge drinking (defined as drinking five or more drinks in a row at least once in the past 2 weeks),

TABLE 14–1. Factors driving college student alcohol and substance use and abuse

Genetics and family history	Genetics and family history are influential in determining susceptibility for student substance use progressing to problem use or a use disorder.
Parental attitudes and behaviors	Students who have parents who abuse alcohol, smoke, or use other drugs or who demonstrate permissive attitudes about substance use are more likely to use substances in college. Parental expectations and perception of mother's approval also influence whether or how much students drink, smoke, or use other drugs, with disapproval being associated with less substance use.
Social influences	Peer groups and direct social pressure to engage in substance use have a considerable influence on student substance use in college (e.g., drinking games where the goal is to consume large amounts of alcohol in a short amount of time). The college years are also marked by social events that are associated with high rates of substance use (e.g., celebrating 21st birthdays, spring break).
Substance use in high school	Students who use and abuse substances in college are more likely to have initiated substance use during high school.
Student engagement	Students who report higher levels of engaged learning and nonrequired campus or community service activities are significantly less likely than those who report less engagement to be binge drinkers or heavy drinkers.
Mental health problems	Students who experience subclinical or clinical symptoms of anxiety or depression, or who report elevated levels of stress, are at higher risk of abusing alcohol and other substances.
Expectation of positive effect	Students are more likely to use or abuse substances if they believe that substance use will lead to positive effects (e.g., enhanced recreational or social experiences, reduced social or sexual inhibitions, enhanced concentration and increased alertness, reduced weight gain, reduced stress, enhanced self-image and feelings of self-worth).

TABLE 14–1. Factors driving college student alcohol and substance use and abuse (continued)

Campus and community environment	Students are more likely to use and abuse substances when there are minimally enforced restrictions on possession on campus and ease of acquisition of substances via friends, classmates, or the Internet. Advertising and promotion of alcoholic beverages at college athletic facilities also lend an air of acceptability to student alcohol use on campus.
Religion and spirituality	Students who report religion is not important to them or who never or rarely attend religious services are more likely than more religious students to drink, use drugs, and smoke.
Sorority and fraternity (Greek) membership	Students in the Greek system are more likely than nonmembers to be current drinkers, binge drinkers, and use other substances including marijuana and nicotine.
Athletic participation	College athletes report higher levels of alcohol use than nonathletes but are less likely to use illicit drugs, including marijuana, or nicotine.

Source.   Adapted from National Center on Addiction and Substance Abuse 2007

with approximately 20% of male students admitting to drinking 10 or more drinks in one occasion in the past month. Students who report frequent binge drinking (binge drinking three or more times within the past 2 weeks) were more likely than those who report infrequent binge drinking to drink at these higher levels (National Center on Addiction and Substance Abuse 2007). In 2005, female college students were noted to have rates of binge drinking that were similar to those of their male counterparts, when the definition of binge drinking was adjusted based on differences in female physiology (i.e., more than four drinks in a row for women vs. more than five drinks in a row for men). From 1993 to 2005, the increase in the proportion of students reporting frequent binge drinking, being drunk three or more times in the past 30 days, and reporting drinking on 10 or more occasions in the past 30 days, was higher among women than among men college students (National Center on Addiction and Substance Abuse 2007).

Although the main substance on college campuses has been alcohol, the proportions of students misusing controlled prescription medications, marijuana, cocaine, and heroin have increased since the early 1990s. In 2005, about 69% (5.4 million) of full-time college students reported drinking, misusing controlled prescription medications, using illicit drugs, or smoking marijuana in the past month; 45% (2.3 million) of current drinkers engaged in two or more other forms of substance use. Students using controlled substances such as pain killers, stimulants, and sedative/hypnotics are at higher risk for binge drinking, which, in turn, increases their risk for accidental overdose (National Center on Addiction and Substance Abuse 2007). Since the passing in several states of ballot measures legalizing the use of marijuana for both medical and recreational uses, the impact of these new laws on trends in use among college students and young adults has yet to be seen. What is known is that college student marijuana use has increased from 3.5% in 2007 to 5.9% in 2014, while rates of perceived risk and personal disapproval of marijuana use have decreased during this time (Johnston et al. 2016). In 2014, an estimated 9.6% of young adults ages 18–25 years reported current marijuana use, with 4.9% of young adults meeting criteria for marijuana use disorder in the past year (Center for Behavioral Health Statistics and Quality 2015).

Screening and Brief Intervention

College health centers and student mental health services can be important venues for screening young adults for high-risk substance use behaviors, because these students are more likely to present for substance use–related injuries or illness (Larimer et al. 2004; Monti et al. 2004–2005). Students with high-risk substance use behaviors are more likely to report significantly lower ratings of their own general health, experience higher rates of injuries, and endorse learning or memory impairment (National Center on Addiction and Substance Abuse 2007). There is also a strong association between substance use and co-occurring mood and anxiety disorders. Among adults age 18 or older in 2014 with any mental illness (defined as having any mental, behavioral, or emotional disorder in the past year that met DSM-IV criteria, excluding developmental disorders and substance use disorders), the percentage of adults who had a co-occurring substance use disorder was highest among those ages 18–25 years (29.3%) (Center for Behavioral Health Statistics and Quality 2015). Unfortunately, only 39.6% of schools report any screening of students for risky alcohol use through health services, and less than 30% report screening for problems with prescription medications (27.1%), illicit drugs (29.9%), or tobacco (29.9%) (National Center on Addiction and Substance Abuse 2007).

The Substance Abuse and Mental Health Services Administration (SAMHSA) supports the use of Screening, Brief Intervention, and Referral to Treatment (SBIRT) as an evidence-based approach to providing universal screening, early intervention, and treatment for people with problematic or hazardous substance use problems (Substance Abuse and Mental Health Services Administration 2013) (Figure 14–1).

The purpose of universal screening is to find students who are having problems with substance misuse, quickly assess the severity of their risk, and identify the appropriate level of intervention. The screening processes typically begin with the use of a single-question item related to alcohol or drug use, which if positive is followed with a validated tool, such as the Alcohol Use Disorders Identification Test (AUDIT; Saunders et al. 1993), the 10-item Drug Abuse Screening Test (DAST-10; Skinner 1982), or the Alcohol, Smoking and Substance Involvement Screening Test (ASSIST; WHO ASSIST Working Group 2002), which are free and available online for easy access (Web sites are provided in note to Figure 14–1). Universal screening allows for the identification of individuals along a full spectrum of use and then provides an opportunity for health care professionals to initiate discussions with patients about their substance use and to provide the appropriate interventions as needed. Students who score low on prescreening or screening tests do not need intervention and generally should receive positive reinforcement for maintaining abstinence or nonrisky use (Substance Abuse and Mental Health Services Administration 2013).

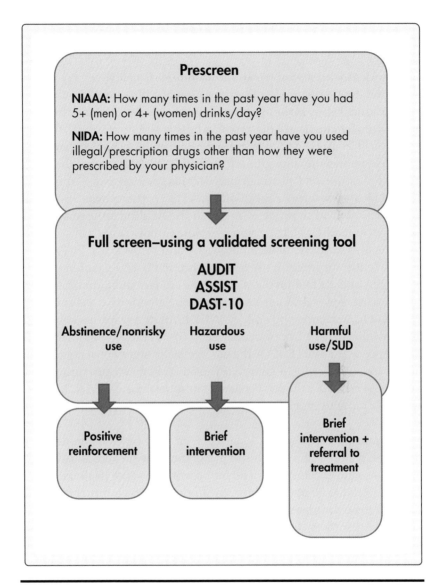

FIGURE 14–1. **Screening, Brief Intervention, and Referral to Treatment (SBIRT) work flow.**

Note. ASSIST=Alcohol, Smoking and Substance Involvement Screening Test (www.who.int/substance_abuse/activities/assist/en/); AUDIT=Alcohol Use Disorders Identification Test (https://www.drugabuse.gov/sites/default/files/files/AUDIT.pdf); DAST-10=10-item Drug Abuse Screening Test (https://www.drugabuse.gov/sites/default/files/dast-10.pdf); NIAAA=National Institute on Alcohol Abuse and Alcoholism; NIDA=National Institute on Drug Abuse; SUD=substance use disorder.
Source. Adapted from Pacific Southwest ATTC 2012.

How to Intervene Once Problematic Substance Use Is Identified

Each student who scores in the "hazardous" risk category may benefit from brief intervention, typically consisting of a time-limited number of motivational intervention sessions (one to five sessions, lasting anywhere from 5 minutes to 1 hour) with a health care professional, focused on increasing insight and awareness about the student's substance use, addressing unhealthy thoughts and behaviors associated with the harmful pattern of use, and eliciting change strategies (Substance Abuse and Mental Health Services Administration 2013). *Motivational interviewing*—a collaborative process in which the health care professional expresses empathy, avoids arguing, explores ambivalence, rolls with resistance, and supports patient autonomy and self-efficacy (SAMHSA-HRSA Center for Integrated Health Solutions 2017)—is often used in brief interventions and involves giving the student individualized feedback regarding level of use and risks associated with it (Monti et al. 2004–2005). Students who engage in harmful or hazardous substance use may also benefit from a challenge to commit to a 30-day period of abstinence as a litmus test for the emergence of signs consistent with a substance use disorder. A commonly used strategy for providing feedback is the FRAMES model: Feedback, Responsibility, Advice, Menu of options, Empathy, and Self-efficacy (Center for Substance Abuse Treatment 1999).

Brief interventions that are done in person utilizing motivational interviewing have been shown to result in significant reductions in risky substance use, with effects maintained for up to 4 years after treatment; however, they tend to be more effective for students with harmful patterns of substance use compared with those who already meet criteria for substance use disorders (Larimer et al. 2004; Monti et al. 2004–2005; Substance Abuse and Mental Health Services Administration 2013). While there are sufficient data to support the use of brief interventions to reduce risky alcohol use among college students, recent research on the efficacy of the SBIRT approach to reducing risky drug use has been promising for cocaine, heroin, amphetamine-type stimulants, and marijuana (Substance Abuse and Mental Health Services Administration 2013). More research is needed to determine the efficacy of brief interventions on reducing nonmedical use of psychoactive substances among non-treatment-seeking, screening-identified college students (Young et al. 2014).

Students in the "harmful use" risk category may also benefit from brief intervention as a bridge to referral to a specialist for more intensive care. Motivational interventional techniques may be helpful in identifying ambivalence toward treatment and facilitating student engagement in substance use treatment (Substance Abuse and Mental Health Services Administration 2013). Student mental health centers should work toward establishing strong referral linkages on campus or in the community in order to improve students' access to appropriate and timely substance use treatment. Other strategies for facilitating student referrals, such as transportation assistance and ongoing follow-up between the student and college health care professional, may encourage student participation and retention in substance use treatment and provide a sense of accountability and continuity for the student (Substance Abuse and Mental Health Services Administration 2013).

In 2014, about 16.3% of young adults needed treatment for a substance use disorder in the prior year (Center for Behavioral Health Statistics and Quality 2015), but only 8% received *specialty substance use treatment* (defined as treatment in a hospital, an inpatient and/or outpatient drug or alcohol rehabilitation facility, or a mental health center). Although there is no one-size-fits-all treatment for students with substance use disorders, the more common treatment modalities are attending self-help groups and other outpatient treatment facilities (Han et al. 2015). The American Society of Addiction Medicine (ASAM) advocates for patient placement into the appropriate levels of care based on the severity of dependence and impairment in level of functioning (Mee-Lee and Schulman 2014) (Table 14–2).

Tools like the ASAM patient placement criteria can assist in determining the appropriate level of "stepped care," using the least restrictive, least invasive, and least costly treatment setting that has the best chance of success (see Figure 14–2). If a patient does not respond to this level of care, then the patient is transitioned to the next level of more intense treatment (Mee-Lee and Schulman 2014; Monti et al. 2004–2005). Student health care professionals can play an important role in identifying students with substance use problems, targeting motivational interventions that aim to move the student toward the appropriate intensity of treatment, and utilizing available campus resources (Monti et al. 2004–2005; Substance Abuse and Mental Health Services Administration 2013).

Policy Approaches to Campus Alcohol and Drug Misuse

As detailed in section "Trends in Substance Use Among College Students," drug and alcohol use on college campuses has become a public

TABLE 14–2. ASAM patient placement criteria (benchmark levels of care)

Level 0.5 Early intervention	Assessment and education
Level I Outpatient services	Less than 9 hours/week, therapeutic interventions and medication management as needed
Level II Intensive outpatient/ partial hospitalization services	More than 9 hours/week, more intensive therapeutic interventions and medication management as needed
Level III Residential inpatient services	24-hour structure, trained counselors and as needed physician care, variable levels of residential intensity, therapeutic interventions
Level IV Medically managed intensive inpatient services	24-hour nursing care and daily physician care, therapeutic interventions

Note. ASAM=American Society of Addiction Medicine.
Source. Adapted from Mee-Lee and Schulman 2014.

health crisis, with rising rates of dangerous alcohol and drug use on campuses nationwide. Almost all 4-year colleges today have alcohol and drug policies and require new students to take a course on the dangers of substance misuse. Many campuses offer substance-free dorm living and have some sort of party monitoring to curb risky substance use, particularly risky drinking. Approximately half of 4-year colleges offer some kind of intervention or treatment program for alcohol misuse. Few colleges, however, are consistently enforcing state laws or even their own drug and alcohol policies. Even where risky drinking is highest—at tailgate parties and other pregame events, at fraternity and sorority houses, and in first-year student dorms—there is widespread indifference to existing policies and laws. Even fewer colleges work to reduce community risk factors, such as restricting the number of outlets selling alcohol or reducing drink specials at bars. The latest trend in campus alcohol policies has been to ban or restrict hard alcohol. Although the effects of these restrictions are still unknown, the theory is that by reducing access to hard alcohol specifically, the school will target dangerous alcohol use. College campus drinking culture today has changed from decades past, in that hard alcohol is ingested more frequently to hasten intoxication and lower the calorie consumption that accompanies ingesting equal amounts of ethanol in beer. Dovetailing with these changes are higher numbers than ever before of female stu-

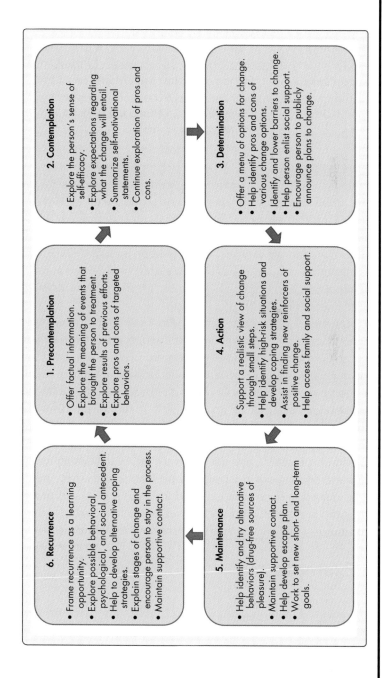

FIGURE 14–2. **Stages of change: intervention matching guide.**

Source. Adapted from Pacific Southwest ATTC 2012.

dents engaging in risky drinking, as well as an increase in campus sexual violence, which has been highly linked to alcohol misuse (Johnston et al. 2016; National Center on Addiction and Substance Abuse 2007).

In the 1990s, a large-scale study of public policy interventions to curb alcohol use among college students was launched by Henry Wechsler, a social psychologist at Harvard University's School of Public Health. Wechsler and colleagues (2000) argued that the environment fuels excessive drinking. A 10-campus experiment to target campus binge drinking was conducted over a 12-year period and referred to as "A Matter of Degree." The researchers set out to work with the local community to change the environment promoting heavy drinking. Early results showed that colleges that made changes to reduce community risk factors showed improvements in drinking behavior. One example of a successful intervention included strong laws to monitor and eradicate fake IDs (Nelson et al. 2005). In another project, called "Safer California Universities," researchers found that enforcing school policy and local laws curbed alcohol misuse, on and off campus; interventions included DUI checks, enforcing underage drinking laws by using underage decoys at parties, more party patrols, and holding hosts liable for disruptions caused by their guests (Saltz et al. 2010).

In 2016, the then U.S. Surgeon General, Dr. Vivek Murthy, released the first Surgeon General's report on alcohol, drugs, and health (the first other than the numerous previous reports on nicotine), called "Facing Addiction in America" (U.S. Department of Health and Human Services 2016). In this report, the Surgeon General identifies multiple public policy measures to tackle risky alcohol and drug use in the community, which parallel interventions that have made a difference on college campuses. These community-level protective factors include regulating the number and concentration of retail outlets selling substances, increasing the costs of substances, enforcing existing laws around substance use (e.g., holding retailers accountable for harms caused by illegal sales), and parental monitoring and support. Community-level risk factors include easy access to substances and low "parental" monitoring and support.

Case Example

Chris, a 19-year-old male student, was referred to student mental health following erratic behavior and multiple requests for stimulant medication. He presented to student health demanding to speak to a doctor about getting treatment for attention-deficit/hyperactivity disorder. While sitting in the waiting room, he was observed to be constantly shifting in his seat, fidgeting with his hands, and tapping his foot on the ground. He appeared easily startled and at times could be heard mumbling to himself. He refused to fill out intake paperwork, stating he didn't want his personal information "in the system." He then accused reception of recording him while he waited for the doctor and stormed out of the clinic. He was found by campus police and taken to the hospital for an evaluation.

Questions: What additional information would you like to know about this student? What would be your differential diagnoses at this point?

When you meet with Chris for an intake, he reports difficulty focusing on his schoolwork due to symptoms of inattention; he is worried about poor grades affecting his ability to maintain his grade point average and keep his scholarship. He is majoring in engineering at the university and expresses significant anxiety related to keeping up with the course work and competition among other students. He worries constantly about his grades and often stays up late into the night trying to keep up with reading assignments and homework. He reports an average of 4–5 hours of sleep, often with early-morning awakening and difficulty falling back asleep. He states that the only thing that helps him calm down and get some sleep is smoking cannabis. Chris started smoking cannabis about 4 months ago, initially on the weekends, but now he smokes every night before he goes to bed. He does not feel that his cannabis use is a problem, but he admits experiencing cravings to use as well as rebound anxiety when he attempts to cut back on his use. He rarely drinks alcohol because he doesn't like the way it makes him feel. He has experimented with other substances in the past and admits to obtaining Adderall (e.g., amphetamine, dextroamphetamine mixed salts) from friends in the past to help him study during finals week.

Questions: How would you screen this student for problematic substance use? What would you take into consideration when coming up with your assessment and plan? If this student refuses a referral to an addiction specialist, what kind of follow-up would you recommend?

Conclusion

Community-level protective and risk factors identified by the Surgeon General's report should be used to inform policy directed at college campus substance use problems. As for most public health crises, the solution lies in a multifocal approach that requires strong leadership on the part of colleges and universities and active engagement of college students, parents, alumni, Greek and athletic organizations, community leaders, and state and federal governments. Student mental health professionals can play an important role in identifying high-risk students through universal screening and facilitating engagement in treatment by providing evidence-based brief intervention and referral to substance use treatment services when appropriate.

KEY CONCEPTS

- High-risk substance use among college students is a public health issue.
- Screening for substance misuse is the first step in identifying risky use and targeting early intervention for individuals at high risk of harmful consequences from substance use.
- Brief intervention utilizing motivational interviewing techniques is a cost-effective and evidence-based strategy for reducing substance use among students identified as having risky patterns of use.

Recommendations for Psychiatrists, Psychologists, and Counselors

1. Universal screening for high-risk substance use among college students using validated screening tools can help identify students who would benefit from targeted early interventions to minimize harmful consequences associated with risky substance use.
2. Motivational interviewing is often used in providing brief interventions, which may consist of a single or multiple sessions, focused on increasing the student's insight and awareness of their substance use and eliciting change strategies for reducing harms associated with risky substance use.
3. Establishing strong referral linkages with available community and campus resources, including self-help groups and outpatient treatment centers, can help to improve access and facilitate student engagement in substance use treatment. If a student refuses referral, offering to follow up with the student provides a sense of accountability and continuity.
4. A stepwise approach to treatment is recommended to ensure that each student receives the appropriate level of care based on the severity of substance use and impairment in level of functioning.

5. It is crucial to become familiar with the specific drug-related policies of your institution and to advocate for increased funding for campus resources and services to help students manage mental health and substance use problems.

Discussion Questions

1. What are the specific drug-related policies at your institution that aim to reduce or prevent student drug use? If someone is caught violating these policies, what are the sanctions? Do you think these policies are effective or well enforced? How well known are these policies to the student body, faculty, and student health care professionals?

2. How accessible are school resources and services for helping college students deal with substance misuse problems, including smoking, drinking, and using drugs? What factors might keep students from getting help for substance misuse problems?

3. What are some barriers to implementing universal screening for high-risk substance use patterns among college students? How can these barriers be addressed?

4. Does your institution collect information to help understand rates and/or consequences of substance use among students? If yes, how is this information used to shape drug-related policies and sanctions? If no, should this kind of information be collected?

Suggested Readings

Center for Substance Abuse Treatment: Enhancing Motivation for Change in Substance Abuse Treatment. Treatment Improvement Protocol (TIP) Series, No 35. HHS Publ No (SMA) 12-4212. Rockville, MD, Substance Abuse and Mental Health Services Administration, 1999

National Center on Addiction and Substance Abuse at Columbia University: Wasting the Best and the Brightest: Substance Abuse at America's Colleges and Universities. New York, The National Center on Addiction and Substance Abuse at Columbia University, March 2007. Available at: http://www.centeronaddiction.org/download/file/fid/1197. Accessed July 21, 2017.

U.S. Department of Health and Human Services, Office of the Surgeon General: Facing Addiction in America: The Surgeon General's Report on Alcohol, Drugs, and Health. Washington, DC, U.S. Department of Health and Human Services, 2016

References

Center for Behavioral Health Statistics and Quality: Behavioral Health Trends in the United States: Results From the 2014 National Survey on Drug Use and Health. HHS Publ No SMA 15-4927, NSDUH Series H-50. Rockville, MD, Substance Abuse and Mental Health Services Administration, 2015. Available at: https://www.samhsa.gov/data/sites/default/files/NSDUH-FRR1-2014/NSDUH-FRR1-2014.pdf. Accessed July 21, 2017.

Center for Substance Abuse Treatment: Enhancing Motivation for Change in Substance Abuse Treatment. Treatment Improvement Protocol (TIP) Series, No 35, HHS Publ No (SMA) 12-4212. Rockville, MD, Substance Abuse and Mental Health Services Administration, 1999

Han B, Hedden SL, Lipari R, et al: NSDUH Data Review. Receipt of Services for Behavioral Health Problems: Results from the 2014 National Survey on Drug Use and Health. Rockville, MD, Substance Abuse and Mental Health Services Administration, 2015. Available at: http://www.samhsa.gov/data/sites/default/files/NSDUH-DR-FRR3-2014/NSDUH-DR-FRR3-2014/NSDUH-DR-FRR3-2014.htm. Accessed July 21, 2017.

Johnston LD, O'Malley PM, Bachman JG, et al: Monitoring the Future National Survey Results on Drug Use, 1975–2015: Vol. 2, College Students and Adults Ages 19–55. Ann Arbor, MI, Institute for Social Research, University of Michigan, 2016. Available at: http://monitoringthefuture.org/pubs/monographs/mtf-vol2_2015.pdf. Accessed July 21, 2017.

Larimer ME, Cronce JM, Lee CM, Kilmer JR: Brief intervention in college settings. Alcohol Res Health 28(2): 98–104, 2004. Available at: https://pubs.niaaa.nih.gov/publications/arh28-2/94-104.pdf. Accessed July 21, 2017.

Mee-Lee D, Schulman GD: The ASAM criteria and matching patients to treatment, in The ASAM Principles of Addiction Medicine, 5th Edition. Edited by Ries R, Miller SC, Saitz R, Fiellin DA. Philadelphia, PA, Wolters Kluwer, 2014, p 428–441

Monti PM, Tevyaw TO, Borsari B: Drinking among young adults: screening, brief intervention, and outcome. Alcohol Res Health 28(4):236–244, 2004–2005. Available at: https://pubs.niaaa.nih.gov/publications/arh284/236-244.pdf. Accessed July 21, 2017.

National Center on Addiction and Substance Abuse at Columbia University: Wasting the Best and the Brightest: Substance Abuse at America's Colleges and Universities. New York, National Center on Addiction and Substance Abuse at Columbia University, March 2007. Available at: http://www.centeronaddiction.org/download/file/fid/1197. Accessed July 21, 2017.

Nelson TF, Weitzman ER, Wechsler H: The effect of a campus-community environmental alcohol prevention initiative on student drinking and driving: results from the "a matter of degree" program evaluation. Traffic Inj Prev 6(4):323–330, 2005 16266941

Pacific Southwest ATTC: SBIRT Curriculum [Powerpoint slides], 2012. Available at: http://attcnetwork.org/resources/resource.aspx?prodID=1046&rcID=21&regionalcenter=*&producttype=*&keywords=sbirt. Accessed on January 24, 2018.

Saltz RF, Paschall MJ, McGaffigan RP, Nygaard PMO: Alcohol risk management in college settings: the safer California universities randomized trial. Am J Prev Med 39(6):491–499, 2010 21084068

SAMHSA-HRSA Center for Integrated Health Solutions: Motivational Interviewing. n.d. Available at: http://www.integration.samhsa.gov/clinical-practice/motivational-interviewing. Accessed on July 21, 2017.

Saunders JB, Aasland OG, Babor TF, et al: Development of the Alcohol Use Disorders Test (AUDIT): WHO collaborative project on early detection of persons with harmful alcohol consumption–II. Addiction 88(6):791–804, 1993 8329970

Skinner HA: The Drug Abuse Screening Test. Addict Behav 7(4):363–371, 1982 7183189

Substance Abuse and Mental Health Services Administration: Systems-Level Implementation of Screening, Brief Intervention, and Referral to Treatment. Technical Assistance Publication (TAP) Series 33, HHS Publ No (SMA) 13-4741. Rockville, MD, Substance Abuse and Mental Health Services Administration, 2013

U.S. Department of Health and Human Services, Office of the Surgeon General: Facing Addiction in America: The Surgeon General's Report on Alcohol, Drugs, and Health. Washington, DC, U.S. Department of Health and Human Services, 2016. Available at: https://addiction.surgeongeneral.gov. Accessed July 21, 2017.

Wechsler H, Lee JE, Kuo M, Lee H: College binge drinking in the 1990s: a continuing problem: results of the Harvard School of Public Health 1999 College Alcohol Study. J Am Coll Health 48(5):199–210, 2000 10778020

WHO ASSIST Working Group: The Alcohol, Smoking and Substance Involvement Screening Test (ASSIST): development, reliability and feasibility. Addiction 97(9):1183–1194, 2002 12199834

Young MM, Stevens A, Galipeau J, et al: Effectiveness of brief interventions as part of the Screening, Brief Intervention and Referral to Treatment (SBIRT) model for reducing the nonmedical use of psychoactive substances: a systematic review. Syst Rev 3(1):50, 2014 24887418

CHAPTER 15

Eating Disorders and Body Image Concerns

Danielle Colborn, Ph.D.
Athena Robinson, Ph.D.

EATING disorders (EDs) and body image concerns are becoming increasingly prevalent on college campuses. The corresponding public health impact is profound because EDs have negative repercussions on students' mental, physical, social, and academic functioning, as well as an impact on the campus community. In general, students without symptomatic attitudes and disordered eating behaviors have more positive self-concept and report less psychological distress than students with such concerns. In this chapter, we provide background on EDs and poor body image and their prevalence on university campuses, draw attention to often underserved groups that experience EDs, describe treatment options including stepped-care approaches, and present guidelines for coordinating ED care on university campuses.

Types of Eating Disorders

There are four main types of EDs described in DSM-5 (American Psychiatric Association 2013) that may manifest among university students. *Anorexia nervosa* (AN) is characterized by restriction of intake leading to excessively low body weight; intense fear of gaining weight; and a distorted view of one's body shape or failure to recognize the seriousness of one's low weight. *Bulimia nervosa* (BN) is characterized by recurrent episodes of binge eating; compensatory behaviors such as purging or excessive exercise; and an overvaluation of one's shape and weight. *Binge-eating disorder* (BED) is characterized by binge-eating episodes—that is, a loss of control over eating while consuming a large quantity of food in a relatively short time period (<2 hours) without compensatory behaviors. Finally, *other specified feeding or eating disorder* (OSFED) may refer to subclinical presentations of the above disorders or to a combination of symptoms that do not meet criteria for the above disorders but that represent an individual's struggles with eating and with shape and weight concerns that interfere with psychological and physical well-being.

Manifestation of Eating Disorders in University Students

PREVALENCE OF EATING DISORDERS ON COLLEGE CAMPUSES

Prevalence of EDs is higher among college students than among other groups. Among college students, ED prevalence rates range from 8% to 32% (Eisenberg et al. 2011; White et al. 2011), and subclinical syndrome rates range from 34% to 67% (Fitzsimmons-Craft et al. 2012). These rates are notably higher than the estimated ED prevalence rate of 2.7% among students ages 13–18 years (Merikangas et al. 2010) and the lifetime prevalence rates for the general population (AN: 0.3% for men, 0.9% for women; BN: 0.5% for men, 1.5% for women; BED: 2.0% for men, 3.5% for women).

Not only are point and lifetime prevalence rates of EDs higher among the college population, but such rates are increasing over time. Over a 13-year period, ED prevalence rates increased from 23% to 32% in female college students and from 7.9% to 25% in male college students (White et al. 2011).

PREVALENCE OF BODY DISSATISFACTION IN COLLEGE SETTINGS

Research over the past several decades has consistently demonstrated that college students have high rates of body image disturbance and body dissatisfaction. Female college students expressed a desire to lose weight and become thinner at a rate of approximately 80%, and reported an increase in body image dissatisfaction with the transition to college (Vohs et al. 2001). Approximately 90% of female college students reported preoccupation with a desire to be thinner (Nelson et al. 1999).

PREVALENCE OF DIETING

Dieting, prevalent across college campuses, is a behavior that may later develop into problematic eating behaviors. A notable portion of college students report that they diet "often" or "always," and 25% of college-age women report bingeing and purging as a method of weight management (Renfrew Center Foundation for Eating Disorders 2003). Although some students who diet will not develop pathological eating, approximately 35% of "normal" dieters ultimately progress to problematic eating, and 20%–30% of this latter group progress to partial or full-syndrome EDs (Shisslak et al. 1995). Such studies highlight that college students are, indeed, often preoccupied with shape, weight, thinness, and dieting—behaviors that research has demonstrated can increase risk for developing EDs.

COLLEGE YOUTH AS A VULNERABLE GROUP

Because the literature highlights the increasing prevalence of disordered eating, body image dissatisfaction, and full-syndrome EDs among college students, there is a need for further investigation into potential contributory factors and correlates. For starters, age in and of itself is correlated with ED onset. Full-syndrome EDs often have an onset between ages 18 and 21 years, the ages at which many youth are attending college. Further, college is a time of major transition in the life of young adults, a time when existing problems may be amplified or exacerbated. For first-year college students, there is a significant change in their immediate living environment, which includes their eating environment. Dining in cafeterias that serve unlimited quantities and a high variety of foods, in combination with the student's increased independence, heightened stress, and more complex social dynamics, can easily lead to difficulties with regulation of eating. These changes during this life and age period likely contribute to an increase in the onset of EDs, in particular BN, BED, and OSFED. Also, a heightened body image culture on college campuses may correlate with ED onset. Internalization of the thin ideal standard of female beauty has been associated with increased body dissatisfaction, which may increase dietary restraint and negative affect, both of which can increase risk for ED behaviors.

UNDERSERVED GROUPS

There has long been a myth that EDs affect a narrow range of sufferers, namely, affluent, white, heterosexual women. Increasingly, data show that EDs do not discriminate and do affect a wide range of people across racial, ethnic, and socioeconomic backgrounds, as well as varying gender identities and sexual orientations. We encourage clinicians working with university populations to be sensitive to signs of disordered eating across a wide variety of student groups.

Male Students

Data suggest that eating problems may be more prevalent among male college students than previously estimated. Although previous data suggested a 10:1 female-to-male ratio of ED, more recent findings indicate that the rate for males is much higher, specifically for males on college campuses, where the female-to-male ratio may be 3:1 (Eisenberg et al. 2011). While symptoms of AN have been found among 20% of female college students, AN symptoms have also been found among 10% of the male students, and 59% of male students endorse preoccupation with the thought of fat on their bodies (Nelson et al. 1999). Also concerning is that male individuals are less likely than female individuals to seek treatment because of shame about having what has traditionally been considered a woman's disease, and they may not be adequately screened on measures that have historically been developed for women; these issues make access to treatment a concern. Additionally, male individuals present with different body image concerns when compared with female individuals. Whereas female individuals tend to focus on being thin and smaller overall, male individuals tend to focus on body composition and the desire for a more muscular and lean appearance, and therefore they may overuse protein supplements or take steroids in addition to restricting their food intake and/or exercising excessively. It is important that clinicians are attentive to these symptoms in male clients and aware of the unique challenges facing men with EDs.

LGBTQ Students

Lesbian, gay, bisexual, transgender, and queer/questioning (LGBTQ) students are also affected by EDs. Gay men are at greater risk of developing EDs than lesbian women; however, individuals at all points along the gender identity and sexual orientation spectra can develop EDs (McClain and Peebles 2016). There is also some indication that transgender youth may be at higher risk for developing EDs compared with the general population (McClain and Peebles 2016). The reasons for these relationships are not entirely clear, but it is likely that social pressures and media influences at the very least play a role.

Ethnic and Minority Students

Although a review of the literature suggests that AN is less common among African Americans, EDs do have the potential to affect all persons regardless of racial or ethnic background. Of note, among ethnic minorities, rates of binge eating are higher than other forms of disordered eating. Also, the rates of EDs among Latina women appear to be rising. In addition, non-white adolescent males appear to be affected by EDs and ED behaviors at a greater rate than the general population (Croll et al. 2002). Despite these concerning trends, ethnic minorities are underrepresented in ED treatment: compared with white individuals, ethnic minorities are less likely to seek treatment for EDs, to be diagnosed with EDs, and to be referred for specialty ED treatment (Sinha and Warfa 2013).

Athletes

ED behaviors and attitudes are prevalent among collegiate athletes, who may be at greater risk for developing full-syndrome EDs than college students who are not athletes. Among female collegiate athletes, the point prevalence of meeting ED criteria was 7%, while 35% were at risk for AN and 38% were at risk for BN (Sundgot-Borgen and Torstveit 2004). Although male collegiate athletes reported experiencing relatively less body weight–related pressure than their female counterparts, about 12% endorsed binge eating; 9.5% were at risk for AN and 38% were at risk for BN (Petrie et al. 2007). Our focus group research with male and female Stanford athletes (12 sports represented) found that 86% and 75% of participants stated that disordered eating and body image concerns, respectively, were a problem in their sport, and 40% reported witnessing water abuse in their sport for weight control. Indeed, even athletes with subclinical EDs typically experience many of the same associated psychological, physical, and behavioral problems found among athletes with diagnostic-level symptoms. Poor body image appears to influence patterns of disordered eating in athletes. Indeed, poor body image and EDs have a multitude of significant negative effects on male and female athletes on the individual (e.g., mental and physical health, performance), team (i.e., teammates, coach), and campus community levels.

Graduate Students

Compared with undergraduate students, graduate students may have different access to levels of care and health-related resources. Variables such as age, often making graduate students independent adults with less parental support, and limited financial resources may restrict their health care options. Graduate students may also be less likely to utilize university health care options or to participate in campus activities, and therefore they may fly under the radar of university screening measures. However, graduate students, compared with younger students, may make up a significant portion of the ED cases seen on campuses and are more likely to have chronic ED symptoms.

Summary

Clinicians working in university settings are encouraged to be sensitive to the signs and symptoms of EDs in underserved groups and to be attuned to their own bias that may lead them to overlook EDs in these groups. Universities would do well to develop outreach, screening, and intervention tools that target all students at risk of EDs, across diverse groups.

Treatment for Eating Disorders and Stepped-Care Approach

University students with eating difficulties may present with varying levels of treatment need. However, all students with EDs require specialized treatment by trained clinicians and programs specifically targeted at EDs. In addition, ED treatment almost always requires multidisciplinary care involving clinicians from mental health, medical care, and nutritional support. We recommend that universities take a stepped-care approach for students, involving appropriate screening, prevention programs, guided self-help, and treatment as indicated.

TREATMENT-SEEKING BEHAVIORS AND SCREENING

Unfortunately, the majority of college students with disordered eating doubt that their concerns warrant intervention, and thus they do not pursue treatment. Given the increased independence of college students and their tendency to avoid seeking treatment, universities would be advised to implement regular screening processes across student bodies to identify potential students in need. Fortunately, a number of accessible and validated screens are available, or universities may choose to develop their own. Screens should be readily accessible and ideally administered as part of a standard, comprehensive, annual health screen. Such screens will increase the likelihood of detecting students in need and triaging them accordingly. For example, the SCOFF Questionnaire (Morgan et al. 2000), while not diagnostic, is brief, well validated, and easy to administer.

Once students in need have been identified, connecting them with appropriate treatment resources is essential. EDs are complex illnesses that require specialized treatment by trained clinicians, and many university counseling centers may not be fully equipped to treat full-syndrome EDs. Thus, knowing when and where to refer out is an essential component of supporting students struggling with eating and weight issues.

PREVENTION AND GUIDED SELF-HELP

Given the high prevalence of full-syndrome EDs and disordered eating symptoms among college students, most college counseling centers are not equipped to fully address and mitigate the demand for traditional forms of interventions. Hence, effective implementation of prevention and guided self-help programs can help to meet a large clinical need while potentially reducing burden on college counseling centers.

Prevention programs can be both universal (aimed at both the general student population and students at high risk of developing EDs) and indicated (geared toward students with subclinical ED symptoms at risk of developing full-syndrome EDs). The Body Project and Reflections Body Image Program are both brief (i.e., fewer than four sessions), in-person, peer-led universal prevention programs that have been shown to reduce ED symptoms and improve body image among college students (Stice et al. 2007). Online prevention programs have also been found effective, the most frequently used being Student Bodies, an eight-session, Internet-based, guided self-help program aimed specifically at women with elevated concerns about shape and weight. Numerous studies have demonstrated the effectiveness of Student Bodies in decreasing shape and weight concerns and preventing the onset of EDs in high-risk groups (Stice et al. 2007). We recommend that universities consider implementing prevention programs such as Student Bodies. Those students who do not improve or whose symptoms worsen can then be referred for traditional forms of clinical treatment in the student counseling center or off campus.

OUTPATIENT CLINICAL TREATMENT

Anorexia Nervosa

As of this writing, there are no empirically validated treatments for adults with AN. The most effective treatment intervention for adolescent AN is family-based therapy (FBT), an intervention that puts parents in charge of managing re-feeding until the young person is able to take on more independence. Obviously, college students may not be in a position to have parents provide full support around eating, because they are typically not living at home and are in a different place developmentally compared with younger adolescents. However, given the medical severity of AN, parental involvement is often indicated for university students, and even when afar, parents can be a great source of support for their child. For example, assuming consent and collaboration of the student, parents can check in regularly with their child, collaboratively create meal plans, and put systems in place for accountability around eating such as text messages or photos at meal times.

Ego-oriented individual therapy, also known as adolescent-focused psychotherapy is effective with young people with AN, and there is reason to believe it could be effective when treating adults for whom family involvement may be limited or not indicated. Ego-oriented individual therapy has its roots in self psychology and focuses on building ego strength and identifying and tolerating emotions, thus reducing the need to rely on AN for overcontrol of affective states.

Finally, cognitive-behavioral therapy (CBT), has shown mixed results when used for the treatment of AN. Many interventions for adults with AN use an integrative mix of CBT skills, interpersonal process, and emphasis on nutritional rehabilitation and increased cognitive flexibility.

Bulimia Nervosa

Unlike AN, BN has a number of strongly empirically validated treatments, with CBT being the most supported and often considered the "gold standard" of treatment for BN. CBT focuses on understanding the cycle of restriction, bingeing, and compensatory behaviors in which patients are caught; development of strategies to promote regulation of eating and reduction of BN behaviors; and use of cognitive restructuring tools to address the relationship between thoughts, feelings, and behaviors associated with BN.

Interpersonal psychotherapy (IPT) is a focused, time-limited treatment that specifically addresses interpersonal problem(s) associated with the onset and/or maintenance of the ED. IPT is an effective treatment for BN. Indeed, IPT and CBT have yielded comparable long-term outcomes. Interestingly, patients in CBT demonstrated higher rates of abstinence from binge eating and lower rates of purging in the shorter-term; however, by follow-up, CBT and IPT patients' behaviors were equivalent (Agras et al. 2000). Despite the relatively slower symptom reduction response rates, IPT patients rated their treatment as more suitable and expected greater success than did CBT patients. IPT is currently recommended as the alternative to CBT for BN, but it has been suggested that therapists inform patients of the slower response time for improvements compared with CBT.

Dialectical behavior therapy (DBT) is a promising intervention that has been shown to be effective in the treatment of BN. DBT integrates Western behavioral therapy with Eastern mindfulness concepts and emphasizes the duality of radical acceptance of oneself at the present moment while also desiring change. DBT may be particularly helpful for individuals with BN who have not responded to standard CBT protocols or for those who have a history of trauma or substance abuse, because DBT is also indicated in the treatment of these conditions.

Binge-Eating Disorder

Similar to BN, BED appears to respond well to CBT, IPT, and DBT, although it should be stressed that none of these psychotherapy interventions appear to lead to weight loss. Psychopharmacological interventions also may be helpful in the treatment of BED.

Other Specified Feeding or Eating Disorders

Because OSFEDs can manifest quite differently, clinicians need to use their best clinical judgment when selecting the appropriate intervention for individual patients. It follows reason that OSFED presentations that appear to be subclinical representations of other EDs would benefit from the treatment indicated for that condition. In general, a combination of focus on nutrition and regulation of food intake, tools to regulate emotions and challenge cognitive distortions, and addressing relapse prevention appear to be indicated.

NOVEL TREATMENTS

A number of developing psychotherapeutic interventions show promise for their use with college-age ED patients. Cognitive remediation therapy (CRT) is a treatment that targets neurocognitive processes with the goal of improving metacognition (how one thinks about one's thinking), cognitive flexibility, and global processing (ability to see the big picture). CRT has shown promise in the treatment of AN, particularly in reducing attrition rates, improving outcomes of concurrent treatments, and improving set-shifting ability (Dahlgren and Rø 2014).

Motivational interviewing is a technique often used in conjunction with other therapies, particularly at the beginning of treatment, to enhance an individual's willingness to participate. In motivational interviewing, the therapist seeks to reduce resistance to treatment by taking the onus of emphasizing and validating reasons for the patient not to engage, thus freeing the patient to explore reasons that treatment may benefit them. Motivational interviewing has been found useful in the treatment of EDs, particularly in regard to enhancing readiness to change.

Finally, acceptance and commitment therapy, an intervention that stresses acceptance of one's thoughts and emotions while emphasizing personal values as motivators of behavior change, has been found useful in the treatment of EDs, particularly in reducing ED symptoms and decreasing likelihood of rehospitalization for ED patients requiring inpatient treatment.

HIGHER LEVELS OF CARE

We always recommend placing students in the lowest level of care that maximizes their recovery and well-being. However, sometimes—despite the best efforts of students and university personnel—individuals struggling with EDs are not able to maintain their health on an outpatient basis and need to be referred to a higher level of care. This may require that a student take a leave of absence from school until the student's health has improved and clinicians are confident that the individual can be maintained on an outpatient basis. The decision to suspend academic goals is a serious one and should involve collaboration between the student, relevant university staff, and appropriate family members.

Medical Hospitalization

An individual who becomes medically compromised because of ED behaviors may require hospitalization at a medical facility specifically designed to treat and care for EDs. A variety of issues such as excessively low body weight (<75% of the median), bradycardia (heart rate <50 BPM during waking hours), hypotension (blood pressure <90/60 during waking hours), orthostatic heart rate changes (change of >20 points in heart rate or blood pressure from lying to standing), or electrolyte abnormalities may lead physicians to recommend inpatient admission until the individual has been stabilized. Medical hospitalization due to ED complications constitutes a medical emergency, and academic institutions are required to coordinate with students requiring this level of intervention. Students may be able to return to outpatient treatment and academic activities once they are discharged, although this is always at the recommendations of their health care team.

Intensive Outpatient Programs and Partial Hospitalization Programs

Intensive outpatient programs typically involve attending a treatment center four to seven times per week for 3–5 hours per day. During this time, patients participate in individual, group, and nutritional therapy and are able to receive in-the-moment support for things like mealtime anxiety and ED cognitions. Partial hospitalization programs are similar to intensive outpatient programs, but typically, patients attend for a full day, having most, if not all, of their meals and snacks at the treatment center. Universities are encouraged to gather information on relevant treatment programs in their area and provide this information to students and families.

Residential Treatment

For students needing further support, residential treatment programs, where patients live for weeks to months at a time, may be indicated. These programs vary in their treatment orientation and philosophy but typically involve a combination of individual, group, and nutritional therapies. We recommend residential programs with strong discharge plans so that patients are transitioned carefully back to outpatient life. In some cases, a step-down approach may be indicated in which patients go from residential treatment, to partial hospitalization programs, to intensive outpatient programs, and then to outpatient care.

COORDINATION OF CARE ACROSS CAMPUS

Although there are high rates of ED onset among college students, universities are in a unique position to be a valuable resource to students in need. When universities are attentive to students' needs and implement early intervention strategies, they can identify and connect students to needed resources and thus decrease the potential impact of EDs on students' academic life. Coordination of care on campuses is most efficient when there is a clearly identified process for identifying students of concern and connecting them to appropriate options for support. It is recommended that universities have designated teams of staff whose purpose is to identify students of concern and coordinate their care. These teams ideally consist of medical, counseling, and dietetic staff members who can collaborate in how to best organize care for individual students. These teams are encouraged to collaborate with other campus personnel, such as resident assistants, resident deans, coaches, trainers, dining room staff, and recreational staff, because these individuals are often the first to have contact with or be in a place to identify students at risk of EDs. Figure 15–1 shows some of the common entities involved in ED treatment on university campuses.

It will likely be important to collaborate with broader campus and community entities, because college counseling centers are often not equipped to treat all patients with full-blown ED cases who present for treatment and because it is essential that individuals with EDs receive specialized treatment from individuals or groups trained specifically in the treatment of eating and weight concerns. Having community resources, whether individual therapists or treatment centers, will be important when outside referrals are indicated. Additionally, collaborating with these entities, or with university medical center staff who may have specialty training in EDs, to provide training and support to counseling center staff can extend the range of students with EDs that counseling centers are equipped to serve.

When working with students with EDs, it is often important to involve families, especially when working with younger students (i.e., first-year students). As discussed in this chapter's section on treatment, families are often an essential source of support for students struggling with EDs. Even though far away, parents are more invested in their child's well-being than any other care provider and can be an important part of treatment plan development. When involving parents in the care of adult children, clinicians must discuss confidentiality and its limits with the student. Students seeking care at university counseling centers should be informed at the outset about confidentiality and its limits. For the vast majority of cases, students must consent in writing prior to involving parents in their health treatment. Exceptions are those students who have become medically and/or psychologically compromised to the point that they are in grave danger; then involving caregivers may become a necessity regardless of the students' wishes. Even in these cases, we recommend that students be informed of the need to break confidentiality before parents are contacted.

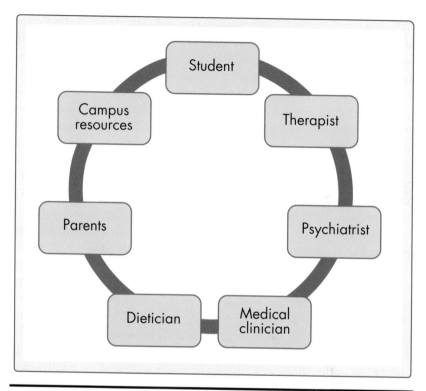

FIGURE 15–1. **Common entities involved in eating disorder treatment and monitoring on college campuses.**

Note. Therapist (e.g., psychologist, licensed clinical social worker) and psychiatrist may be someone on campus at counseling and psychological services, or in the department of psychiatry or psychology, or someone at an off-campus private practice. All clinicians involved in the treatment should have eating disorder specialty training. Campus resources may include student disability services (if the student needs to take a medical leave of absence or a reduced course load) and/or a social worker in counseling and psychological services.

Case Example

Emily, a college sophomore, self-identified as female, presented for treatment for her ED. Emily struggled with restriction during her first year at college and consequently lost approximately 15 pounds during that year, yielding her lifetime lowest weight (with a body mass index [BMI] of 17.6). During that first year, she met with a medical physician at her student health center who advised her that she was low weight and needed to gain weight immediately. Despite her low weight, Emily was not hospitalized because her vital signs (e.g., pulse, temperature, ortho-static heart rate changes) were stable enough to attempt refeeding on an outpatient basis. The physician referred Emily to a psychologist in the college's counseling and psychological services. After one meeting, Emily discontinued treatment prematurely. Nonetheless, Emily met with the original physician weekly for weight and vital sign checks and also with a dietician approximately five times. Emily was able to gain weight, and she focused on this especially while she was at home during the summer between her freshman and sophomore years. Unfortunately, binge eating developed during Emily's refeeding. By the time of her presentation to the clinic midway through her sophomore year, she had restored weight (BMI of 19.6) but was binge eating three to four times per week and had been doing so for approximately 6 months. In one binge episode, for example, Emily ate the following: dinner (1 large chicken and cheese enchilada with chips), 4 packets of cheese crackers (10 crackers in each), approximately 2 cups of chocolate chips, 1 large handful of M&Ms, 5 Red Vines, and 3 Reese's Peanut Butter Cups. Emily endorsed experiencing a sense of loss of control over these episodes and distress related to the binge eating. She also endorsed all of the associated features of binge eating, including eating much more rapidly than normal during the episode, eating until she was uncomfortably full, eating in the absence of physical hunger, eating alone because she was embarrassed by the amount of food she was eating, and guilt regarding the eating episodes. She was diagnosed with current BED and AN in full sustained remission.

Treatment consisted of CBT for BED. The CBT allowed initial therapeutic focus on Emily's current patterns of eating, with the goal being to normalize them (i.e., eating three meals and three snacks daily, not going too long without eating, etc.). Emily recorded her intake on food logs and over time was able to notably improve her daily pattern of eating. Per the CBT for BED protocol, therapy also focused on developing alternative activities to manage binge urges as well as psychoeducation about the nature and consequences of binge eating.

Emily was able to obtain abstinence from binge eating after 12 sessions of CBT for BED. Her abstinence was sustained for an additional 2 months, after which point treatment was terminated successfully.

Conclusion

An ED is a serious, complex illness that affects an individual's physical, mental, and emotional well-being. EDs affect university students at a higher rate compared with the general public, and these rates are increasing over time. Increased incidences of body image dissatisfaction and dieting behavior in the context of significant life transitions make university students particularly vulnerable to the development of EDs, and their tendency to avoid seeking treatment puts them at risk of serious health consequences. Although women continue to experience EDs at higher rates than men, ED rates in male individuals are increasing rapidly. Many groups that experience EDs, including men, ethnic minorities, and LGBTQ individuals, are underserved in regard to ED treatment. The implementation of appropriate screening measures will improve the likelihood of accurate detection of EDs among university students. Empirically validated prevention and guided self-help programs can address a significant clinical need while ameliorating much of the burden placed on university counseling centers. When further treatment is indicated, interventions should be evidence based and tailored to an individual's need and presentation. Coordination of care across the university will enhance the likelihood of accurate detection and appropriate referral for students in need.

KEY CONCEPTS

- Eating disorders are serious illnesses that impact physical and psychological well-being and are becoming increasingly prevalent on university campuses.

- Body image concerns and dieting behaviors are highly prevalent among university students and may lead to the development of problematic eating behaviors.

- The unique setting of college has the potential to exacerbate or contribute to disordered eating given the period of life transition, increased independence, and change in eating environment that most university students experience.

- Underserved groups on university campuses are often overlooked and do not receive appropriate screening or treatment for disordered eating.

- Specialized treatment for students presenting with eating disorders is always indicated. It is recommended that treatment be evidence based, and that referrals be provided to the local community and higher levels of care when indicated.

Recommendations for Psychiatrists, Psychologists, and Counselors

1. A stepped-care approach to the treatment of eating disorders includes appropriate screening, prevention programs, guided self-help, and treatment as indicated.
2. University staff should be sensitive to the signs and symptoms of eating disorders in underserved groups, such as male students, minority students, athletes, graduate students, and LGBTQ students and should use or develop outreach, screening, and intervention tools to target all students at risk of eating disorders.
3. Implementation of appropriate screening measures, such as the SCOFF Questionnaire (Morgan et al. 2000), will enhance detection of students in need and allow for triaging to appropriate services.
4. The implementation of evidence-based treatments for eating disorders will enhance the likelihood of positive outcomes.
5. The use of prevention and guided self-help programs for eating disorders can practically meet a large clinical need and potentially reduce the burden on university counseling centers.
6. Universities should have a clearly identified process for identifying students of concern that involves a multidisciplinary team to coordinate care across campus.
7. Universities should be aware of when to refer students to outside resources, including higher levels of care, and have a solid referral base established.
8. Families are often essential sources of support for students, and university staff are encouraged to be thoughtful about when and how to involve parents in the care of students with eating disorders.

Discussion Questions

1. Who are the key entities on your university campus that would ideally be involved in identifying and reaching out to students of concern for the development of eating disorders?
2. What are the signs and symptoms of eating disorders among students that you want your university to be on the lookout for?
3. What are the risks to your university of not adequately identifying students at risk of eating disorders and connecting them to appropriate resources?

4. How can your university organize and coordinate outreach to the underserved groups on your campus that are at risk of developing eating disorders?

Suggested Readings

Fairburn C: Overcoming Binge Eating: The Proven Program to Learn Why You Binge and How You Can Stop, 2nd Edition. New York, Guilford, 2013

Sandoz EK, Wilson KG, Du-Frene T: Acceptance and Commitment Therapy for Eating Disorders: A Process-Focused Guide to Treating Anorexia and Bulimia. Oakland, CA, New Harbinger, 2010

Schaefer J, Rutledge T: Life Without Ed: How One Woman Declared Independence From Her Eating Disorder and How You Can Too. New York, McGraw Hill Education Products, 2004

References

Agras WS, Walsh T, Fairburn CG, et al: A multicenter comparison of cognitive-behavioral therapy and interpersonal psychotherapy for bulimia nervosa. Arch Gen Psychiatry 57(5):459–466, 2000 10807486

American Psychiatric Association: Diagnostic and Statistical Manual of Mental Disorders, 5th Edition. Arlington, VA, American Psychiatric Association, 2013

Croll J, Neumark-Sztainer D, Story M, Ireland M: Prevalence and risk and protective factors related to disordered eating behaviors among adolescents: relationship to gender and ethnicity. J Adolesc Health 31(2):166–175, 2002 12127387

Dahlgren CL, Rø O: A systemaic review of cognitive remediation therapy for anorexia nervosa—development, current state and implications for future research and clinical practice J Eat Disorder 2(1): 26, 2014 25254110

Eisenberg D, Nicklett EJ, Roeder K, Kirz NE: Eating disorder symptoms among college students: prevalence, persistence, correlates, and treatment-seeking. J Am Coll Health 59(8):700–707, 2011 21950250

Fitzsimmons-Craft EE, Harney MB, Koehler LG, et al: Explaining the relation between thin ideal internalization and body dissatisfaction among college women: the roles of social comparison and body surveillance. Body Image 9(1):43–49, 2012 21992811

McClain Z, Peebles R: Body image and eating disorders among lesbian, gay, bisexual, and transgender youth. Pediatr Clin North Am 63(6):1079–1090, 2016 27865334

Merikangas KR, He JP, Burstein M, et al: Lifetime prevalence of mental disorders in U.S. adolescents: results from the National Comorbidity Survey Replication—Adolescent Supplement (NCS-A). J Am Acad Child Adolesc Psychiatry 49(10):980–989, 2010 20855043

Morgan JF, Reid F, Lacey JH: The SCOFF questionnaire. West J Med 172(3):164–165, 2000

Nelson WL, Hughes HM, Katz B, Searight HR: Anorexic eating attitudes and behaviors of male and female college students. Adolescence 34(135):621–633, 1999 10658869

Petrie TA, Greenleaf C, Carter JE, Reel JJ: Psychosocial correlates of disordered eating among male collegiate athletes. Journal of Clinical Sport Psychology 1:340–357, 2007

Renfrew Center Foundation for Eating Disorders: Eating Disorders 101 Guide: A Summary of Issues, Statistics, and Resources. Philadelphia, PA, The Renfrew Center Foundation for Eating Disorders, 2003

Shisslak CM, Crago M, Estes LS: The spectrum of eating disturbances. Int J Eat Disord 18(3):209–219, 1995 8556017

Sinha S, Warfa N: Treatment of eating disorders among ethnic minorities in western settings: a systematic review. Psychiatr Danub 25 (suppl 2):S295–S299 2013 23995197

Stice E, Shaw H, Marti CN: A meta-analytic review of eating disorder prevention programs: encouraging findings. Annu Rev Clin Psychol 3:207–231, 2007 17716054

Sundgot-Borgen J, Torstveit MK: Prevalence of eating disorders in elite athletes is higher than in the general population. Clin J Sport Med 14(1):25–32, 2004 14712163

Vohs KD, Heatherton TF, Herrin M: Disordered eating and the transition to college: a prospective study. Int J Eat Disord 29(3):280–288, 2001 11262506

White S, Reynolds-Malear JB, Cordero E: Disordered eating and the use of unhealthy weight control methods in college students: 1995, 2002, and 2008. Eat Disord 19(4):323–334, 2011 22352972

CHAPTER 16

Stress and Trauma

Ryan B. Matlow, Ph.D.
Victor G. Carrion, M.D.

ALTHOUGH experiences of intense stress and, in particular, trauma are not regularly addressed in our everyday discourse in working with students at the university level, such experiences are prevalent and ubiquitous. Stressors tax our resources and place a burden on our systems. Stress and trauma impact all of us. Ninety percent of all individuals will experience a traumatic event at some point in their lifetime (Kilpatrick et al. 2013). *Trauma* entails the experience of a direct or perceived uncontrollable threat to the safety or well-being of the individual in question, their loved ones, or their community. Specific categories of trauma experiences include noninterpersonal threat (e.g., injury, accident, illness, natural disaster) and interpersonal harm (e.g., physical or emotional abuse, physical and sexual assault, neglect, exposure to crime and violence). Trauma implies both an objective component and a subjective component. Even if a clinician may not consider a given event to be traumatic, if the individual found it to be traumatic or extremely threatening, the event is considered a trauma. Every one of us likely has experienced at least one traumatic event in our lives or cares about someone who has. The stress of traumatic experiences reverberates, having a ripple effect in various (and often unexpected) areas of our lives and in the lives of the individuals, communities, and systems around us.

Although not everyone exposed to trauma will develop a diagnosable psychological condition as a result of stresses and traumatic experiences, trauma affects everyone in one way or another. We may experience traumatic stress and/or changes in perspective or functioning that fall below the threshold required for diagnosis. We may be at increased risk for developing psychopathology or other stress-related disorders in the future. Or we may experience other physical or mental health difficulties indirectly related to the trauma experience—we now know that the prevalence and severity of major public health concerns (e.g., cancer, cardiovascular disease, autoimmune illness, suicide) increase with trauma exposure (Substance Abuse and Mental Health Services Administration 2014). Also, trauma impacts the manifestation of any psychiatric condition. For example, individuals with bipolar disorder cycle more rapidly when exposed to traumatic events (Post and Miklowitz 2010). Prevention of trauma and early efforts to intervene can counter the negative effects. Therefore, it is paramount that we consider and address trauma in our work at universities.

Considering Stress and Trauma When Working With University Students

For students, the university experience can be a time of vulnerability when it comes to dealing with stress and trauma. University students are required to function independently but are often still developing their skills in self-awareness, self-regulation (including emotion and cognitive regulation), and interpersonal effectiveness. For many students, the university experience entails a major step in emerging from the protective guidance and oversight of the home environment (family and community), making this a delicate transitional period. It is an important academic, social, and developmental period highlighted by increased independence and decision-making experience. Although development during the university experience provides new opportunities to learn and apply skills for managing stressors, these efforts require support, preparation, and guidance from the surrounding community. Given their newly increased level of independence and autonomy, university students often engage in developmentally appropriate behaviors involving individuation, exploration, experimentation, and risk taking. While important for personal development, these behaviors may leave students at increased risk for trauma exposure, whether due to accident or interpersonal violation. Additionally, it is important to remember that many forms of psychopathology (e.g., psychosis, mood disorder, personality disorder) typically emerge during the developmental stages that, for many, coincide with university attendance; as clinicians, we need to be sensitive to the stress an individual feels when receiving a mental health diagnosis and seek collaboration or consultation from individuals with experience in traumatology in order to sensitively manage potentially negative reactions.

In addition, distress from previous life traumas (e.g., those occurring earlier in childhood) may be exacerbated or may resurface during the university experience. The normal stressors of the university experience can place additional burden on individuals with histories of trauma and may elicit posttraumatic stress reactions that were previously dormant. With skills, supports, and guidance in place, university students have opportunities for healing through "corrective experiences" and attainment of self-confidence. It is expected and normal for trauma experiences to take on different meanings (and elicit different emotional and cognitive reactions) for individuals as they progress through stages of their life and development; the university experience marks one of the significant developmental stages during which individuals may experience a shift in their understanding and responses to previous traumatic events. In addition, some experiences associated with being a student at a university may trigger traumatic stress because they are reminders of past traumas. For example, being alone, feeling hungry or tired, feeling overwhelmed, and experiencing a loss of routine or change in daily structure are all experiences that are common for university students yet are also common elements of traumatic events. Awareness of these commonalities and triggers can be explicit and/or covert. With less conscious awareness, there is greater risk that one will respond to these triggers in an automatic way, without much thought or preparation. Gaining insight into the relevance of past experiences can help prevent or diminish maladaptive responses.

Finally, the increased risk for trauma exposure and posttraumatic stress is exacerbated by the loss or absence of multiple support resources and protective factors. As mentioned above, university students are commonly removed from the typical family, community, and social supports that have provided scaffolding and protection at earlier stages of development. As students enter into the university experience, there is commonly a loss of confidence and of the sense of safety, security, and stability that they felt in the home environment. Therefore, the process of going to university may, in itself, be experienced as intensely stressful or traumatic given the potential for the experience to be perceived as threatening to individual safety, security, and stability. In addition, given the loss of their previous structure and support, many responsible students may see this time as an opportunity to challenge their need for previous ongoing treatment and may experiment with stopping or reducing pharmacological and/or psychosocial interventions and therapies; although such decisions may be developmentally appropriate, it is important that university clinicians monitor potential risks and provide appropriate guidance.

Keeping in mind that 1) stress and trauma affect everybody and 2) university students may be at increased risk for trauma exposure and post-traumatic stress, it is important that we, as service professionals in higher education, be prepared to address these issues in our roles. Preparation involves awareness of the impact of trauma; intentional thought about how we will recognize and address student trauma experiences and reactions; and knowledge of the skills, practices, and resources that can be applied to support students experiencing traumatic stress.

Considerations for Special Student Groups

Although stress and trauma are ubiquitous, some student groups may experience disproportionately high rates of exposure to adversity and/ or increased risk for trauma-related distress. University clinicians should consider and be attuned to the needs of these special student groups, while also taking care to prevent making assumptions about trauma exposure that may serve as a source of stigma for students from such groups.

GENDER IDENTITY

Societal expectations to uphold traditional male versus female gender categories can be a source of stress for university students with nonconforming gender identities. Such students may have experienced victimization and stigma in the past and, in many cases, are likely to have experienced family or social conflict around gender identity; these past stressors (and the associated emotional and behavioral reactions) may surface or be triggered by course content, class discussions, and social interactions at the university. Unfortunately, in many universities (and in general public settings), students face multiple, continuous reminders that there is little, if any, space for acknowledgment of or acceptance of nonconforming gender identities (e.g., gender-specific bathrooms and dormitories). In addition, the university experience may be a time when students explore and expand their gender (and sexual) identity (see Chapter 26, "Lesbian, Gay, Bisexual, Transgender, and Queer/Questioning Students").

Clinicians should be sensitive to the stigma and adversity that students may face as they conduct natural and healthy exploration. It is important within the context of both clinical service and general everyday practice to cultivate physical and psychological spaces that allow individuals to express and explore their gender identity without judgment, that acknowledge the stresses associated with presenting a nonconforming gender, and that enhance each individual's sense of safety and security. In particular, peer support and ally groups provide communities of support that can serve as resources to mitigate the potential distress and trauma resulting from society's early stage of readiness to adopt and accept a flexible and fluid spectrum of gender identity.

IMMIGRATION STATUS

Student (and family) immigration status can serve as an additional source of stress at the university. Some immigrant students may have higher rates of previous trauma exposure, because reasons for leaving the home country may include exposure to traumatic events, processes of migration can be traumatic, and many immigrants settle in communities that experience disproportionately high rates of trauma and adversity. Students who have immigrated are also likely to be experiencing acculturative stresses that include conflicts related to integrating home and adopted cultures, experiencing discrimination, and developing language fluency. Similarly, separation from home cultures, traditions, and communities can serve as a source of distress, which can be exacerbated during the university experience, which often inherently entails additional separation from family and community. These stresses can be compounded with legal concerns related to legal status, immigration status, and threats of deportation (against the student or family members). In many cases, unstable or uncertain legal status can result in the experience of added pressure to perform well academically so as not to jeopardize the legal status.

In response, university clinicians and officials can adopt and proliferate policies that protect the rights of immigrant students and support the development of a safe, allied, and protective university community. Making sure that immigrant students are aware of their legal rights—and the legal steps they can take to advocate and protect themselves—also helps to bolster security and stability. Finally, immigrant students may need spaces to process past traumas, to process the stresses of acculturation and discrimination, and to process any anxieties or worries related to legal status, potentially with university mental health professionals or in peer support groups.

"HARD-TO-REACH" STUDENTS

Many students at the university do not readily access or engage with student social groups or campus health services. These groups and services can help to mitigate the negative impact of stress and trauma exposure during the university experience; therefore, students who do not access these resources may be at greater risk for experiencing traumatic stress. Such students may feel isolated in their experience of distress and may have difficulty initiating the social supports and relational engagement that is important for building a feeling of safety and stability.

University messaging, mental health campaigns, and psychoeducation delivery through wellness programming can help to deliver important information and resources to these "hard-to-reach" students. For example, general wellness programming for all students that includes instruction and practice of self-care and coping skills can help these students develop the resources to manage distress in their university experience. In addition, providing education and resources to dorm resident advisors, professors and teachers, and administrative staff (who will naturally have contact with all students) on the impact of stress and trauma is important so that these professionals can serve as additional supports and points of entry for students who do not typically access traditional services.

Impact of Trauma: Symptoms and Presentation

Traumatic stress can manifest in a variety of ways. Most classically, we refer to posttraumatic stress disorder (PTSD). PTSD requires exposure to a traumatic stressor (through direct experience or witnessing in person or through indirect exposure to the aversive details of trauma experienced by a loved one or by individuals serving in professional capacities), as well as the presence of each of four symptom clusters (American Psychiatric Association 2013): *Intrusion symptoms* involve the reexperiencing or replaying of aspects of the trauma in undesired (often uncontrollable) ways, such as through unwanted thoughts and memories, nightmares, flashbacks, unintentional reenactment, and prolonged distress or emotional reactivity following exposure to trauma reminders. *Avoidance symptoms* involve persistent, active efforts to avoid trauma-related stimuli, including thoughts, feelings, and external reminders (e.g., people, places, objects, situations). *Negative alterations in cognitions or mood* following the traumatic event include difficulty remembering features of the experience, negative (often distorted) beliefs about oneself or the world (e.g., "this happened to me because I am a bad person," "the world is a dangerous place"), negative emotions, persistent blame toward self or others, and loss of interest in or connection to significant activities or relationships. Finally, *marked alterations in physiological arousal* following the traumatic event include experiences of hypervigilance, exaggerated startle, sleep disturbance, concentration difficulty, and irritability. To meet criteria for PTSD, these symptoms must be present for at least 1 month and must cause regular interference and impairment in social, occupational, educational, or independent functioning.

Trauma experiences can be expressed through other forms of psychopathology or distress, in addition to PTSD. Symptoms of depression and anxiety often emerge, resurface, or become stronger following trauma exposure. Symptoms of other psychological disorders are often exacerbated by trauma exposure. In addition, the apparent presence of other psychological or developmental disorders can often be explained by trauma. For example, experiences of concentration, memory, or learning difficulties that may look like attention-deficit/hyperactivity disorder (ADHD) can be the result of trauma exposure. (In these cases, it is important to distinguish true neurodevelopmental ADHD symptoms from distraction or inattention due to anxiety, worry, or reexperiencing.) Also, trauma exposure occurring during the course of development (which is known to proceed through the mid-20s) can impact basic skills, abilities, and competencies (D'Andrea et al. 2012; Teicher and Samson 2016). Across development, individuals build skills in neurocognitive functioning (executive functioning, language, attention, and memory), regulatory functioning (including homeostatic, physiological, and emotional regulation), intrapersonal functioning (sense of self and independent functioning), and interpersonal functioning (relationships). However, trauma exposure during development diverts resources away from these competency and skill-building tasks and toward tasks of survival. In this way, developmental trajectories can be derailed, and individuals may experience lasting deficits in various developmental domains as a consequence of trauma exposure in childhood and adolescence. These impairments are not necessarily permanent, but considerable consistent practice and scaffolding may be required to build skills outside the typical developmental trajectory.

Addressing Student Trauma Experiences

It is important that we, as leaders and professionals in higher education, not only know the signs and symptoms of traumatic stress, but also be prepared to address trauma in the setting and context in which we are working. As mentioned in the description of PTSD above, avoidance is a core trauma symptom, and we often see avoidance playing out on the service professional and systems level as well as the student or client level. Clinicians sometimes hesitate to bring up traumatic experiences out of fear that the ensuing distress will be harmful for the client. However, in actuality, the opposite is true: the more we avoid talking about trauma, the stronger the related distress becomes (we often say that PTSD feeds on avoidance). Therefore, there is a need to "avoid avoidance" and to challenge ourselves to acknowledge, recognize, and address the impact of traumatic experiences on the students and clients with whom we interact. The experience of the emotions stemming from traumatic events (e.g., fear, anger, sadness) is therapeutic when we are able to tolerate the distress within a safe, supportive setting. Establishing a context of safety and support requires that we approach the topic of trauma carefully and sensitively and that we come prepared to address the distress that may naturally arise.

First, in addressing student trauma experiences, we need to recognize and normalize the range of responses to traumatic experiences. Not all trauma experiences result in distress, psychopathology, or impairment; therefore, it is important for us to reflect on whether a student's current functioning is negatively impacted by a trauma experience before delving deeply into a dialogue about trauma. In fact, the literature refers to "posttraumatic growth" as a potential response to trauma in which highly stressful or traumatic events result in positive change and personal growth (Tedeschi and Calhoun 2004). Nonetheless, it is also common and normal for students exposed to trauma to experience the posttraumatic stress and other psychological symptoms described previously, and individuals may experience a combination of both distress and growth in their responses to trauma. Trauma symptoms stem from a biological stress reaction. In many cases, acute stress symptoms after a recent trauma or threat will naturally resolve within 1–2 months, in which case our main role as clinicians is to ensure ongoing safety and to support the student in tolerating distress while their system adjusts and reacclimates to a safe environment. Symptoms persisting for 3 or more months following trauma exposure are indicative of an injury or insult to the typical stress response, likely warranting clinical attention and more in-depth processing. Regardless of trajectory, providing information and psychoeducation is paramount: helping students and clients to understand that their trauma-related symptoms are normal and expected, given exposure to adversity and traumatic life experiences, is one of the most powerful interventions we can make as mental health care professionals.

Second, as we enter into conversations with university students about trauma, we need to be prepared to actively participate and provide support within this interaction. One component of this preparation is the anticipation and acceptance of the fact that the conversation is likely to be stressful and difficult. As mentioned earlier, the theme of trauma elicits feelings of fear, anger, and sadness; addressing and processing trauma involve being able to tolerate the negative emotions connected with the trauma experience as they arise. As mental health professionals, we are in a key role to provide support, assistance, and scaffolding to help university students and clients tolerate their trauma-related distress. To do this, we must anticipate their distress, be attentive and watchful for when distress surfaces, and have a sense of how we will respond when distress arises in the interaction.

Third, when we ask about traumatic experiences and their impact, it is important to know what we are going to do if and when trauma and traumatic stress are present. We need to be ready to provide support and resources. One form of support is an exploration or offering of tools and practices for coping with distress. Helping individuals identify the supports and (internal and external) resources they can access when experiencing trauma-related distress helps empower them to tolerate and cope with the distress. We can also offer and introduce new skills and practices, such as mindfulness and relaxation skills, and we can help students and clients to develop healthy habits when it comes to exercise, diet, sleep, and hygiene. In addition, it is important to be familiar with trauma-focused counseling resources and/or treatment approaches in case further support is needed. Recommended treatment approaches are discussed in the following section, "Core Components of Psychological Intervention for Trauma."

Finally, in addressing student trauma experiences, we need to recognize and be aware of the impact of secondary traumatic stress and vicarious traumatization. As mental health care professionals, we also feel the distress affecting our traumatized students and clients, and it is not uncommon for clinicians to experience the same trauma symptoms (PTSD and otherwise) as our clients through a parallel process. Therefore, it is important to be on the lookout for signs of secondary stress and vicarious trauma in ourselves, which may include exhaustion, overinvolvement, hopelessness, anger, and cynicism, to name a few. In anticipating the expected impact of vicarious stress, we should also know how we plan to manage this stress; this entails accessing support and consultation from peers and supervisors and engaging in proper self-care. As we do with our students and clients, we must adopt an accepting approach toward our experiences of (secondary) traumatic stress, keeping in mind that we experience this stress because we are caring individuals who, in our efforts to provide support and healing, feel what others feel. This is an expected part of the work we do (and is not a sign of weakness).

Core Components of Psychological Intervention for Trauma

In addressing university student experiences of trauma and traumatic stress, clinicians should be familiar with recommended, evidence-based treatment approaches. Although numerous therapies have been identified as effective for addressing trauma and PTSD, readers are referred to the leading structured, trauma-focused intervention approaches for adults, including cognitive processing therapy (Resick et al. 2016) and prolonged exposure therapy (Foa et al. 2007). In addition, leading evidence-based, trauma-focused interventions for children and adolescents may be suitable for adaptation for transition-age youth in the university setting. These include trauma-focused cognitive-behavioral therapy (Cohen et al. 2016); cue-centered therapy (Carrion 2016); and attachment, self-regulation, and competency training (Blaustein and Kinniburgh 2010).

Although the specific details, activities, and theoretical approaches of the various interventions may differ, each of the listed treatments (and other effective treatments for traumatic stress) entails a set of core components that are essential for trauma treatment (Table 16–1). Some of these components are discussed in greater detail below.

ESTABLISHING A SENSE OF SAFETY AND SECURITY

To process and address traumatic stress, individuals must not feel threatened in their current context or situation; in other words, a safe

---

TABLE 16–1. Core components of interventions for stress and trauma

---

Trauma-focused assessment, including trauma history and trauma symptoms

Crisis intervention and stabilization: establishing a sense of safety and security

Psychoeducation about responses to stress and trauma: normalizing traumatic stress reactions

Skill development in the identification, expression, and regulation of distressing thoughts and feelings

Trauma processing through approach and exposure

Trauma experience integration: understanding and redefining the impact of stress and trauma on the individual's life and functioning

Building empowerment, optimism, and resilience

---

space is required. Although many individuals may experience ongoing threats or ongoing trauma in their lives, their sense of safety can be enhanced by developing safety plans and/or identifying resources that can be accessed in case of threat. In addition, the individuals must feel safety and trust in their relationship with their clinician. Trauma treatment is reliant on a positive, supportive relationship; most trauma experiences are interpersonal in nature and inherently involve a violation of trust or social norms. Therefore, the clinician must work with the student to establish trust, a sense of security, and a sense of control through an empathic, supportive relationship.

PSYCHOEDUCATION

As discussed in earlier sections, psychoeducation on the stress response, the impact of trauma, and expected reactions and symptoms is important for normalizing experiences of trauma and traumatic stress and for helping clients to understand the reasons behind their emotions, behaviors, and symptoms. It can be important to review prevalence rates of specific types of traumas (e.g., physical or sexual abuse) so individuals do not feel that they are alone in their experience. Psychoeducation is also important for instilling hope and optimism—for instance, by letting the client know that people can heal from trauma and that we as clinicians know how to work to make things better.

SKILL DEVELOPMENT

Traumatic stress, particularly when experienced in childhood or adolescence, often results in difficulties in identifying, expressing, and regulating trauma-related cognitions (thoughts) and emotions (feelings). Therefore, building skills in these areas is an important part of trauma intervention. As clinicians, we can help clients develop awareness of distressing thoughts and feelings and help them learn how these experiences are connected to their trauma experience and trauma reminders. We can also help them to identify and expand their skill set (or "toolbox") of practices for coping with distress; there are likely many coping practices or tools they have at hand (but are unaware of), and there are many coping, relaxation, and grounding practices that we can introduce and teach. An important aspect of skill development involves increasing clients' confidence in their own resources and helping them to feel empowered in their ability to tolerate and master the distressing trauma-related thoughts and feelings that have often come to dominate them. Development of emotion identification, expression, and regulation skills also provides an important foundation that sets the stage for further work in trauma processing.

APPROACH AND EXPOSURE

With an adequate mastery of coping skills, clients can begin to approach their trauma experience via exposure techniques. Exposure can take many forms (e.g., narrative storytelling, writing, imaginal exposure, in vivo exposure), but the essential elements are that the client combats avoidance, gains practice in using skills to tolerate distress, and learns new patterns of responding to trauma cues and trauma triggers. It is important to remember that the goal of exposure is not to reenact or reintroduce a traumatic experience but to help the client effectively engage with and process the thoughts, feelings, and formerly neutral trauma reminders or cues that are disrupting their everyday functioning. When coupled with effective application of coping skills, exposure techniques increase clients' sense of empowerment in dealing with their trauma.

TRAUMA EXPERIENCE INTEGRATION

Another useful intervention is to redefine the role of the trauma in the individual's life through the active processing of the trauma and its impact. Individuals with posttraumatic stress often experience fragmented or disorganized cognition and emotions related to their trauma(s), but the skills and exercises practiced in earlier stages of intervention allow a more coherent experience of trauma memories and a new perspective on the trauma experience. It is important to take time to reflect on these changes and to help facilitate the shifts in perspective and self-identity. Trauma integration can occur through narrative exposure, reframing of cognitive distortions or attributions, and future-oriented value and goal setting. This process can enable clients to move from seeing themselves as helpless victims to seeing themselves as empowered survivors. Through trauma experience integration, clients often experience a positive shift in their self-perception and identity development.

Case Example

Maria is a 19-year-old student who enters the university counseling center following a recommendation from the resident assistant in her dorm, who noticed that she has been increasingly withdrawn, isolated, and irritable. Maria reports that she began to notice changes in her mood when she began "pulling all-nighters" to handle a heavy academic load and slipping grades this past quarter. However, her difficulties got much worse after she was robbed one night following a concert in the city. She states that this experience brought back memories of her childhood when her family was threatened after their house was broken into; she recalls a difficult period in her childhood when her family lived in an unstable and violent neighborhood, and they spent many nights awake after hearing gunshots outside their home. Since her recent mugging, Maria has been having difficulty sleeping, finds herself feeling nervous and on edge, and is constantly watching her surroundings, especially at night. She also has found herself to be short-tempered, and Maria describes a recent specific incident in which she got into a heated argument with a classmate in her political science class, stating that she felt her emotions got "out of control" and that she said things she wishes she hadn't said.

After conducting this initial assessment, Maria's university therapist works to normalize Maria's difficulties by discussing common responses to stress and trauma, including the symptoms of negative mood, irritability, emotion dysregulation, and hypervigilance that Maria has endorsed. Maria's therapist also works to place Maria's current stresses in context and learns that Maria feels a great deal of pressure around her academic performance. She is the oldest sibling in an immigrant family and is the first person in her family to attend college. Maria wants to establish a successful career for herself so she can support her family and help to fulfill her parents' hopes for their family. She also worries about her parents' undocumented legal status and hopes that her academic success can be used as an argument in her parents' ongoing case for citizenship. After acknowledging the various stresses and pressures she is carrying, Maria states that she feels better knowing why she has been feeling so down and irritable.

Maria and her therapist explore the ways Maria has coped with stress and adversity in the past. Maria states that when she was at home as a child and young adult, her mother and her sisters would comfort one another when they were stressed or anxious; she misses having this close family support. Maria and her therapist set a goal for Maria to visit home more frequently and to have regular phone calls with her parents and sisters. In addition, they explore and practice ways Maria can cope with distress and anxiety in the moment through deep breathing, progressive muscle relaxation, and yoga. Maria especially uses these practices when walking on campus at night and in the dark—which, in working with her therapist, she identified as being a trauma trigger—and she makes plans to walk with friends at night to help increase her sense of safety. Over time, these activities and practices contribute to a gradual reduction in the frequency and severity of Maria's experience of nervousness, anxiety, irritability, and low mood.

Finally, Maria's therapist helps her to locate a university student group that is active in advocating and rallying for immigrants' rights. Maria starts to attend group meetings, makes friends with group members (many of whom are from immigrant families), and begins to participate in campus events and rallies. Maria enjoys her involvement with the student group and states that it helps her feel more connected with her community.

Conclusion

While the university experience may be a time of stress and potentially increased risk for many students, it is also a time of growth, opportunity, and redefinition. The importance of providing support for students in managing stress and trauma cannot be understated, and it is equally important to view the university experience as an opportune time to engage students and clients in acknowledging and addressing the impact that stress and trauma have had in their lives. The maturation, growth, and learning that naturally occur for students while at university may provide an optimal point of entry to help reshape students' perspectives and make new meaning of their trauma experience. To do this, we, as clinicians, must consider the stresses and traumas affecting students, recognize the signs of posttraumatic stress, and be prepared to provide the trauma-focused support and resources that students need and deserve. With these components in place, we will contribute to a university experience that promotes healing, resilience, and growth for students.

KEY CONCEPTS

- Stress and trauma affect the lives of all university students, yet these issues are not commonly addressed in the university setting. Supporting university students requires attention to the stressors and traumas impacting their development and functioning.

- As clinicians, we can help students address stress and trauma by providing information and education, providing safe and supportive spaces, promoting skill building in stress management, and providing opportunities for positive identity development.

- Universities should offer resources that facilitate the identification of stressors and trauma, as well as the prevention and treatment of trauma-related distress—for example, hotlines, support groups, counseling services, or university ambassadors or ombudspersons specifically focused on addressing stress and trauma.

Recommendations for Psychiatrists, Psychologists, and Counselors

1. Stress and trauma affect us all and are part of the human experience. Clinicians can help to normalize the wide range of reactions to stress and trauma by providing information and psychoeducation, as well as opportunities for skill development and practice.

2. A common reaction to stress and trauma (in individuals, communities, and systems) is avoidance of trauma-related content and trauma reminders. Clinicians can help counter avoidance by acknowledging the presence of stress and trauma and by helping students and communities approach trauma content in a structured and supported way.

3. Clinicians should be aware that for many students, the university experience can be a time of vulnerability, involving increased independence at a stage when self-regulation and interpersonal skills are still developing. This can leave some students at risk for trauma-related distress (stemming from previous traumatic experiences or from new experiences of trauma exposure).

4. Student stress and general functioning is contextualized by previous life experiences and adversity. Clinicians should make efforts to consider the context for challenges experienced and observed at the university.

5. Building and promoting skills and practices for emotion identification and emotion regulation (e.g., coping, mindfulness, relaxation skills) are important for helping students feel supported in addressing reactions to stress and trauma.

6. Attending to student stress and trauma impacts clinicians. It is important for clinicians to recognize, accept, and process their own secondary stress reactions to better serve students.

Discussion Questions

1. What are ways that traumatic stress impacts the lives and performance of university students with whom you work? Where and how does traumatic stress come up in your interactions with students?

2. How do you see students dealing with and responding to traumatic stress in their lives? In what ways might you be able to support them in building their skills for addressing trauma?

3. How can you (in your role) facilitate the feeling of belonging and promote dialogue and conversation about the prevalence and impact of trauma to increase awareness and responsiveness to these issues?

4. How does student traumatic stress impact your functioning in your role at the university and in your personal life? How do you take care of yourself in dealing with secondary traumatic stress?

Suggested Readings

Foa EB, Keane TM, Friedman MJ, Cohen JA (Eds.): Effective Treatments for PTSD: Practical Guidelines From the International Society for Traumatic Stress Studies, 2nd Edition. New York, Guilford, 2008

van der Kolk B: The Body Keeps the Score: Brain, Mind, and Body in the Healing of Trauma. New York, Penguin, 2014

van Dernoot Lipsky L: Trauma Stewardship: An Everyday Guide to Caring for Self While Caring for Others. Oakland, CA, Berrett-Koehler Publishers, 2009

References

American Psychiatric Association: Diagnostic and Statistical Manual of Mental Disorders, 5th Edition. Arlington, VA, American Psychiatric Association, 2013

Blaustein ME, Kinniburgh KM: Traumatic Stress in Children and Adolescents: How to Foster Resilience Through Attachment, Self-Regulation, and Competency. New York, Guilford, 2010

Carrion VG: Cue-Centered Therapy for Youth Experiencing Posttraumatic Stress Symptoms: A Structured, Multimodal Intervention. New York, Oxford University Press, 2016

Cohen JA, Mannarino AP, Deblinger E: Trauma-Focused CBT for Children and Adolescents: Treatment Applications. New York, Guilford, 2016

D'Andrea W, Ford J, Stolbach B, et al: Understanding interpersonal trauma in children: why we need a developmentally appropriate trauma diagnosis. Am J Orthopsychiatry 82(2):187–200, 2012 22506521

Foa EB, Hembree EA, Rothbaum BO: Prolonged Exposure Therapy for PTSD: Emotional Processing of Traumatic Experiences: Therapist Guide. New York, Oxford University Press, 2007

Kilpatrick DG, Resnick HS, Milanak ME, et al: National estimates of exposure to traumatic events and PTSD prevalence using DSM-IV and DSM-5 criteria. J Trauma Stress 26(5):537–547, 2013 24151000

Post RM, Miklowitz DJ: The role of stress in the onset, course, and progression of bipolar illness and its comorbidities: implications for therapeutics, in Understanding Bipolar Disorder: A Developmental Psychopathology Perspective. Edited by Miklowitz DM, Cicchetti D. New York, Guilford, 2010, pp 370–413

Resick PA, Monson CM, Chard KM: Cognitive Processing Therapy for PTSD: A Comprehensive Manual. New York, Guilford, 2016

Substance Abuse and Mental Health Services Administration: SAMHSA's Concept of Trauma and Guidance for a Trauma-Informed Approach. Rockville, MD, Substance Abuse and Mental Health Services Administration, 2014

Tedeschi RG, Calhoun LG: Posttraumatic growth: conceptual foundations and empirical evidence. Psychol Inq 15:1–18, 2004

Teicher MH, Samson JA: Annual Research Review: Enduring neurobiological effects of childhood abuse and neglect. J Child Psychol Psychiatry 57(3):241–266, 2016 26831814

CHAPTER 17

Sleep Disorders

Shannon S. Sullivan, M.D.

FOR many adolescents and young adults, meeting the heightened academic, athletic, work-study employment, and social challenges and opportunities of the university environment can put the squeeze on healthy sleep. Such demands on time, when encountered by students who may be quite new to self-directed time management without the supports of a more structured home environment, may render students vulnerable to serious sleep loss and to potential impacts on studies, health, and well-being. Therefore, consideration of sleep disorders must start with an assessment of sleep sufficiency—that is, whether adequate sleep times are available to, and prioritized by, the student.

While young adults ages 18–25 are thought to require 7–9 hours of sleep per day, individuals at the younger end of this age group may require closer to 8–10 hours (Hirshkowitz et al. 2015). It is probable that many undergraduates arrive on campus already sleep deprived: recent data from the Centers for Disease Control and Prevention (CDC) indicate that 68.4% of high school students received 7 hours or less per night (Wheaton et al. 2016), and 75% of 17-year-olds report that they habitually do not get enough sleep (Keyes et al. 2015). Lack of knowledge about the importance of sleep and best habits may lead to further sacrifice of sleep when students are away from home. Considering the challenges noted above, chronically insufficient sleep may be a near-universal phenomenon at some point in the university student's time on campus, with attendant consequences for well-being, health, and safety. Studies show that short sleep in adolescents is associated with poor school performance, obesity, metabolic dysfunction and cardiovascular morbidity, increased depressive symptoms, suicidal ideation, risk-taking behaviors, and athletic injuries (Watson et al. 2017).

While there is substantial literature about the biological changes to sleep-wake (circadian) cycles occurring in adolescence, the campus environment presents an additional host of unique challenges. The sleep environment itself may be complicated by high-density housing, including the presence of one or more roommates, disturbing background noise and light, personal electronic devices, and omnipresent social opportunities, with sleep, study, and recreation occurring in the same small space. Beyond challenges to total sleep hours and environmental degradation of sleep spaces, irregular timing of sleep brought on by variable class schedules, assignment deadlines, and "cramming," as well as substance use—including stimulants such as caffeine and energy drinks as well as use of prescription and recreational drugs, alcohol, and sedatives—may further complicate the sleep picture.

The challenge for sleep evaluation and treatment, then, is twofold: it involves assessing both quantity and quality of sleep. Assessing *quantity* starts with a basic determination of how much time the student has allotted for sleep, and how variable that time is, across weekdays and weekends, and evaluating whether unrealistic expectations regarding sleep requirements are present. It is equally important to know about sleep patterns before onset of symptoms and to learn what coping strategies and compensations the student employs to address sleep shortfalls. Problems with sleep *quality*, in terms of subjective sleep complaints, can be broadly divided into three distinct categories: 1) daytime sleepiness or fatigue, 2) insomnia or disturbed sleep, and 3) nocturnal behaviors. Although individual disorders can be associated with more than one of these broad categories, clinical evaluation and workup are tuned for each of these complaints uniquely. This chapter summarizes sleep disorders that are common among university students, with a discussion of presenting features and treatments, and discusses consequences of sleep disorders on students' performance, health, and well-being.

Common Sleep Disorders

CIRCADIAN RHYTHM SLEEP-WAKE DISORDERS AND DELAYED SLEEP PHASE TYPE

Circadian rhythms are endogenous, near-24-hour biological rhythms entrained or synchronized to the 24-hour light-dark cycle. Circadian rhythm disorders arise when any of the following occur: alterations of the circadian time-keeping system, problems with its entrainment mechanisms, or a misalignment with the external environment. General criteria for a circadian rhythm sleep-wake disorder include 1) a chronic or recurrent pattern of sleep-wake disruption is due primarily to alteration of the endogenous circadian timing system or misalignment between this rhythm and the sleep-wake schedule desired or required by an individual's physical environment or by school, work, or social schedules; 2) circadian rhythm disruption leads to symptoms of insomnia, daytime sleepiness, or both; and 3) these sleep-wake disturbances cause significant distress or impairment in mental, physical, social, educational, or other important areas of functioning (American Academy of Sleep Medicine 2014).

In delayed sleep phase type (DSPT), there is significant delay—often by greater than 2 hours—in the phase of the major sleep episode relative to required sleep time and wake time. Students with DSPT have a chronic (>3 months), recurrent complaint of inability to fall asleep and difficulty awakening at a required clock time. Onset is typically in adolescence. When allowed to choose their own ad libitum schedule, such as during a school break, students exhibit improved sleep quality and duration for age and maintain a "night owl" sleep-wake pattern. Weekend oversleep is common. Individuals with DSPT may have extreme sleep inertia (difficulty awakening and confusion) in the morning, resulting both from insufficient sleep time and from awakening at a time of high sleep propensity in their rhythm. It should be noted that individuals with this disorder may have increased rates of other mental disorders, such as depression, bipolar disorder, obsessive-compulsive disorder, or attention-deficit/hyperactivity disorder. Evening activities and later sleep timing have also been associated with greater alcohol and marijuana use among adolescents ages 12–21 years (Hasler et al. 2017).

The association between onset of adolescence and a shift toward evening circadian phase preference was described over 20 years ago (Carskadon et al. 1993). This preference is mediated in part by genetic influence—for example, polymorphism in the circadian clock gene *hPer3*—and reinforced by behavioral activities such evening exposure to bright light or electronic use, schoolwork, and social, exercise, and dining activities, as well as low morning light exposure. Increased intake of caffeine or stimulants used to combat daytime sleepiness may further exacerbate delayed nocturnal sleep time. Although the exact prevalence of DSPT is not known in the general population, the disorder appears to be greater in adolescents and young adults, with a reported prevalence of 7%–16% (American Academy of Sleep Medicine 2014). No studies have assessed racial or ethnic differences in DSPT.

Objective findings, including recordings of sleep logs and/or actigraphy over an interval of at least 1 and preferably 2 weeks, demonstrate delayed sleep onset and sleep offset relative to required or acceptable times. For many affected individuals, sleep onset times may be between 1 A.M. and 6 A.M., with wake times in the middle to late morning or early afternoon. Polysomnography is not required for the diagnosis, but if performed, the study should optimally occur at preferred (i.e., delayed) times to avoid prolonged sleep onset times and to best capture rapid eye movement (REM) sleep on the second half of the study. Importantly, individuals with DSPT who undergo a conventionally timed polysomnography followed by mean sleep latency testing may demonstrate REM sleep in naps occurring at their typical home sleep times, increasing potential for false-positive test results. Other tests used in workup of DSPT include measures of core body temperature nadir and dim-light melatonin onset (DLMO), although these are not routinely performed at most centers. Questionnaires aimed at determining chronotype, such as the Morningness-Eveningness Questionnaire, can also be helpful in identifying individuals with a strong evening chronotype, although many normal sleepers also score high on eveningness.

A variety of behavioral strategies, most often in association with properly timed exposure to light and darkness, have been proposed in the treatment of DSPT. Use of exogenous melatonin is one recommendation. Prescribed wake time, with or without prescribed sleep time, involves setting a fixed wake time (usually starting near the individual's current best wake time) with outside-type light exposure (light boxes have been suggested in some settings) at wake time for at least 30–45 minutes, with serial advancement to an earlier wake time (e.g., advancement by 20 minutes every 3–5 days), to the goal required wake time. Such prescribed wake times require adherence 7 days per week to be optimally effective, which may be problematic for many students. *Chronotherapy*, a sleep-wake timing prescription involving more rapid serial delay of sleep time and wake time, has been used for individuals with a more pronounced phase delay. As is the case with many behaviorally based therapies, follow-up and regular contact during treatment is important. Referral to a behavioral sleep medicine specialist is often very helpful for young adults suffering with circadian rhythm disorders and is recommended whenever such resources are available; there is growing evidence that DSPT can be treated successfully using cognitive-behavioral therapies (Blake et al. 2017). (A list of behavioral sleep medicine specialists is available at www.behavioralsleep.org.)

There are numerous reports of melatonin contributing to phase advancement of sleep onset and/or circadian markers in DSPT patients, with ingestion occurring across a range of time, typically anywhere from 5 hours before bedtime to present sleep onset time (Wyatt 2011). Various doses have been studied, with low-dose melatonin (e.g., 0.3–0.5 mg) being as effective as higher doses (e.g., 5 mg) as long as the exogenous melatonin is given before the endogenous release of melatonin, which is typically about 2–3 hours before habitual sleep onset (Wyatt et al. 2006). Timed physical activity and exercise and mealtimes have also been proposed to be helpful in establishing a change in sleep-wake timing. In recent practice parameters, the American Academy of Sleep Medicine notes insufficient evidence to give recommendation for or against 1) prescribed timing of sleep-wake and/or physical activity/exercise, 2) strategic receipt and/or avoidance of light, 3) use of medications other than melatonin to phase shift and/or to promote sleep or wakefulness, and 4) other interventions that exert effects by altering bodily functions to impact sleep-wake behaviors (i.e., somatic interventions) (Auger et al. 2015). These practice parameters note positive endorsement at a second-tier degree of confidence of strategically timed melatonin for the treatment of DSPT.

Detection and management of DSPT is important because affective disorders are associated with sleep-wake and circadian disturbances (Lewy 2009). Dysfunction of the circadian system has been implicated in onset, maintenance, and recurrence of mood symptoms (Naismith et al. 2014), and in young people with mood disorders, circadian misalignment such as delayed circadian phase is present early on in the development of the disease (Robillard et al. 2013a). Both unipolar and bipolar depression subtypes have been associated with lower evening melatonin secretion and phase delay (Robillard et al. 2013b). More recently, therapies targeting sleep-wake cycle and circadian system dysfunction have been proposed to improve the course of depression in young people exhibiting this profile (Hickie et al. 2013).

Although DSPT is thought to be the most common type of circadian rhythm disturbance in young adults, other circadian rhythm disorders may be present in the university student population. These should be considered in patients presenting with consistent sleep timing complaints.

INSOMNIA

Insomnia is best thought of as a group of disorders featuring common symptoms, including one or more of the following sleep symptoms on a regular basis—classically, 3 or more nights per week: 1) difficulty initiating sleep, 2) difficulty maintaining sleep and 3) waking up earlier than desired. Insomnia may be accompanied by resistance to going to bed on appropriate schedule and difficulty sleeping without intervention (medication, substance use, etc.). In addition, the individual reports daytime consequences related to the sleep disturbance, including fatigue and/or sleepiness; attention, concentration, or memory impairment; impaired social, athletic, job, or academic performance; mood disturbance; behavioral problems (hyperactivity, impulsivity, aggression, etc.); reduced motivation or drive; proneness for errors or accidents; and increased worry about sleep. Insomnia can be short term (less than 3 months) or chronic (greater than 3 months) in duration. Symptoms should not be better explained by another sleep disorder, such as restless leg syndrome or sleep apnea. They should also not be explained purely by inadequate opportunity (i.e., not enough time allotted for sleep) or inadequate circumstances (i.e., lack of quiet, dark, safe sleep environment), although clearly both of these elements may be modifying factors in the university setting.

Common subtypes include psychophysiological insomnia, in which heightened arousal and sleep concern, as well as maladaptive sleep associations, are present; individuals with this subtype demonstrate an excessive focus on sleep and often exhibit high sleep effort, as well as insomnia due to another mental disorder and insomnia due to substance use. Inadequate sleep hygiene is classified as an insomnia subtype in *The International Classification of Sleep Disorders*, Third Edition (ICSD-3; American Academy of Sleep Medicine 2014), and the university environment is uniquely outfitted to lead to poor sleep hygiene, whose features include daytime napping; maintaining a highly variable sleep-wake schedule; frequently using sleep-disrupting substances such as caffeine, tobacco, alcohol, and recreational drugs; engaging in mentally, emotionally, or physically activating activities close to bedtime; using the bedroom for activities other than sleep, such as eating or studying (a virtual given in many dormitory settings); and failing to maintain a comfortable environment for sleep.

Workup for the complaint of insomnia in the collegiate student requires careful assessment of contributing factors—medical, psychological, mental, and behavioral—as well as consideration of substance use, the possibility of an unsafe sleep environment, and history of violence or trauma. Because the insomnia complaint may be an expression of a different underlying disorder or experience, the importance of a careful history and the art of listening cannot be underappreciated. The sleep history should include assessing the characteristics of premorbid sleep, and questioning how the student was accustomed to sleeping at home prior to campus life as well as how the student's sleep changes while on school breaks and/or when off campus. It is important to assess for prescription, over-the-counter, or other substances employed as remedies by the student to address sleep complaints or daytime symptoms.

Sleep diaries and actigraphy may be helpful in the workup of insomnia. Polysomnography is not necessary unless a physiological or medical disorder is thought to be associated with insomnia symptoms (e.g., the possibility of sleep-disordered breathing with primarily sleep maintenance difficulties).

Insomnia is the most prevalent sleep disorder among adolescents (Auger et al. 2015). Identifying and treating insomnia are critical to university students, because sleep disturbance is an important contributor to, and possibly even a cause of, cycles of increasing vulnerability and risk among young people (Harvey 2015). Common factors may be shared between sleep disturbance and mental health disorders, including problems with stress and/or arousal, emotion processing, and cognitive factors (Cowie et al. 2014). Additionally, chronic insomnia increases the subsequent risk for somatic health problems, interpersonal problems, psychological and emotional problems, high incidence of anxiety, and risk-taking behavior (Roberts et al. 2008).

The mainstay of insomnia treatment is identifying and addressing contributing and perpetuating factors. When appropriate, a referral for cognitive-behavioral therapy for insomnia (CBT-I) should be made. Cognitive-behavioral sleep interventions are typically short-term, multicomponent, and goal oriented. CBT-I techniques aim to modify the patterns of thinking and behavior that may be underlying the sleep disturbance, such as poor sleep hygiene, irregular sleep-wake schedules, delayed bedtimes, presleep hyperarousal, and maladaptive sleep-related cognitions. This modality has been well established in adult populations, and a recent meta-analysis of cognitive-behavioral sleep interventions in adolescents demonstrated subjective and objective improvement in sleep times, as well as improvements in global sleep quality, daytime sleepiness, depression, and anxiety (Wyatt et al. 2006).

In young adults with no other mental health disorders, hypnotic therapy should be used with great caution, particularly on a chronic basis. This is partly due to relatively insufficient data evaluating the effectiveness of prescription hypnotics in college-age young adults (e.g., 17- to 22-year-olds), with typical studies lumping young adults over age 18 with middle-aged adults. There are no high-quality large adolescent studies of the most commonly used hypnotics (e.g., zolpidem). Additionally, the side-effect profiles of such agents give rise to concerns about vulnerabilities among this population, including risks of parasomnias, significant morning sedation, dependence, and use with other substances. The university environment is one in which new skills and knowledge are mastered at a laudable clip; the approach to improving sleep should be one of skills acquisition. Good sleep is something that can, in most cases, be practiced and achieved in the absence of chronic hypnotic therapy.

SLEEP-DISORDERED BREATHING

Sleep-disordered breathing involves physiological abnormalities in sleep due to the presence of increased airway resistance (and possible collapse), which increases the effort of breathing. Sleep-disordered breathing may encompass sleep fragmentation and poor sleep stability, oxygen desaturation and/or hypoventilation, and frank apneas. Its prevalence in college student populations has not been distinctly determined; however, sleep-related breathing disorders are common in both school-aged pediatric (3%–4%) and middle-aged adult (up to 49.7%) populations (Heinzer et al. 2015). Sleep-disordered breathing may be increased by alcohol or other sedative use before sleep, as well as by weight gain, both of which have been reported with heightened frequency among university students.

Although sleepiness is a common presenting complaint for middle-aged individuals, this may be less true for the young adult student population. Fatigue, unrefreshing sleep despite adequate hours, poor sleep quality, sleep fragmentation, and mental fog may be experienced by university students. Insomnia, in particular difficulty maintaining sleep, is not uncommon. Inattention, impairment in concentration and mood, and behavioral changes have been linked to sleep-disordered breathing as well. The daytime symptoms of sleep-disordered breathing may mimic or overlap those of attention-deficit disorders, so history and clinical evaluation of the airway is prudent, and consideration of a sleep study is encouraged if symptoms suggesting a breathing disorder are present. Quality of life is generally adversely affected, and bed partners or roommates may also notice the other person's sleep disruption, excessive movement, or noisy breathing in sleep (which may not be reported as classic snoring). In addition to excess weight and alcohol use, chronic nasal obstruction (either inflammatory or structural), large tonsils or neck, a narrow jaw structure (associations include long face, chronic mouth breathing, and open bite), or mandibular retrusion may be present. Family history should always be solicited, because sleep-related breathing disorders are often familial.

Workup includes polysomnography—preferably with electroencephalography—to assess frequency of sleep disturbance associated with breathing abnormalities. Management options include upper airway surgery, including oropharyngeal, nasal, and skeletal, as well as orthodontic appliances, weight loss, and continuous positive airway pressure (CPAP) therapy. Timing of surgery is worth consideration, because students may miss about 7–14 days of school following soft tissue surgery, and much longer following jaw surgery. Positive airway pressure (PAP) therapy can be an excellent noninvasive treatment option, but there may be embarrassment or social stigma associated with it. Also, although special housing is not a priori required for PAP, top bunks may be a challenge to manage power cords, the device, and the humidifier. The issue has not been well studied, but experience indicates that some university housing offices are open to special consideration for rooming based on CPAP use.

PARASOMNIAS

Parasomnias are undesired physical events that occur during entry into sleep, within sleep, or during arousal from sleep. They encompass abnormal sleep-related movements, behaviors, dreams, and autonomic nervous system activity, over which there is no conscious, deliberate control. Commonly encountered parasomnias in young adults include the REM parasomnia; nightmare disorder; and the non–rapid eye movement (NREM) disorders of arousal, the presence of which peak earlier in childhood but may manifest or persist into the late teens and early twenties, such as sleepwalking, confusional arousals, sleep terrors, and sleep-related eating disorder, among others. Sleep enuresis is another parasomnia that may manifest or recur in the young adult.

The NREM disorders of arousal share common features. They classically arise out of Stage N3 (slow-wave) sleep. The individual's eyes may be open and in a glassy stare, and the individual is usually very hard to awaken and, if awakened, is confused and may even be combative. Amnesia is typically present, with poor or no recall of behaviors the next day. Events typically occur in the first half of the sleep period, but they may also increase or occur at nontypical times in response to recovery sleep after deprivation.

Although disorders of arousal often involve routine behaviors, at times dangerous behaviors may be present. Such behaviors include urinating in a wastebasket, climbing out of a window, bumping into objects, falling down, leaving one's domicile, or driving. A sleep terror may transition into agitated sleepwalking or running; self-injury, ranging from minor cuts and bruises to life-threatening injury, can occur. Violence to others has also been reported, with potential legal or forensic implications. Sleep-related abnormal sexual behaviors, a subgroup of NREM parasomnias, can have major interpersonal, clinical, and criminal consequences.

The prevalence of NREM parasomnias in college-aged young adults has not been definitely studied, but rates are reported to be about 3%–4% for confusional arousals and sleepwalking and about 2% for sleep terrors (American Academy of Sleep Medicine 2014). A genetic predisposition has been hypothesized, and several priming factors have been identified, most of which are quite common in the collegiate environment. These factors include sleep deprivation, situational stress, sleep-disordered breathing, travel or sleeping in a different location than usual, external stimuli such as phone calls or electronic messaging, and internal stimuli such as distended bladder or migraine headache. Alcohol has also been proposed to be a potential trigger. However, the ICSD-3 emphasizes that disorders of arousal not be diagnosed in the presence of alcohol intoxication, because the behaviors of alcohol intoxication may superficially resemble those of a sleepwalker. That said, alcohol promotes slow-wave sleep early in the sleep period, and other γ-aminobutyric acid (GABA)ergic sedative hypnotics such as zolpidem have been associated with parasomnia activity. Clinically, it is important to advise patients identified as at risk for NREM parasomnia against alcohol intake as well as use of non–benzodiazepine receptor agonists (e.g., zolpidem) before sleep. It is worth noting that although NREM parasomnias have in the past been linked to mood disorders such as anxiety or depression, it is believed that the overwhelming majority of individuals with disorders of arousal do not have psychological or neurological pathology.

Workup for NREM parasomnia requires a careful history and physical examination; although polysomnography is not required in clear-cut cases, a sleep test may be undertaken to evaluate for other diagnoses in the differential, such as seizure disorder, or to evaluate for priming co-diagnoses such as sleep-disordered breathing. In particular, if behaviors are stereotyped in nature and occur with equal frequency at any time of night, rather than in the first half of the sleep period, seizure disorder must be considered.

Treatment involves supportive care whenever possible—especially safeguarding of the sleep environment. When appropriate, useful modifications include heavy drapes or other window coverings, avoidance of top bunks or upper-floor rooms with balconies, and safeguarding keys. Door alarms have been used in some cases to alert others to a sleepwalking event in progress, although alarms may prove troublesome in a group living situation. Importantly, avoiding sleep deprivation and taking strides toward stress management are critical. When an individual has a history of frequent or ongoing events or unintentional injury to self or others, it is important to notify and educate roommates and hallmates of potential parasomnia episodes. Notification is essential because there is some degree of safety risk to roommates attempting to awaken a sleepwalker. Additionally, advance notice also may help mitigate social embarrassment potentially associated with noninjurious parasomnia behaviors.

CENTRAL HYPERSOMNIAS

Central hypersomnias include narcolepsy with cataplexy, narcolepsy without cataplexy, and the very rare Kleine-Levin syndrome, among others. They should be considered in cases of excessive daytime sleepiness despite routinely attaining adequate hours of sleep and may be associated with weight gain or coincident onset of behavioral or mood disorders. If bona fide cataplexy is present, narcolepsy with cataplexy should be highly considered. Referral to an accredited sleep center is recommended if these disorders are suspected. A number of more common disorders associated with hypersomnia, among them insufficient sleep, sleep-disordered breathing, and circadian rhythm disorders, should be carefully considered during the diagnostic process. Other sources of central hypersomnia include posttraumatic hypersomnia and hypersomnia secondary to a brain lesion. Additionally, chronic infectious processes have also been linked to daytime fatigue and to a lesser extent sleepiness and should therefore be considered as well.

Consequences: Performance, Health, and Well-Being

Ultimately, significant sleep difficulties can jeopardize health in the short run and the long run. In adults, short sleep duration (<7 hours per night) is associated with increased risk of obesity, high blood pressure, diabetes, coronary heart disease, stroke, frequent mental distress, and death (Itani et al. 2017); sleep-disordered breathing at moderate to severe levels has also been associated with many of these outcomes (St-Onge et al. 2016). In a meta-analysis of over 5 million individuals from 153 studies, the CDC recently estimated that short sleep duration is associated with mortality (risk increased 12%; with a linear association between mortality and sleep duration <6 hours) and risk increase for diabetes (increased 37%), obesity (increased 38%), hypertension (increased 17%), cardiovascular diseases (increased 16%), and coronary heart diseases (increased 26%) (Liu et al. 2016). It can be argued that away at college for the first time, many students are laying down sleep habits that may last a lifetime—for better or worse.

Not all health outcomes associated with poor sleep take years to develop. Youth ages 14–18 years were more likely to be overweight if they slept <8 hours per night during the school week, and odds of being overweight increased by more than 2.5-fold for youth sleeping 5–7 hours on school nights (Seicean et al. 2007). When young healthy volunteers who typically sleep 8–9 hours are allowed to sleep only 4–6 hours, insulin resistance and glucose intolerance occur (Grandner et al. 2016). From a mental health perspective, inadequate sleep has been associated with depression, anxiety, and suicidal ideation in adolescents (Gangwisch et al. 2010; Lee et al. 2012; Moore et al. 2009). Poorer sleep quality is correlated with worsening levels of depression symptoms in adolescents ages 14–20 years (Dağ and Kutlu 2017), further underscoring the importance of identification and treatment. In a recent large study of over 370,000 adolescent students, depression, stress, and sleep satisfaction significantly predicted suicidal ideation (Im et al. 2017). Also compounding the proposed bidirectional relationship between poor sleep and mood disorders, sleep deprivation has been associated with enhanced reactivity toward negative stimuli and can impair the accurate recognition of human emotions (Gujar et al. 2011; van der Helm et al. 2010).

The mental health impacts of poor sleep can be far-reaching, and students presenting with complaints of poor sleep should be screened for symptoms of depression and other mood disorders. Safety, too, must be considered. The National Highway Traffic Safety Administration estimates that over 80,000 accidents per year are due to drowsiness behind the wheel (U.S. Department of Transportation 2011), likely an underestimate due to underreporting; both short sleep duration and snoring are risk factors associated with drowsy driving (Centers for Disease Control and Prevention 2013). Young people may be the most vulnerable to the effects of sleep loss; in a study of fall-asleep vehicle crashes, peak age for crashes was 20 years, and 55% of drivers were under age 25 (Pack et al. 1995).

Not surprisingly, performance also is impacted by poor sleep. Academic performance has been shown to be negatively affected by sleep deprivation (Beebe et al. 2017). Sleep loss is associated with subjective affective, cognitive, and physical symptoms and objective differences on tasks of visual memory, reaction time, and visual motor speed (Stocker et al. 2017). Risk-taking behavior may also follow. In particular, compared with adolescents who sleep 9 hours, those sleeping 7 hours or less per night were more likely to report several injury-related risk behaviors (infrequent bicycle helmet use, infrequent seatbelt use, riding with a driver who had been drinking, drinking and driving, and texting while driving).

Case Example

Maya is a first-year, 18-year-old student who presents in March with a 3-month history of excessive daytime sleepiness, difficulty falling asleep at night, and difficulty waking in time for an 8 A.M. chemistry class. She gets into bed at 11 P.M. but does not fall asleep for several hours. She denies racing thoughts but reports she does not feel sleepy. To avoid feeling frustrated, she often picks up her phone and updates social media until she can fall asleep. She reports feeling stressed about her performance in chemistry, and lately, she has stopped exercising and greatly curtailed social activities because of "being out of energy." Once asleep, she states that she is "dead to the world" until the morning. She frequently sleeps through her alarms. She has a dry mouth in the morning and reports feeling foggy and slow moving until 10 A.M. She is tired during the day, and when possible takes a 20-minute nap in the library around 3 P.M. At around 9 P.M., she often feels less tired. On the weekends, she has a work-study job at a campus cafe until 1:30 A.M. and goes to bed between 2:00 and 2:30 A.M. with sleep onset within 20 minutes. She sleeps in until 11 A.M. or later.

Maya lives in a dormitory with one roommate, with whom she has a good relationship. She occupies the bottom bunk; the room is dark and quiet. Her roommate leaves for sports practice at 5:30 A.M. Maya reports feeling safe in her environment. She denies use of alcohol, recreational drugs, or tobacco. She drinks 4–6 cups of coffee or energy drinks per day. Over the recent winter break, she returned home (which is located in a different time zone from her university) and slept from 1:00–9:30 A.M. daily, similar to her younger brother. Her sleepiness resolved when home, and her fatigue largely, but not completely, improved. In high school, she recalls "always having to be dragged out of bed by my mom" for school but denies prolonged difficulty falling asleep or daytime sleepiness.

Questions: What diagnoses should be considered for Maya? What types of assessments are appropriate? What types of treatment would you recommend for this student?

Conclusion

Along with nutrition and exercise, sleep is a pillar of health. Unique challenges are faced by students who are new to managing their sleep solo, in a sensorily rich, busy, and often-stressful campus environment in which they have competing demands on time. Adequate hours reserved for sleep may be sacrificed for athletic, academic, and social obligations; such opportunities extend from the early morning hours to late night. In addition, sleep disorders are not rare in this age group, and symptoms may become more evident as compensations are compromised. The burden of parasomnias may range from inconvenience and social embarrassment to serious harm and legal consequences. On the other hand, insomnia, sleep apnea, and the sleep loss associated with circadian rhythm disorders may each differentially contribute to poor sleep quality in ways that directly impact student mental health. Poor sleep is a risk factor for depression, suicidal ideation, declines in performance, and accidents. Fortunately, the vast majority of sleep disorders are readily manageable with adequately trained clinicians and resources, and healthy sleep practices can be learned and reinforced with beneficial results.

KEY CONCEPTS

- Sleep disorders such as delayed sleep phase type, insomnia, sleep-disordered breathing, and parasomnias are not uncommon in college-age students. While a careful history and physical examination are key to recognizing the diagnosis, referral to a sleep center may be required.

- Sleep is not a waste of time. Inadequate hours of sleep can lead to a host of negative consequences, and good sleep hygiene and protected time and space to sleep should be emphasized.

- Good sleep practices can be learned and mastered.

Recommendations for Psychiatrists, Psychologists, and Counselors

1. Sleep disorders may be associated with co-occurring mood or other mental health disorders. If one is present, evaluate for the other.
2. Assess quantity and variability of sleep throughout the week. In general, 8–10 hours of sleep is optimal for younger university students, whereas 7–9 hours is recommended for older students.
3. Assess quality of sleep: Does the student exhibit difficulties falling asleep, difficulty staying asleep, or both?
4. Assess behaviors in sleep: Ask about substance use, and assess the student's perception of safety.
5. Discuss daytime symptoms: Ask about sleepiness, fatigue, accidents, and/or mood disruption, as well as changes in grades or social or athletic performance.
6. Assess the sleep environment: Include questions about electronics, roommates, noise, and exogenous light.
7. Insomnia and circadian rhythm disorders respond well to distinct cognitive and behavioral therapies. Consider referral for these therapies.
8. Impart tips for healthy sleep, such as the following: schedule enough time for sleep; take naps in a pinch, but keep them short and sweet, and aim for the early afternoon; curtail substances—caffeine, tobacco, and other stimulants, as well as alcohol and other recreational substances, all of which negatively impact sleep; keep a regular sleep schedule 7 days a week; turn off electronics an hour before bed and keep them off during sleep.

Discussion Questions

1. What factors should be considered when a first-year male student reports inability to fall asleep before midnight for his 8:00 A.M. class the next morning? What history is needed?
2. What might be the appropriate steps to take for a third-year undergraduate student with a history of sleepwalking?
3. What are best sleep practices for college athletes who are on the road across time zones up to once per week during the season and/ or who have early morning team practice requirements?

Suggested Readings

American Academy of Sleep Medicine: International Classification of Sleep Disorders, 3rd Edition. Darien, IL, American Academy of Sleep Medicine, 2014
Hirshkowitz M, Whiton K, Albert SM, et al: National Sleep Foundation's sleep time duration recommendations: methodology and results summary. Sleep Health 1(1): 40–43, 2015

References

American Academy of Sleep Medicine: International Classification of Sleep Disorders, 3rd Edition. Darien, IL, American Academy of Sleep Medicine, 2014
Auger RR, Burgess HJ, Emens JS, et al: Clinical practice guideline for the treatment of intrinsic circadian rhythm sleep-wake disorders: advanced sleep-wake phase disorder (ASWPD), delayed sleep-wake phase disorder (DSWPD), non-24-hour sleep-wake rhythm disorder (N24SWD), and irregular sleep-wake rhythm disorder (ISWRD). An update for 2015. J Clin Sleep Med 11(10):1199–1236, 2015 26414986
Beebe DW, Field J, Miller MM, et al: Impact of multi-night experimentally induced short sleep on adolescent performance in a simulated classroom. Sleep 40(2), 2017 28364497
Blake MJ, Sheeber LB, Youssef GJ, et al: Systematic review and meta-analysis of adolescent cognitive-behavioral sleep interventions. Clin Child Fam Psychol Rev 20(3):227–249, 2017 28331991
Carskadon MA, Vieira C, Acebo C: Association between puberty and delayed phase preference. Sleep 16(3):258–262, 1993 8506460
Centers for Disease Control and Prevention: Drowsy driving—19 states and the District of Columbia, 2009–2010. MMWR Morb Mortal Wkly Rep 61(51–52):1033–1037, 2013 23282860
Cowie J, Alfano CA, Patriquin M, et al: Addressing sleep in children with anxiety disorders. Sleep Med Clin 9:137–148, 2014
Dağ B, Kutlu FY: The relationship between sleep quality and depressive symptoms in adolescents. Turk J Med Sci 47(3):721–727, 2017 28618721
Gangwisch JE, Babiss LA, Malaspina D, et al: Earlier parental set bedtimes as a protective factor against depression and suicidal ideation. Sleep 33(1):97–106, 2010 20120626
Grandner MA, Seixas A, Shetty S, Shenoy S: Sleep duration and diabetes risk: population trends and potential mechanisms. Curr Diab Rep 16(11):106, 2016 27664039
Gujar N, Yoo SS, Hu P, Walker MP: Sleep deprivation amplifies reactivity of brain reward networks, biasing the appraisal of positive emotional experiences. J Neurosci 31(12):4466–4474, 2011 21430147
Harvey AG: A transdiagnostic intervention for youth sleep and circadian problems. Cognit Behav Pract 23(3):341–355, 2015

Hasler BP, Franzen PL, de Zambotti M, et al: Eveningness and later sleep timing are associated with greater risk for alcohol and marijuana use in adolescence: Initial findings from the NCANDA study. Alcohol Clin Exp Res 41(6):1154–1165, 2017 28421617

Heinzer R, Vat S, Marques-Vidal P, et al: Prevalence of sleep-disordered breathing in the general population: the HypnoLaus study. Lancet Respir Med 3(4):310–318, 2015 25682233

Hickie IB, Naismith SL, Robillard R, et al: Manipulating the sleep-wake cycle and circadian rhythms to improve clinical management of major depression. BMC Med 11:79, 2013 23521808

Hirshkowitz M, Whiton K, Albert SM, et al: National Sleep Foundation's sleep time duration recommendations: methodology and results summary. Sleep Health 1(1):40–43, 2015

Im Y, Oh WO, Suk M: Risk factors for suicide ideation among adolescents: five-year national data analysis. Arch Psychiatr Nurs 31(3):282–286, 2017 28499568

Itani O, Jike M, Watanabe N, Kaneita Y: Short sleep duration and health outcomes: a systematic review, meta-analysis, and meta-regression. Sleep Med 32:246–256, 2017 27743803

Keyes KM, Maslowsky J, Hamilton A, Schulenberg J: The great sleep recession: changes in sleep duration among U.S. adolescents, 1991–2012. Pediatrics 135(3):460–468, 2015 25687142

Lee YJ, Cho SJ, Cho IH, Kim SJ: Insufficient sleep and suicidality in adolescents. Sleep 35(4):455–460, 2012 22467982

Lewy AJ: Circadian misalignment in mood disturbances. Curr Psychiatry Rep 11(6):459–465, 2009 19909668

Liu Y, Wheaton AG, Chapman DP, et al: Prevalence of healthy sleep duration among adults—United States, 2014. MMWR Morb Mortal Wkly Rep 65(6):137–141, 2016 26890214

Moore M, Kirchner HL, Drotar D, et al: Relationships among sleepiness, sleep time, and psychological functioning in adolescents. J Pediatr Psychol 34(10):1175–1183, 2009 19494088

Naismith SL, Lagopoulos J, Hermens DF, et al: Delayed circadian phase is linked to glutamatergic functions in young people with affective disorders: a proton magnetic resonance spectroscopy study. BMC Psychiatry 14:345, 2014 25496061

Pack AI, Pack AM, Rodgman E, et al: Characteristics of crashes attributed to the driver having fallen asleep. Accid Anal Prev 27(6):769–775, 1995 8749280

Roberts RE, Roberts CR, Duong HT: Chronic insomnia and its negative consequences for health and functioning of adolescents: a 12-month prospective study. J Adolesc Health 42(3):294–302, 2008 18295138

Robillard R, Naismith SL, Rogers NL, et al: Delayed sleep phase in young people with unipolar or bipolar affective disorders. J Affect Disord 145(2):260–263, 2013a 22877966

Robillard R, Naismith SL, Rogers NL, et al: Sleep-wake cycle and melatonin rhythms in adolescents and young adults with mood disorders: comparison of unipolar and bipolar phenotypes. Eur Psychiatry 28(7):412–416, 2013b 23769680

Seicean A, Redline S, Seicean S, et al: Association between short sleeping hours and overweight in adolescents: results from a US suburban high school survey. Sleep Breath 11(4):285–293, 2007 17440761

St-Onge MP, Grandner MA, Brown D, et al; American Heart Association Obesity, Behavior Change, Diabetes, and Nutrition Committees of the Council on Lifestyle and Cardiometabolic Health; Council on Cardiovascular Disease in the Young; Council on Clinical Cardiology; and Stroke Council: Sleep duration and quality: impact on lifestyle behaviors and cardiometabolic health: a scientific statement from the American Heart Association. Circulation 134(18):e367–e386, 2016 27647451

Stocker RPJ, Khan H, Henry L, Germain A: Effects of sleep loss on subjective complaints and objective neurocognitive performance as measured by the immediate post-concussion assessment and cognitive testing. Arch Clin Neuropsychol 32(3):349–368, 2017 28431034

U.S. Department of Transportation, National Highway Traffic Safety Administration: Traffic Safety Stats. 2011. Available at: https://crashstats.nhtsa.dot.gov/Api/Public/ViewPublication/811449. Accessed May 5, 2017.

van der Helm E, Gujar N, Walker MP: Sleep deprivation impairs the accurate recognition of human emotions. Sleep 33(3):335–342, 2010 20337191

Watson NF, Martin JL, Wise MS, et al; American Academy of Sleep Medicine Board of Directors: Delaying middle school and high school start times promotes student health and performance: an American Academy of Sleep Medicine position statement. J Clin Sleep Med 13(4):623–625, 2017 28416043

Wheaton AG, Olsen EO, Miller GF, Croft JB: Sleep duration and injury-related risk behaviors among high school students—United States, 2007–2013. MMWR Morb Mortal Wkly Rep 65(13):337–341, 2016 27054407

Wyatt JK: Circadian rhythm sleep disorders. Pediatr Clin North Am 58(3):621–635, 2011 21600345

Wyatt JK, Dijk DJ, Ritz-de Cecco A, et al: Sleep-facilitating effect of exogenous melatonin in healthy young men and women is circadian-phase dependent. Sleep 29(5):609–618, 2006 16774150

Intervening Early in First-Episode Psychosis in a College Setting

Kate V. Hardy, Clin.Psych.D.

Brenda Gonzalez-Flores, M.S.

Jacob S. Ballon, M.D., M.P.H.

SERIOUS *mental illness* (SMI) is a broad term that includes psychiatric disorders with severe symptomatology and functional impairment when untreated. Although these disorders can be a great source of distress and disability, treatment is now based on a recovery model in which expectations of successful treatment include maintaining a positive expectation of future functioning. With appropriate and effective treatment, individuals with SMI can resume their quality of life and expect to meet social and occupational milestones.

This chapter focuses primarily on issues related to people with psychotic disorders, considered to be among the potentially most disabling forms of SMI. *Psychosis* refers to a cluster of symptoms associated with various psychiatric, neurological, and medical conditions that lead to an impairment with reality testing. Predominant features include *hallucinations* (sensorial perceptions without the presence of an external or physical stimulus that can occur in any of the five senses) and *delusions* (unusual thoughts or false beliefs that are inconsistent with the cultural norm and that are held despite contrary evidence). In addition, psychosis can be accompanied by disorganized thinking and speech, grossly disorganized or abnormal motor behaviors, catatonia, and negative symptoms (e.g., diminished emotional expression, avolition, alogia, anhedonia). The most common primary psychotic disorder is schizophrenia; however, in this chapter, we consider the term *psychosis* broadly because symptoms are generally still emerging in college students, often resulting in diagnostic uncertainty at the initial point of identification and treatment. Students presenting with first onset of psychotic symptoms may go on to develop schizophrenia or schizoaffective disorder, but the symptoms could also be due to substance use, affective disorders such as bipolar disorder or depression, trauma, or certain medical conditions. Because the etiology of psychosis can vary, a comprehensive assessment is essential.

Universities often struggle with how to respond ethically and legally to students presenting in crisis with psychosis. While college is an exciting time for students, it involves a major life transition with numerous demands and challenges. Academic stress, social pressures, continuous sleep disruptions, separation from family, and an increase in responsibilities can leave students more vulnerable to substance use and other mental health problems. Given these demands, college students may experience their first onset or exacerbation of mental health problems. Consider the following example:

> Mark enrolled at a small college where he was looking forward to majoring in English. The college was 1,500 miles from home, and he made the transition to dorm living easily, including making new friends. The first year passed uneventfully, and Mark got straight As. As a sophomore, Mark started to notice that he was having difficulty concentrating in class and was experiencing decreased motivation. For the first time, he received a B. After winter break, Mark began to put in extra hours in the library, often working all night. His friends noted a change because Mark

was not socializing as before. Late one night while studying, Mark heard voices whispering. At first, he thought they were noises coming from outside, but soon he became convinced that he was hearing an angel speaking to him. Mark became more isolated and started missing classes. In the spring, the resident advisor (RA) in the dorm observed Mark mumbling to himself. The RA sought advice from his resident dean. The resident dean dismissed the RA's concerns and suggested that Mark's behavior was due to the stress of studying for upcoming exams. Mark became more isolated and convinced that he was engaged in a spiritual battle that could herald the end of the world if ignored. He stopped communicating with his family, which worried them to the point of contacting the college for information. His parents were told, however, that Mark "is an adult now and he has the right to choose with whom he communicates" and therefore no information can be provided. By summer, Mark became convinced that he was losing the spiritual battle and began performing "rituals" in the parking lot, which involved pacing around in a small square for several hours; this behavior prompted a call to the police. Mark resisted talking to the police and became agitated when they tried to stop him from pacing. The police took him involuntarily to a hospital. Upon discharge from the hospital, Mark was told to take a medical leave or risk disciplinary action for his recent behavior. He returned home and has yet to complete college 3 years later.

Unfortunately, this example presents a common description of how the onset of psychosis, and access to treatment, occurs for thousands of young adults in the United States each year. Symptoms of psychosis typically emerge in late adolescence and early adulthood (Perkins et al. 2006), the period during which young people are starting college. Nearly 70% of high school students enrolled in college in 2015 (Bureau of Labor Statistics 2017). With 100,000 new cases of psychosis occurring each year in the United States, it can be expected that each year a significant number of students will experience their first episode of psychosis while on a college campus.

Identification of Psychosis in the College Setting

Recent advances in the treatment of psychotic disorders include the rise of dedicated services for early intervention in psychosis that aim to provide a number of evidence-based interventions to support young people in recovery and their families. However, before early intervention can be provided, there must be effective early identification. Research has shown that the *duration of untreated psychosis* is an important factor in the long-term prognosis of individuals experiencing a first episode of psychosis. The World Health Organization (WHO) recommends a duration of untreated psychosis of no more than 12 weeks, and Birchwood and colleagues (2013) suggest that there is a "critical period" for intervention within the first 6 months of psychosis, after which there is a plateau in the effectiveness of interventions. A recent multicenter study in the United States, funded by the National Institute of Mental Health, found that the median duration of untreated psychosis was 74 weeks (Addington et al. 2015)—well beyond the WHO-recommended 12 weeks.

Challenges in the identification of psychosis exist in all settings but may be particularly acute in a college setting, where students present with a range of mental health problems. During early adulthood, individuals are also experiencing increased autonomy and decreased oversight as they transition to a college campus or as they spend less time with family members through engagement in education and work activities. Increased anonymity can result in mental health difficulties going unrecognized and untreated. Psychotic disorders often have a *prodromal period*, or a time preceding the onset of fully psychotic symptoms. Broadly speaking, symptoms are considered to be fully psychotic when they are experienced with 100% conviction and have an impact on the behavior or functioning of the individual. During the prodromal stage, the symptoms are often nonspecific and may be ascribed to other diagnoses, such as depression, anxiety, or attention-deficit/hyperactivity disorder, or the symptoms may simply be considered a normative reaction to the stressors of college life. However, a deeper look will often reveal accompanying "attenuated" (or subthreshold) symptoms or even brief, full psychotic symptoms that may indicate the imminent onset of full psychosis. Early symptoms often include distressing and impairing perceptual disturbances, such as hearing or seeing things that others do not experience, unusual thoughts, or suspiciousness. Importantly, these symptoms should be assessed, because early identification will help to identify the most appropriate treatment plan for the young person.

One of the first signs that a student is struggling with a mental health problem is a change in academic performance. Faced with possible hallucinations or preoccupying thoughts in the form of delusions, as well as possible cognitive symptoms, the academic performance of a student struggling with psychosis may be characterized by declining grades, incomplete assignments, or missed classes. Additionally, there are often observable changes in behavior, which are atypical for the young person. However, when considering behavior, it is important to consider the cultural and environmental context. For example, although the vignette described Mark's "spiritual battle," this language would not be immediately indicative of a potential problem if this language could be normative for the student's religious background. As in Mark's case, there should also be associated distress and impaired functioning before a diagnosis of a psychotic disorder can be made.

Studies have demonstrated the impact of psychosis on cognitive functioning, which may consequently have an effect on school functioning. In the North American Prodromal Longitudinal Study, people at clinical high risk for schizophrenia were compared with healthy control subjects and people diagnosed with schizophrenia. Cognitive changes were seen in the high-risk group and are a key component of the composite risk score that has been developed from this work (Cannon et al. 2016). Cognitive changes in early psychosis typically relate to processing speed, verbal learning, and working memory. Deficits in these areas put students at a great disadvantage compared with their peers. Further, many students look to psychoactive substances, prescribed or not, including psychostimulants, to help remedy these deficits. These medications unfortunately can worsen nascent psychotic symptoms.

Beyond cognitive changes, social changes are also typically seen at the onset of illness. Many students become withdrawn and begin to isolate socially. Withdrawing into one's own thoughts often further separates the student from peers, making detection more difficult. However, this change also presents an opportunity for early detection, because any behavior that is atypical for a particular student may be a red flag for further investigation. Screening tools for early signs of psychosis exist and may aid in the detection of symptoms indicative of a risk of developing psychosis (Loewy et al. 2005; Miller et al. 2004).

Barriers to Treatment Among College Students With Serious Mental Illness

Individuals with serious mental illness are often challenged by stereotypes, prejudice, and discrimination from the general public and even from health care professionals. They are often depicted as dangerous, violent, and unreliable in media reports and popular culture. These stigmatizing attitudes delay the seeking of help and are a significant barrier to treatment. There are three distinct forms of stigma: 1) public stigma, 2) perceived stigma, and 3) personal stigma. *Public stigma* is defined as the collective negative views about mental illness held by a community; *perceived stigma* refers to one's beliefs of how society views individuals with mental illness; and *personal stigma* is defined as one's endorsed adverse attitudes and beliefs about mental illness toward oneself (Kosyluk et al. 2016). Stigma impacts a person at multiple levels, including academic performance, self-esteem, employment, housing retention, and overall quality of life. Feelings of guilt and shame are often associated with stigma. Because of the fears of being labeled "mentally ill," many with serious mental illness withdraw from their inner social circles, especially during the early stages of psychosis when unchallenged delusions begin to become more deeply held. Furthermore, students who isolate have lower levels of community engagement and social relationships. Withdrawal from social networks may make identification even more challenging.

Research has found that unfamiliarity with serious mental illness is a strong predictor of stigmatizing attitudes. A major obstacle in connecting students with mental health services is lack of familiarity with the symptoms and early warning signs of psychosis (Feeg et al. 2014). In a survey conducted by the University of South Carolina, 87 faculty members were asked about their familiarity with mental disorders (Brockelman and Scheyett 2015). The researchers found that the least familiar mental disorders included personality disorders (43.5%), schizophrenia (42.3%), and paranoia (41.7%). Faculty often struggle with how to respond to students in distress. Brockelman and Scheyett (2015) found that the most common approach was to extend a deadline and discuss mental health concerns with the student. Nearly 80% of faculty consulted with the office of disability resources or counseling centers to gather more information about the resources available on campus. Although that number is encouraging, it is not known how many of those consultations result in referral to a coordinated specialty care (CSC) program, which is recommended for first-episode psychosis, for further management.

Another barrier to initiating psychiatric treatment is the difficulty front-line student health professionals have empathizing with students with psychosis, especially during active symptoms. Too often individuals with serious mental illness feel blamed for their disorder or worry that their psychotic symptoms will be viewed as a sign of weakness or that they are "crazy." To address this issue, Bunn and Terpstra (2009) had medical students simulate the auditory hallucinations of a voice-hearer by listening to headphones. The participant had to continue with daily activities while listening to the voices. The study found that this experience led to higher levels of empathy toward individuals with serious mental illness. A similar approach can be adapted to health professionals and faculty training on campus.

Given its distinct environment, college presents a unique opportunity to identify and treat serious psychopathology. Early intervention leads to better academic, social, health, and occupational outcomes. Attempts must be made to reduce stigma and other treatment barriers in order to improve the trajectory for students with serious mental illness.

Management of Psychosis in College Students

After identification of a person with early psychosis, the next step is to determine the appropriate treatment and management. The gold standard for treatment of early psychosis is to engage the client in a CSC program (Heinssen et al. 2014). These clinics present a recovery-oriented approach to care through shared decision making, and they provide at least the following evidence-based services: medication management, individual psychotherapy (particularly cognitive-behavioral therapy [CBT] for psychosis), supported education and/or employment, and family psychoeducation. According to evidence from the National Institute of Mental Health's Recovery After an Initial Schizophrenia Episode (RAISE) study, these support services increase adherence to treatment and improved quality of life (Kane et al. 2016). Although these clinics are being rapidly developed and implemented in communities around the United States, there are still many areas that do not have such services available. A regularly updated list of early intervention for psychosis services across the United States, including many that fit the CSC model, can be found at the Prodrome and Early Psychosis Program Network (PEPPNET) Web site (https://med.stanford.edu/peppnet.html).

Medication management of early psychosis is best done within the shared decision-making framework of a CSC. Shared decision making helps the clinician join with the student, and the student's family, to consider treatment options. Some young people may resist antipsychotic medications, because of a lack of agreement about the diagnosis or need for medication, unpleasant side effects, or general lack of efficacy. Therefore, working together to develop a shared treatment plan that the student will adhere to, and be honest about, is paramount. A low dose of second-generation antipsychotic medication is best offered first, and effort should be made to give an adequate trial of lower doses of medication before moving to higher doses. Nonpharmacological treatments are also important to include, because they help to reinforce the potential benefits of pharmacotherapy and address issues not tackled through medication—for example, coping with symptoms and managing stress or developing plans for returning to school. Including CBT for psychosis and supported education services within a student health center's offerings may improve overall treatment outcomes. More frequent interactions with students with psychosis give universities additional points of contact to help in identification and intervention with potential relapse behaviors.

Treatment Accommodations to Maintain Students With Serious Mental Illness in School

College administrators and health officials often face a significant dilemma when considering how best to help a student once an episode of psychosis has been identified. As seen in the case example about Mark, there are often concerns about student privacy. Privacy laws can be difficult to understand and can present limitations, especially because college students are generally over the age of majority and can make decisions for themselves, yet students are often still dependent on parents financially and emotionally. The two privacy laws at the center of the discrepancy are the Family Educational Rights and Privacy Act (FERPA), which protects student privacy, and the Health Insurance Portability and Accountability Act (HIPAA), which concerns privacy of medical information. In 2008, the Department of Health and Human Services and the Department of Education issued joint guidelines on the intersection of FERPA and HIPAA. Student health records are specifically covered under FERPA; however, a mechanism exists for alerting parents to potential mental health crises. The exceptions for privacy, outlined in 34 CFR § 99.31(a), include that information may be shared with parents in an emergency situation. As in the case example, when Mark was noted to be having psychotic symptoms—particularly those that warranted an involuntary hospitalization—this threshold was likely met and parents could, and likely should, have been notified. Application of this rule appropriately would have allowed Mark's parents to help coordinate with the college to provide the necessary referral to provide him treatment and reduce his duration of untreated psychosis.

Once identification of a student with psychosis has been made, along with the determination of appropriate care resources, administrators face a difficult decision regarding whether the student is healthy enough to remain in school. At the heart of the dilemma is trying to find the best long-term solution for the student in relation to continuing in a potentially high-pressure academic environment or the pursuit of other life goals. Many schools have de facto policies mandating (or strongly recommending) medical leave after an initial episode; however, these policies are often detrimental to the student. Sending students home is not without risk to the student, because there may not be adequate mental health resources, such as a CSC clinic, in the hometown. Further, many college students returning home find themselves socially isolated because their peers remain at their respective universities. Students sent home may not have further opportunities to sustain their academic progress.

The Judge David L Bazelon Center for Mental Health Law (2007) proposed a set of guidelines for campus mental health treatment. The nearly 50 guidelines suggest that schools create a policy to support students to maintain their academic progress while supporting them with counseling and voluntary leaves of absence when needed. In addition, schools should provide education to students and student health leaders on campus about mental health issues. College counseling centers should be available to students 24/7, including during school holidays. There should be access to emergency services when needed, but student health centers should make provisions for ongoing care to prevent crises from developing. When students need to take time away from school, they should be allowed to maintain contact with peers and professors and to continue coursework remotely if possible. When involuntary leave is necessary, the head of the counseling center should be included in any committee making these case-by-case decisions. Ultimately, schools should provide the resources needed to help maintain students as close to the university as possible.

When students are able to stay enrolled, the college or university has further obligations under federal disability rights law—the same as would apply to students with physical disabilities. These accommodations may take the form of students' being given increased time for examinations or being allowed to take exams in a private area. Students should be allowed to retroactively withdraw from classes if their performance was significantly impacted by their psychiatric symptoms and they were unable to complete the necessary course work to pass the class. Housing accommodations should also be taken into consideration, including whether or not students should have roommates, depending on their specific psychiatric needs. These accommodations should be considered in consultation with the treatment clinician for the student, and the university may require documentation of the illness and needs from a mental health professional (U.S. Department of Education 2015).

Case Example Revisited

Had supports been in place to identify psychosis earlier in the example of Mark, his trajectory could have been different, as illustrated below:

Mark is enrolled at a small university where he is looking forward to majoring in English literature. The university has recently undertaken an early-psychosis education initiative and has trained all student support staff and wellness center staff in how to recognize and respond to the early signs of psychosis. Mark's first year passes uneventfully, and he and his family are pleased with his first-year grades. As a returning sophomore, however, Mark starts to notice difficulty concentrating in class and feeling less motivated. For the first time at college, he receives a B on one of his class finals. On returning to school after the winter break, Mark begins to put in extra hours in the library and finds himself working through the night on several occasions. The RA in his dorm notices this change in his behavior and talks to Mark about this, and although Mark reassures the RA that everything is fine, they agree to touch base again in a couple of weeks. The RA informs the resident dean of the concerns and they agree to monitor the situation. When the RA reconnects with Mark 2 weeks later, Mark confides in the RA that he has been hearing things and that he feels confused and frightened by this. The RA provides Mark with some information about auditory hallucinations, including information on how common these phenomena are and different reasons they might occur (e.g., stress, sleep deprivation, psychosis, drugs). They set up an appointment with a psychiatrist at the student wellness center, and the RA accompanies Mark to this appointment.

The wellness center psychiatrist conducts an assessment in which Mark reports that he has been hearing voices and thinks it is the voice of his angel talking to him. The psychiatrist recommends that Mark receive further evaluation at the local early intervention in psychosis service and reiterates the normalizing message provided by the RA regarding hallucinations. He also provides further information on the importance of early intervention and suggests that Mark also reach out to his family for additional support. Mark does so, and his family travels to the area to attend the appointment with the early-intervention team. Mark is accepted into the service to commence treatment, which includes meeting with an educational and vocational support worker. This support worker coordinates with Mark, his family, and the college to establish a plan to support Mark with his studies, including an amended schedule for the remainder of the semester.

Conclusion

Students presenting with a recent onset of psychosis are heterogeneous and present with many different needs. Although many will have cognitive and social deficits at the onset of illness, this is not the case for all students. The overall panoply of symptoms that one can have—from hallucinations and delusions to primarily negative symptoms, including cognitive difficulties and social isolation—means that careful attention must be paid to the specific needs of each individual. Successful treatment of students in this age group requires an appreciation of the common symptoms, as well as a unique and personalized approach to treatment. There is no "one size fits all" approach to treatment of psychotic illnesses. Providing strong institutional support, easily accessible and free of stigma, gives students the best chance of continued academic success. Once treatment has commenced, students should be supported to maintain their education at the level that best fits their current functioning. When a medical leave is necessary, a plan for return to the college, or completion of studies, should be in place. With early identification and intervention and appropriate educational supports, young people experiencing an onset of psychosis while enrolled in college can be assisted to access the treatment they need and to progress toward their educational goals (see section "Recommendations for Psychiatrists, Psychologists, and Counselors").

KEY CONCEPTS

- College presents a unique opportunity to identify and help students with serious mental illness. With early identification and intervention and appropriate educational supports, young people experiencing an onset of psychosis while enrolled in college can be supported to access the treatment they need and to progress toward their educational goals.

- Providing strong institutional support that is easily accessible and free of stigma gives students with serious mental illness the best chance of continued academic success.

- Forced medical leaves should be used minimally after all other options have been exhausted. When students need to take time away from school, they should be allowed to maintain contact with peers and professors and to continue coursework remotely if possible. When involuntary leave is necessary, the head of the counseling center should be included in any committee that makes these case-by-case decisions.

Recommendations for Psychiatrists, Psychologists, and Counselors[1]

Basic Principles

1. Universities should make extra efforts to ensure that faculty and college counseling staff are trained in early identification of the signs of psychosis and the use of early psychosis screening measures (e.g., Prodromal Questionnaire, Yale PRIME Screen—Revised, Structured Interview for Psychosis-Risk Syndromes).
2. College faculty and staff members should encourage students to utilize on-campus mental health services if students exhibit academic, behavioral, and/or emotional difficulties that could be related to an underlying mental health condition.
3. College counseling centers should make direct efforts to engage and encourage students to access mental health services.
4. College counseling center and emergency psychiatric services should be available 24/7.

Treatment Planning

5. Appropriate treatment and management should follow the coordinated specialty care model, which emphasizes shared decision making and an individualized treatment plan.
6. Treatment care should involve a comprehensive approach that includes evidenced-based psychotherapy, medication management for first-episode psychosis, family psychoeducation and support, case management, and housing and academic accommodations.
7. If the student has been hospitalized, college counseling centers should try to work closely with the hospital treatment team to ensure aftercare planning (the student must consent first).

Accommodations and Leaves of Absence

8. Colleges and universities should provide reasonable housing and academic accommodations to allow students to maintain their academic progress and social relationships.

---

[1]Recommendations are based on "Supporting Students: A Model Policy for Colleges and Universities" (Judge David L. Bazelon Center for Mental Health Law 2007).

9. If medical leave of absence is necessary, students should be allowed to remain in contact with peers and professors to maintain a strong social support network.

10. Absences for treatment and hospitalization should count as excused absences. Students should not be sanctioned or punished for missing classes due to a mental health condition.

Discussion Questions

1. How do students at your university ordinarily find their way to psychiatric treatment? What can be done to help lower the barriers for students seeking treatment for potential psychotic disorder?

2. How does your university typically handle a new-onset psychotic disorder? How is the family contacted? What are the treatment options for students?

3. How does your university help students maintain their academic progress when a psychotic disorder emerges?

Suggested Readings

Heinssen RK, Goldstein AB, Azrin ST: Evidenced-based treatments for first episode psychosis: components of coordinated specialty care. April 14, 2014. Available at: http://www.nasmhpd.org/sites/default/files/ Summary%20of%20Evidence-BasedTreament%20Components %20for%20FEP_14APR_2014_Final.pdf. Accessed July 21, 2017.

Judge David L Bazelon Center for Mental Health Law: Supporting Students: A Model Policy for Colleges and Universities. Washington, DC, Bazelon Center for Mental Health Law, 2007

Stanford University Prodrome and Early Psychosis Program Network (PEPPNET). Available at: https://med.stanford.edu/peppnet.html. Accessed July 21, 2017.

References

Addington J, Heinssen RK, Robinson DG, et al: Duration of untreated psychosis in community treatment settings in the United States. Psychiatr Serv 66(7):753–756, 2015 25588418

Birchwood M, Connor C, Lester H, et al: Reducing duration of untreated psychosis: care pathways to early intervention in psychosis services. Br J Psychiatry 203(1):58–64, 2013 23703317

Brockelman KF, Scheyett AM: Faculty perceptions of accommodations, strategies, and psychiatric advance directives for university students with mental illnesses. Psychiatr Rehabil J 38(4):342–348, 2015 26053532

Bunn W, Terpstra J: Cultivating empathy for the mentally ill using simulated auditory hallucinations. Acad Psychiatry 33(6):457–460, 2009 19933888

Bureau of Labor Statistics: College enrollment and work activity of 2015 high school graduates. April 27, 2017. Available at: https://www.bls.gov/news.release/hsgec.nr0.htm. Accessed July 21, 2017.

Cannon TD, Yu C, Addington J, et al: An individualized risk calculator for research in prodromal psychosis. Am J Psychiatry 173(10):980–988, 2016 27363508

Feeg VD, Prager LS, Moylan LB, et al: Predictors of mental illness stigma and attitudes among college students: using vignettes from a campus common reading program. Issues Ment Health Nurs 35(9):694–703, 2014 25162192

Heinssen RK, Goldstein AB, Azrin ST: Evidence-based treatments for first episode psychosis: components of coordinated specialty care. April 14, 2014. Available at: http://www.nasmhpd.org/sites/default/files/Summary%20of%20Evidence-BasedTreament%20Components%20for%20FEP_14APR_2014_Final.pdf. Accessed July 21, 2017.

Judge David L Bazelon Center for Mental Health Law: Supporting Students: A Model Policy for Colleges and Universities. Washington, DC, Bazelon Center for Mental Health Law, 2007

Kane JM, Robinson DG, Schooler NR, et al: Comprehensive Versus Usual Community Care for First-Episode Psychosis: 2-year outcomes from the NIMH RAISE Early Treatment Program. Am J Psychiatry 173(4):362–372, 2016 26481174

Kosyluk KA, Al-Khouja M, Bink A, et al: Challenging the stigma of mental illness among college students. J Adolesc Health 59(3):325–331, 2016 27324577

Loewy RL, Bearden CE, Johnson JK, et al: The Prodromal Questionnaire (PQ): preliminary validation of a self-report screening measure for prodromal and psychotic syndromes. Schizophr Res 79(1):117–125, 2005 16276559

Miller TJ, Chicchetti D, Markovich PJ, et al: The SIPS Screen: a brief self-report screen to detect the schizophrenia prodrome. Schizophr Res 70(supp l1):78, 2004

Perkins DO, Lieberman JA, Lewis S: First episode, in The American Psychiatric Press Textbook of Schizophrenia, edited by Lieberman JA, Stroup TS, Perkins DO. American Psychiatric Press, 2006, pp 353–364

U.S. Department of Education: Students with Disabilities Preparing for Postsecondary Education. Revised 2015. Available at: https://ed.gov/about/offices/list/ocr/transition.html. Accessed July 21, 2017.

U.S. Department of Health and Human Services, U.S. Department of Education: Joint Guidance on the Application of the Family Educational Rights and Privacy Act (FERPA) and the Health Insurance Portability and Accountability Act of 1996 (HIPAA) to Student Health Records. November 2008. Available at: https://www2.ed.gov/policy/gen/guid/fpco/doc/ferpa-hipaa-guidance.pdf. Accessed July 21, 2017.

CHAPTER 19

Autism Spectrum Disorder

Lawrence K. Fung, M.D., Ph.D.

NEURODEVELOPMENTAL disorders are a group of disorders that involve disruption of brain development. This group of disorders is broadly defined and includes a wide range of psychiatric and neurologic disorders. Psychiatric disorders that belong to this group include autism spectrum disorder (ASD), attention-deficit/hyperactivity disorder (ADHD), intellectual disabilities, and learning disorders. Neurologic disorders such as epilepsy and cerebral palsy are considered neurodevelopmental disorders. Neurogenetic disorders (e.g., fragile X syndrome, tuberous sclerosis, neurofibromatosis type 1) also are among the neurodevelopmental disorders. Among these neurodevelopmental disorders, ASD and ADHD are the most common in the university setting. ADHD is covered in Chapter 13 of this book, so this chapter focuses on autism spectrum disorder.

This chapter is tailored for psychiatrists, psychologists, and leaders of higher education who interact with individuals with ASD. I begin by describing the presentation of ASD in college students. Then I discuss the strengths as well as the challenges of students with ASD. Because the college years represent a critical time for identity formation, I critically analyze the ASD identity as it is perceived by students with ASD and their neurotypical peers. A summary of mental health needs is presented with an analysis of current services provided to college students with ASD. I discuss career development resources and opportunities for college students with ASD. I conclude with a case example that illustrates some of the concepts discussed throughout the chapter.

ASD in College Students

ASD is characterized by challenges with social interactions, restricted interests, cognitive inflexibility, stereotyped behaviors, and sensory aberrations. The prevalence of ASD has increased over the past 30 years. According to the most recent study by the Centers for Disease Control and Prevention (Christensen et al. 2016), 1 in 68 children age 8 years carries a diagnosis of ASD. In a sample of 7,461 adults in the community who participated in a national survey of psychiatric morbidity in England, the prevalence of ASD in adults was estimated to be 1 in 102 (Brugha et al. 2011). In the United States, approximately one-third of individuals with ASD attend a 2- or 4-year college (Shattuck et al. 2012). The prevalence of ASD in college students in a single institution was estimated to be 1 in 52 to 1 in 143 (White et al. 2011).

College students with ASD are often challenged by sociocommunicative differences. Key hurdles these individuals face before entering college include atypical social-emotional reciprocity, aberrant nonverbal communicative behaviors used for social interaction, and difficulties in developing, maintaining, and understanding relationships; these issues commonly persist in college. A common example of difficulty in social-emotional reciprocity is failure of typical back-and-forth conversation. Often, students with ASD have a disproportionate tendency to talk about their topics of interest, and this behavior impedes fluid conversational exchanges. The development of nonverbal communicative abilities, such as understanding and using body language, is often delayed in students with ASD. The immature development of nonverbal communicative abilities puts students with ASD in a disadvantaged situation, because college students often communicate with each other in subtle and nonverbal ways. Consequently, initiating and deepening friendships are often challenging for students with ASD. Compounded by previous adverse experience in social interactions, the lack of rewarding social experience can initiate and precipitate social isolation for some individuals with ASD.

Many students with ASD have a history of highly restricted, fixated interests that are unusual in intensity or focus. When these individuals are younger, the circumscribed or perseverative interests may be quite different from the typical range of interests at their chronological age. As they grow older and become young adults, their restricted interests may become more similar to the interests of their neurotypical peers. However, the level of focus on their fixated interests may be noticeably higher than that of most other students. The activities associated with the restricted interests of many students with ASD are important parts of their daily routines. These students tend to have inflexible adherence to routines; sticking with their schedule is often beneficial for them. Although the consequence of following their schedule can be predictably advantageous, their rigid cognitive thinking style can sometimes prevent them from performing other tasks. Some students with ASD are hypersensitive to noise and therefore have trouble attending large classes, whereas others have a tendency to seek certain sensory inputs. These sensory aberrations can lead to other issues. The former may cause students to avoid going to classes and other social activities, whereas the latter may cause the students to get into trouble, especially when their actions are not welcome by others and the students with ASD are not consciously aware of their actions. Stereotyped or repetitive motor movements are classic symptoms of ASD that are noticeable by most people. When students with ASD are younger, they might flap their hands, line up their toy cars, or repeat television commercials verbatim. When they become young adults, repetitive behaviors tend to become subtler in high-functioning individuals with ASD.

Inasmuch as there are discrete diagnostic criteria for ASD, each student with ASD is unique. College students with ASD tend to have at least average intellectual abilities. A subset of them have very high IQs. Although some students with ASD are not inherently motivated to seek friendships in college, others do have a strong desire to build social relationships. Those who are motivated to make friends in college often struggle with social interactions. Few students with ASD are socially savvy, even if they had years of deliberate social skills training during childhood and adolescence.

Overall, the behavioral phenotype of ASD is highly heterogeneous. One contributing factor to the heterogeneity of the ASD phenotype may be associated with the diverse etiological factors of the disorder. The heritability of ASD has been found to range from 40% to 80% (Hallmayer et al. 2011; Sandin et al. 2014; Tick et al. 2016). Over 1,000 genes have been shown to be associated with ASD (SFARI Gene 2018); about 65 of them are strongly linked to the ASD phenotype (Sanders et al. 2015). Many environmental factors have also been found to be associated with ASD. Another contributing factor to the heterogeneity of the ASD phenotype is related to the developmental nature of the disorder. Although most human beings are able to start walking by age 12–15 months, some take a shorter time and some take a longer time to achieve this important basic motor milestone. When a 16-month-old child is not able to walk, it does not mean that the child will never walk. It only means that the child might have a delayed motor milestone. This child may start walking at 17 months or later, but most children are able to walk sometime in their toddlerhood. Similarly, individuals with ASD may not be socially mature when they enter college at age 18, but they may become more socially capable as they grow older. However, the rates of maturation in their sociocommunicative abilities vary greatly, which contributes to the heterogeneity of the ASD phenotype. Finally, early intervention is believed to be beneficial in reducing symptoms in ASD. Depending on multiple factors, including duration of the treatment and effectiveness of the therapist, the residual ASD symptoms can be highly variable.

In addition to the heterogeneity of the ASD phenotype, the presence of psychiatric comorbidities can make the clinical picture of students with ASD unclear for practitioners who have less experience assessing these individuals. Anxiety, depression, and ADHD are very common in students with ASD. Often, the mental health needs of individuals with ASD revolve around the comorbidities instead of the core symptoms of ASD.

Strengths of University Students With ASD

It is important to recognize that students with ASD are differently abled, illustrated by the following anonymous quote: "Autism is not a processing error. It's a different operating system." In fact, some students with ASD have outstanding abilities to perform specific tasks. Students with ASD who have apparent developmental disabilities can also display strong, sometimes extraordinary, specific talents (e.g., music performance, complex mathematical computations). Depending on the nature of their interests, students with ASD may use a learning style different from that of their neurotypical peers. Qian and Lipkin (2011) proposed a learning-style theory for understanding behaviors of individuals with ASD. They theorized that learning is about fitting training materials (data) with functions that can be generalized to similar situations. Whereas neurotypical individuals tend to use an "interpolation" learning style, individuals with ASD often use a "look-up table" learning style. The latter learning style allows students with ASD to memorize many facts effectively, but they often find making inferences from facts challenging. The look-up table learning style also enhances ASD students' abilities on lexical processing of individual words, but these students may not be very strong in their grammar. Because of their tendency to focus on the facts, students with ASD are very good at hyperfocusing on specific tasks in which they are interested. However, they may not see the big picture of their learning, which is related to weak central coherence, a classic feature of ASD.

Weak central coherence can become an advantage for students with ASD. The restricted interests and rigid cognitive thinking style of many students with ASD can enhance their perseverance on very challenging tasks. These students then are in a great position to focus on their tasks of interest, obtain deeper understanding, and even break new ground with unprecedented discoveries. Many psychiatrists believe that Albert Einstein and Isaac Newton would have been deemed to be on the ASD spectrum if they had been formally assessed. These scientists changed all of our lives because they saw the world very differently from others. Their repetitive behaviors and restricted interests led to discoveries that touch all of our lives. Similarly, when the restricted interests and talents of students with ASD coincide, and if the people around them support their explorations without prejudice, they may be able to excel in what they do and contribute to the community at large.

Specific unusual abilities have been found in some individuals with ASD. One example is visuospatial abilities. For instance, Stephen Wiltshire, a savant with ASD, has drawn exquisite details of landscapes after a single helicopter tour (Mottron 2011). Other examples of remarkable abilities in some individuals with ASD include superior judgment of absolute pitch, memory tasks such as memorizing numbers in phone books, and computations such as calendrical calculations. Many individuals with ASD are better at processing large amounts of perceptual information than their neurotypical peers (Mottron 2011). With hyperfocus on tasks of interest, high level of attention to details, extensive vocabulary, and strengths in visual memory, many students with ASD excel in school. Some students with ASD are strong in science, technology, engineering, and medicine—the STEM fields. One recent study found that children with ASD and superior mathematical information processing possessed a unique pattern of brain organization. These children with ASD were found to utilize in novel ways cortical regions typically involved in perceptual expertise (Iuculano et al. 2014). This finding may explain the atypical and even desirable learning approach used by individuals with ASD.

Challenges of College Students With ASD

Among the various challenges faced by college students with ASD, the most common areas of difficulty include limited interpersonal competence, managing competing demands in postsecondary education, and poor emotion regulation, as revealed by a survey completed by primary stakeholders (including parents, educators and support staff from secondary and postsecondary institutions, and students) (S. W. White et al. 2016). Results from a comprehensive survey of current and former college students with ASD indicate that academic supports appeared to be adequate; however, support in social and emotional domains was found to be suboptimal.

Psychosocial stressors and psychiatric comorbidities are very common in adults with ASD. Transitioning from high school to college is hard for all adolescents but especially for students with ASD. The structure and routines that helped students with ASD be more comfortable in high school are no longer available to them during the transition. The new structure and routines in the college setting may not be easily established, especially when students are not living at home and parents are no longer closely involved in their education. Students with ASD often have Individualized Education Program (IEP) teams of teachers and professionals supporting them before college. Members of IEP teams typically include special education teachers, mainstream teachers, speech therapists, occupational therapists, school psychologists, and parents. An IEP team sets goals to enhance a student's education. Most colleges do not have the resources to form similar teams of professionals to set personalized educational goals for students with ASD. Without the support from a team of professionals, students with ASD entering college are usually not ready to set their own educational goals. This apparent gap in supporting the student in the transition to college can cause tremendous anxiety.

In addition to having academic challenges, entering college students often face challenges living in their new environment. Some students may not have previously shared a room or attended college parties. With deficits in social interactions, these novel experiences can cause extreme anxiety. The cumulative challenges in transitioning to a novel environment, handling a heavy academic load, and maneuvering the complex social settings can cause debilitating anxiety, isolation, withdrawal, and even depression.

Poor executive functioning is very common in students with ASD. Although they may be intellectually capable of learning course materials, they may not be able to get to class or exams on time or to complete their homework because of poor time management skills. They may be able to learn the course materials well, but some students may need more time to complete their tests (sometimes due to slower processing speed). If students with ASD are not able to arrange accommodations with their professors, they may end up receiving poor grades in their classes.

Many students with ASD have significant challenges in interacting socially with their peers. They often have difficulties with interpreting social cues and understanding new social contexts. Owing at least partially to restricted interests, they can sometimes talk about their subjects of interest for a long time without knowing that others have lost interest in the topic. Contrary to most people's perception of ASD, most students with ASD are motivated to make new friends in college, but not all are able to successfully establish true friendships. Furthermore, like their peers, students with ASD are interested in pursuing romantic relationships. Intimate relationships are important in development and are very salient in emerging adulthood. Secure romantic attachment in adulthood is associated with greater commitment, trust, and satisfaction. However, the growth of the capacity for sexual feelings during puberty may not be accompanied by a parallel growth of knowledge in sexual issues.

Individuals with ASD often have challenges in monitoring their own emotions and understanding other people's emotions. Emotion dysregulation can be triggered by a variety of external factors. For individuals with ASD, the triggers may be associated with sensory hyperreactivity or sociocommunicative difficulties. Emotion dysregulation can lead to anger, or even more serious consequences such as self-injurious behaviors and aggressive behaviors toward others.

During the formative years in college, students establish their individual identities. The diagnosis of ASD, the ways in which students with ASD view themselves, and the ways in which other students and teachers perceive ASD can collectively affect the well-being of students with ASD.

The ASD Identity and College Students' Perceptions of ASD

Identity formation is a complex developmental task for adolescents and young adults in general. For individuals with ASD, disability identification and self-efficacy can positively or negatively affect this developmental stage. Individuals with ASD may not have the strongest sense of their own emotions, but they are often sensitive to the ASD label. In the fifth edition of the *Diagnostic and Statistical Manual of Mental Disorders* (DSM-5), the American Psychiatric Association (2013) formally created the new ASD diagnosis, merging the DSM-IV diagnoses of autistic disorder, Asperger's disorder, and pervasive development disorder not otherwise specified. Before DSM-5 was published, many students with ASD had the diagnosis of Asperger's disorder. Individuals with Asperger's disorder have at least average intelligence and do not have language development delays. Some students with Asperger's disorder are quite gifted, and some excel in school. Therefore, for some individuals with ASD and their families, the Asperger's diagnosis may mean a better prognosis, and consequently a lot of students with the Asperger's diagnosis relate to this identity more than to an ASD diagnosis. Students with Asperger's disorder may not want the ASD label because they are sometimes concerned about peer reactions if they disclose their ASD diagnosis and peer acceptance of their atypical behaviors when they disclose their ASD diagnosis.

Using data collected from the National Longitudinal Transition Study–2 involving 11,000 students, 920 of whom were diagnosed with ASD, Shattuck and colleagues (2014) reported that 69% of college students with ASD considered themselves to have a disability or special need. Yet, 72% of college students with ASD reported a high level of confidence in their ability to get information they need and to get school staff and other adults to listen to them. In this study, students were asked to rate various statements including "You can handle most things that come your way," an item that was rated lower among students majoring in STEM. Notably, 41% of students with ASD were STEM majors.

Interestingly, in a recent study to investigate the affective responses of college students toward potential peers with ASD, neurotypical students appeared to show more positive responses or less negative responses when they were aware of a peer's ASD diagnosis (Brosnan and Mills 2016). In another study examining the knowledge of and attitudes toward students with ASD, neurotypical students who identified a high number of incorrect traits categorized as aggressive or misleading were more likely to have less positive attitudes toward their peers with ASD (D. White et al. 2016). Matthews and colleagues (2015) examined the attitudes toward students with ASD among college students in a single 4-year university in the United States. Using vignettes with characters manifesting behaviors characteristic of ASD, the authors assessed the attitudes of neurotypical college students toward characters in three labeling conditions: 1) characters labeled as high-functioning college students with ASD, 2) characters labeled as neurotypical college students, and 3) characters without labels. Students assigned to the ASD label condition reported more positive attitudes toward the vignette characters than students assigned to the no label condition. These results indicate that knowledge of the ASD diagnosis can improve neurotypical college students' attitudes toward college students with ASD. Matthews and colleagues also studied the relationships between the attitudes toward students with ASD and the study participants' gender, knowledge about ASD, and level of broad autism phenotype (BAP) characteristics. Higher BAP scores indicate the presence of more ASD-like characteristics. Male students and students with lower scores on the BAP Questionnaire reported more positive attitudes across the three labeling conditions.

The findings described above have important practical implications for college students with ASD. They imply that within a university environment, disclosing the ASD diagnosis to peers could help students with ASD reduce their own level of perceived stigma. This reduced stigma can potentially lower the anxiety of students with ASD in the college environment and increase their willingness to seek help from the school's disability support services and health professionals.

D. White and colleagues (2016) also found that college students who personally knew someone with ASD would be more likely to have positive attitudes toward peers with ASD. On the contrary, those who had no prior personal relationships with an individual with ASD were more likely to notice observable traits commonly seen among those with ASD (e.g., flat facial expression, poor eye contact).

An important consideration is how college campuses can disseminate knowledge about ASD to improve college students' attitudes toward students with ASD. To improve students' understanding of college students with ASD, Gillespie-Lynch and colleagues (2015) developed online training about ASD and piloted the training with 365 undergraduate students taking psychology courses in a 4-year university. Participants completed a pretest, online training, and a posttest. Participation in the training was associated with increased knowledge about ASD. Misconceptions about ASD were common among the participants. For example, they confused ASD with other disorders, such as learning disabilities. This study demonstrated that online training in knowledge about ASD is a feasible approach to increasing college students' understanding and acceptance of their peers with ASD.

Mental Health Services for College Students With ASD

Students with ASD need to have access to mental health services. Despite having intact cognitive skills, most college students with ASD struggle with independence and interactions with others. These difficulties can be stressful and predispose these students to depression and anxiety. A systematic review of the literature describing experience and supports of individuals with ASD enrolled in college and university programs revealed that anxiety was the most commonly reported experience (71%), followed by loneliness (53%) and depression (47%) (Gelbar et al. 2014).

Cognitive-behavioral therapy (CBT) is a promising treatment for depression and anxiety in the general population. Accumulating evidence has also supported that this therapeutic modality is effective in treating anxiety and depression in high-functioning adolescents with ASD. Although no large trials have been reported about use of CBT in college students or high-functioning young adults with ASD, case series and case reports have suggested that CBT is helpful in treating depression and anxiety in this population (Lake et al. 2014).

The precipitation of anxiety and depression in individuals with ASD is in part related to their stressful social interactions with others. Although many college students have already received some social skills training before they enter college, they often still struggle with communicating with peers in social settings. Most studies of social skills training in high-functioning adults with ASD involve CBT and/or parent involvement. Cognitive enhancement therapy (CET) is an emerging treatment for ASD. Originally developed for treatment of schizophrenia, CET employs computer-based and/or group-based exercises designed to improve both social and nonsocial cognitive function through strategic training and repetitive practice. An 18-month feasibility study demonstrated that CET improved both cognitive function and social behavior in adults with ASD (Eack et al. 2013). A systematic review of psychosocial interventions for adults with ASD found six studies of social cognition training in high-functioning individuals on the spectrum (Bishop-Fitzpatrick et al. 2013). Social cognition training seeks to improve patients' ability to understand social cues, thereby improving social functioning. Four of these studies utilized computer-based training, which teaches patients to detect facial expressions and emotions in the eyes. Five of the six studies reported significant improvements in social cognition, communication, and social skills.

Pharmacological treatments of anxiety and depression are typically indicated when psychotherapeutic treatments are partially or minimally effective. Antidepressants such as selective serotonin reuptake inhibitors can potentially be helpful for reducing depression and anxiety. It is important to note that beneficial effects from these treatments typically take several weeks to emerge. Some students with ASD have a history of irritability and associated aggressive behaviors. If these behaviors are severe, treatment with atypical antipsychotic medications may be indicated. Because individuals with ASD are often more sensitive to medications than their neurotypical peers, a more conservative approach, including slower titration schedule and lower starting dose, is recommended.

Academic Support for College Students With ASD

In summarizing what needs to be done to maximize the potential of college students with ASD, it is helpful to consider the "Seven Vectors of Development" during the college years, as articulated by Chickering and Reisser (1993). The seven vectors are developing competence, managing emotions, moving through autonomy toward interdependence, developing mature interpersonal relationships, establishing identity, developing purpose, and developing integrity. Using the seven vectors as a construct, Table 19–1 summarizes the various tasks that students with ASD, school officials and disability professionals, and mental health professionals need to do to support these students during this important and formative period in their lives.

Although mental health resources are crucial for college students with ASD, optimal academic support can also reduce their anxiety and improve their quality of life (Pinder-Amaker 2014). College officials who know that they have students with ASD need to proactively reach out to these students and create more structure and predictability for them. Counseling supports (e.g., developing checklists for assignments, prioritizing tasks), modifications in the classroom (e.g., decreasing distractions, providing written instructions), and accommodations for testing (providing a separate location with less distraction and extra time) should be available to students with ASD. Because of difficulties in cognitive flexibility, students with ASD need to be provided with advance notice of meetings, topics to be discussed, and changes in schedules. Resident advisors of residence halls should be alerted to the presence of a student with ASD. Peer mentors may help students with ASD acclimate to the new school environment. Resident advisors and peer mentors should be trained to detect warning signs of depression or anxiety in students with ASD. Without such proactive supports, these students are at increased risk for anxiety, depression, and even suicide.

Various universities have implemented innovative programs to support college students with ASD. These programs aim to address the difficulties in executive functioning and social-emotional regulation in students with ASD. They can be categorized under five common service

TABLE 19–1. Developmental tasks for students with autism spectrum disorder (ASD) and support they need during college

Vectors of development during college[a]	Strategies for students with ASD	Support from school officials/disability professionals	Support from mental health professionals
Developing competence	Seek help from professionals; develop strengths and interests through college courses; continue to develop nonacademic interests such as music and sports.	Tutoring; academic coaching	
Managing emotions	Seek help from professionals; acquire skills to manage a variety of emotions (both positive and negative); develop support system in college setting; maintain support from family and close friends.	Reaching out to students with ASD	Psychotherapy; pharmacological treatments
Moving through autonomy toward interdependence	Develop interpersonal competence (e.g., active listening, collaborating); begin separation from parents on emotional needs, and start relying on peers and other adults in school; participate in social activities.	Organizing group activities; establishing a mentoring program	Social skills group
Developing mature interpersonal relationships	Participate in social activities; develop more in-depth sharing but less clinging; accept imperfect relationships; nurture relationships.	Cultivating inclusion; educating neurotypical students and teachers about ASD; educating individuals with ASD about intimacy	

TABLE 19–1. Developmental tasks for students with autism spectrum disorder (ASD) and support they need during college (*continued*)

Vectors of development during college[a]	Strategies for students with ASD	Support from school officials/disability professionals	Support from mental health professionals
Establishing identity	Accept the ASD identity; disclose their identity to peers; accept identity with respect to physical appearance, cultural influence, ethnic heritage, and sexual orientation.	Understanding the needs of students with ASD	Individual counseling
Developing purpose	Explore career options and long-term personal interests.	Providing vocational counseling and programs designed to bring students with ASD to the workforce	
Developing integrity	Develop values that incorporate various subtle factors (e.g., gestures in social interactions) and accommodate ambiguities and uncertainty (this is especially hard for students with ASD because of their cognitive style).		Individual counseling

[a]Chickering and Reisser 1993.

models: those with a clinical focus, social skills focus, and academic skills focus; research-based models; and mixed models (Gerhardt et al. 2014). The services involved with a program having a clinical focus include individual counseling, group therapy, and supported living and transportation. Therapists may be licensed social workers, psychologists, or psychiatrists. Sometimes, the students needing such programs may live in off-campus residential program housing. In programs with the social skills focus, a mentoring program, social skills group, and social activities are the key activities; these services are provided by disability services professionals, as well as by neurotypical students and professors in the university. Programs focusing on support of academic skills are typically offered by disability services offices, tutoring centers, or agencies in the community; these programs offer tutoring and academic coaching. In some universities, psychosocial and other novel interventions are being studied; the researchers offer assessments and treatments for students who participate in the research studies. When students are applying for college, parents should consider assessing the needs of their students and strive to find a college that can provide the services that individual students need.

Students with ASD often receive significant support from IEP teams while they are in elementary, middle, and high schools. Vanbergeijk and colleagues (2008) proposed that students with ASD also should be supported by an individualized college plan (ICP). They recommend that the ICP should define academic modifications, social skills training goals, independent living skills, vocational goals, and mental health supports. The ICP team would be composed of the student, a disability services professional, a mental health professional, a peer mentor, and a faculty member or academic advisor. The main goals of the ICP team are to facilitate the transition of students with ASD from high school to college, as well as to guide them academically and socially during their time in college. They may even collaborate with other professionals to help students transition from college to the workforce.

Career Development Opportunities for College Students With ASD

One major overall goal for college students with ASD is to start establishing independence. The transition from school to a work setting is one of the biggest hurdles for individuals with ASD. Approximately 50%–75% of high-functioning adults with ASD are unemployed (Smith et al. 2015). Even students with ASD who excelled academically often have trouble understanding what it takes to get a job. Individuals with ASD often have difficulties identifying the right jobs for which they should apply and with the stress involved with handling job applications. After getting a job, keeping the job requires good communication with supervisors, colleagues, and customers. Some jobs require flexibility. The lack of routine can create tremendous distress for some adults with ASD.

Supported employment programs have been shown to significantly increase the success rate in obtaining a job for individuals with ASD. Mawhood and Howlin (1999) conducted a study in the United Kingdom to assess a supported employment program for high-functioning individuals with ASD. The program involved employment specialists who were responsible for identifying appropriate job sites, providing guidance to the worker with ASD for the first 2–4 weeks of the program, ensuring that the participant could cope with the social and work-related requirements of the job, educating employers about ASD and the focus of supportive employment, and advising coworkers and supervisors on how to deal with problems that might arise during participants' employment. The support was tapered down to weekly visits within the second month, and then further decreased to only occasional visits by the fourth month. The supported employment program was shown to result in successful offers for two-thirds of participants, compared with only 25% of participants in the control group.

With advances in artificial intelligence, virtual reality job interview training (VR-JIT) has become a reality. In an efficacy trial, VR-JIT was shown to improve interviewing skills among trainees with ASD (Smith et al. 2015). At a 6-month follow-up, VR-JIT trainees had a greater chance of attaining a competitive position than control subjects. These results suggest that VR-JIT is a promising method to enhance vocational outcomes among high-functioning adults with ASD.

Because high-functioning individuals with ASD appear to do well in the STEM fields, some technology companies have embraced the opportunity to recruit young adults with ASD to their workforce. Companies such as Specialisterne (http://usa.specialisterne.com) have a mission to match the talents of people with ASD with employment opportunities. Pilot projects have been successful in demonstrating the positive impact of empowering individuals with ASD in many countries around the world. Furthermore, using novel methods for assessing, training, and managing neurodiverse talent, companies such as SAP are demonstrating that the neurodiverse approach to their workforce is yielding significant innovations by teams with employees with ASD (Austin and Pisano 2017).

Case Example

Ed is a 16-year-old incoming first-year college student with an IQ of 140 and intense interest in aeronautics. He was able to master calculus when he was 11; he knows the periodic table by heart; he knows all the factoids about space shuttles. Ed was accepted at a prestigious university to study aerospace engineering through its early decision program. His dream is to become an astronaut one day.

Ed has carried a diagnosis of Asperger's disorder since he was 4 years old. He has never lived away from home. Before starting college, his parents provided everything he needed. He has never cooked, done his laundry, or paid any bills. He has never developed a habit of cleaning up his room or anywhere he has lived. His social skills have been very limited since he was young. During high school, Ed had one best friend, Harry, who likes aeronautics as well. Harry was accepted to another prestigious university to study mechanical engineering. Ed and Harry saw each other twice in the summer before matriculating to college.

Like most first-year students, Ed chose to live in the dormitory in his first year of college. He was assigned to a double room in a coed dormitory. His first roommate, Garrett, was a friendly 18-year-old majoring in history. Garrett invited Ed to attend activities in the dormitory, but Ed declined all opportunities. Ed did not make any friends in his first year of college. He focused on his studies, but his forgetfulness led to late submission of his assignments. Furthermore, he took on a very large course load, which became increasingly more overwhelming for him. Ed believed that he was too busy, so he was not motivated to do even basic personal care, including taking a shower and doing his laundry. His roommate complained about Ed's personal hygiene. This issue was even discussed among others in the dormitory, and Ed became an infamous character of the dormitory. Several students posted threatening notes on the door of his room.

In the second semester, Ed began missing classes, gained 30 pounds, slept 15 hours a night, and stayed in his room most of the time. He was not able to focus on his studies and had no support of any kind near him. For the first time in his life, his grades dropped and he even failed two classes. One day, while thinking about how to explain his grades to his parents, he crossed the road in front of his dormitory without looking and was hit by a car. He sustained significant injuries of his lower extremities, and was hospitalized for 3 weeks. After the accident, Ed's parents visited the university's dean of students, and found out that Ed had not received any support from the university in his first year. The dean recommended that Ed take a leave of absence for a semester and then receive counseling from a school psychologist after returning to school.

While Ed was recovering from his injuries, his parents visited 10 universities with programs that were designed to serve individuals with neurodevelopmental disorders. They found that these programs have dedicated staff members to help students with ASD transition from high school to college. These programs also have academic coaches who help students determine their learning styles, optimize learning objectives, and learn how to advocate for themselves. Furthermore, these programs have staff members assigned to assist students with ASD to gain independent living skills. These programs also recruit and train typically developing students to engage with students with ASD and help them with connecting to the rest of the college community. Importantly, the cultures of these universities support neurodiversity.

With his parents' involvement, Ed decided to transfer to one of the universities with dedicated programs for students with ASD. Ed did extremely well in his new school. He made several close friends in his class. He graduated with honors in aerospace engineering and was accepted to a master's degree program of a top university. He continues to pursue his dream of becoming an astronaut someday.

This case example demonstrates that high-functioning individuals with ASD often struggle with challenges in executive function, social interactions, and living independently. The lack of support for these individuals is very common. Very few schools have dedicated programs supporting the transition from high school to college. However, when the support is available, individuals with ASD can excel academically and their social skills can grow steadily.

Conclusion

In this chapter, I have described the presentation of high-functioning college students with ASD, summarized their strengths and challenges in the formative years in college, and provided guidelines of what support they need in the university setting. The environment these students face in college can shape their formation of and perception of their own identity as individuals with ASD. I have provided evidence on the desirable outcomes of disclosing the ASD diagnosis to peers as well as the benefits of educating neurotypical students in the university setting. In addition to the interactions with neurotypical students, the college experience of students with ASD is also influenced by the mental health services, academic, and career development support they receive. Currently, most tertiary education institutions do not have programs providing such support tailored for students with ASD. Much is yet to be done to help students with ASD to succeed and contribute to society.

KEY CONCEPTS

- College students with autism spectrum disorder (ASD) are differently abled. They tend to be hyperfocused on tasks of interest. They can have a high level of attention to details, extensive vocabulary, and strengths in visual memory.
- Poor executive functioning and sociocommunicative abilities are major challenges for high-functioning adults with ASD.
- Students on the autism spectrum are sometimes reluctant to disclose their ASD diagnosis, but studies have found that disclosing the ASD diagnosis to peers could help them to reduce the level of perceived stigma.
- College officials should take a proactive approach to help students with ASD and establish programs that can help the students to overcome anticipated academic and social difficulties.
- While it is important to help students transition from high school to college, it is also important for college officials to prepare students to transition from college to the workforce.

Recommendations for Psychiatrists, Psychologists, and Counselors

1. A proactive approach to helping students with ASD in overcoming their challenges socially and academically in various stages of their time in college is necessary. Mental health professionals are encouraged to participate in additional training programs to strengthen their skills for working with individuals with ASD.
2. A major measure of success for students with ASD is their ability to live independently. In assessing students' mental health needs, clinicians should inquire how the students are doing in the following domains of transition: housing, general health, academic performance, social interactions with peers, interactions with faculty and staff, and employment.

3. Enhancing students' skills to advocate for themselves is recommended.
4. Liaising with school officials to facilitate students' use of supportive, nonstigmatizing, and developmentally appropriate programs at school is strongly encouraged.

Discussion Questions

1. What are the strengths of students with ASD?
2. What challenges do students with ASD face?
3. How can the university address the needs of students with ASD?
4. What are some of the services that mental health professionals offer to support and treat students with ASD?
5. How can companies use the talents of individuals with ASD?

Suggested Readings

Mottron L: Changing perceptions: the power of autism. Nature 479(7371):33–35, 2011
Pinder-Amaker S: Identifying the unmet needs of college students on the autism spectrum. Harv Rev Psychiatry 22(2):125–137, 2014
Vanbergeijk E, Klin A, Volkmar F: Supporting more able students on the autism spectrum: college and beyond. J Autism Dev Disord 38(7):1359–1370, 2008

References

American Psychiatric Association: Diagnostic and Statistical Manual of Mental Disorders, 5th Edition. Arlington, VA, American Psychiatric Association, 2013
Austin RD, Pisano GP: Neurodiversity as a competitive advantage. Harv Bus Rev May-June:96–103, 2017
Bishop-Fitzpatrick L, Minshew NJ, Eack SM: A systematic review of psychosocial interventions for adults with autism spectrum disorders. J Autism Dev Disord 43(3):687–694, 2013 22825929
Brosnan M, Mills E: The effect of diagnostic labels on the affective responses of college students towards peers with 'Asperger's syndrome' and 'autism spectrum disorder'. Autism 20(4):388–394, 2016 26045542
Brugha TS, McManus S, Bankart J, et al: Epidemiology of autism spectrum disorders in adults in the community in England. Arch Gen Psychiatry 68(5):459–465, 2011 21536975
Chickering AW, Reisser L: Education and Identity. San Francisco, CA, Jossey-Bass, 1993

Christensen DL, Baio J, Van Naarden Braun K, et al: Prevalence and character-istics of autism spectrum disorder among children aged 8 years—Autism and Developmental Disabilities Monitoring Network, 11 sites, United States, 2012. MMWR Surveill Summ 65(3):1–23, 2016 27031587

Eack SM, Greenwald DP, Hogarty SS, et al: Cognitive enhancement therapy for adults with autism spectrum disorder: results of an 18-month feasibility study. J Autism Dev Disord 43(12):2866–2877, 2013 23619953

Gelbar NW, Smith I, Reichow B: Systematic review of articles describing expe-rience and supports of individuals with autism enrolled in college and uni-versity programs. J Autism Dev Disord 44(10):2593–2601, 2014 24816943

Gerhardt PF, Cicero F, Mayville E: Employment and related services for adults with autism spectrum disorders, in Adolescents and Adults With Autism Spectrum Disorders. Edited by Volkmar FR, Reichow B, McPartland JC. New York, Springer, 2014 pp 104–119

Gillespie-Lynch K, Brooks PJ, Someki F, et al: Changing college students' con-ceptions of autism: an online training to increase knowledge and decrease stigma. J Autism Dev Disord 45(8):2553–2566, 2015 25796194

Hallmayer J, Cleveland S, Torres A, et al: Genetic heritability and shared envi-ronmental factors among twin pairs with autism. Arch Gen Psychiatry 68(11):1095–1102, 2011 21727249

Iuculano T, Rosenberg-Lee M, Supekar K, et al: Brain organization underlying superior mathematical abilities in children with autism. Biol Psychiatry 75(3):223–230, 2014 23954299

Lake JK, Perry A, Lunsky Y: Mental health services for individuals with high functioning autism spectrum disorder. Autism Res Treat 2014:502420, 2014 DOI: 10.1155/2014/502420 25276425

Matthews NL, Ly AR, Goldberg WA: College students' perceptions of peers with autism spectrum disorder. J Autism Dev Disord 45(1):90–99, 2015 25070469

Mawhood L, Howlin P: The outcome of a supported employment scheme for high-functioning adults with autism or Asperger syndrome. Autism 3(4):229–254, 1999

Mottron L: Changing perceptions: the power of autism. Nature 479(7371):33–35, 2011 22051659

Pinder-Amaker S: Identifying the unmet needs of college students on the autism spectrum. Harv Rev Psychiatry 22(2):125–137, 2014 24614767

Qian N, Lipkin RM: A learning-style theory for understanding autistic behav-iors. Front Hum Neurosci 5:77, 2011 21886617

Sanders J, He X, Willsey AJ, et al: Insights into autism spectrum disorder genomic architecture and biology from 71 risk loci. Neuron 87(6):1095–1102, 2015 26402605

Sandin S, Lichtenstein P, Kuja-Halkola R, et al: The familial risk of autism. JAMA 311(17):1770–1777, 2014 24794370

SFARI Gene: Human Gene Module. Available at https://gene.sfari.org/database/human-gene/. Accessed January 18, 2018.

Shattuck PT, Narendorf SC, Cooper B, et al: Postsecondary education and employ-ment among youth with an autism spectrum disorder. Pediatrics 129(6):1042–1049, 2012 22585766

Shattuck PT, Steinberg J, Yu J, et al: Disability identification and self-efficacy among college students on the autism spectrum. Autism Res Treat 2014:924182, 2014 24707401

Smith MJ, Fleming MF, Wright MA, et al: Brief report: vocational outcomes for young adults with autism spectrum disorders at six months after virtual reality job interview training. J Autism Dev Disord 45(10):3364–3369, 2015 25986176

Tick B, Bolton P, Happe F, et al: Heritability of autism spectrum disorders: a meta-analysis of twin studies. J Child Psychol Psychiatry 57(5):585–595, 2016 26709141

Vanbergeijk E, Klin A, Volkmar F: Supporting more able students on the autism spectrum: college and beyond. J Autism Dev Disord 38(7):1359–1370, 2008 18172747

White D, Hillier A, Frye A, Makrez E: College students' knowledge and attitudes towards students on the autism spectrum. J Autism Dev Disord, May 26, 2016 [Epub ahead of print] 27230760

White SW, Ollendick TH, Bray BC: College students on the autism spectrum: prevalence and associated problems. Autism 15(6):683–701, 2011 21610191

White SW, Elias R, Salinas CE, et al: Students with autism spectrum disorder in college: results from a preliminary mixed methods needs analysis. Res Dev Disabil 56:29–40, 2016 27262124

CHAPTER 20

The Suicidal Student

Michele S. Berk, Ph.D.
Molly Adrian, Ph.D.

SUICIDE is the second leading cause of death among individuals ages 15–24 years in the United States (Centers for Disease Control and Prevention 2014). Among college students, 9.8% reported seriously considering suicide in the past 12 months, 6.7% reported engaging in intentional self-injury, and 1.5% reported attempting suicide (American College Health Association 2016). Rates are higher among students who have sought help from college counseling centers. Data collected from college counseling centers in the 2015–2016 academic year showed that 25.5% of students seen reported having engaged in intentional self-injury, 33.2% had seriously considered suicide, and 9.3% had previously attempted suicide (Center for Collegiate Mental Health 2017). As shown in Table 20–1, both suicide attempts and nonsuicidal self-injury are robust risk factors for future suicidal behavior (Shain 2016). Taken together, these data demonstrate the need for effective suicide prevention strategies for college students. In this chapter, we address this need by reviewing the extant data related to college students on suicide risk factors, risk assessment, safety planning, and treatment approaches.

Risk Factors for Suicidal Behavior in College Students

Numerous risk factors for suicide and suicide attempts have been identified in the research literature and are similar across adolescent and adult populations. Risk factors include 1) prior suicidality and self-harm behavior (e.g., suicidal ideation, nonsuicidal self-injury, prior suicide attempts); 2) psychiatric disorders (e.g., mood disorders, substance abuse and dependence, conduct disorder, borderline personality disorder, anxiety, psychotic disorders); 3) cognitive, emotional, and behavioral states and traits (e.g., hopelessness, poor problem-solving skills, perception of being a burden to others, emotion dysregulation, impulsivity, risk-taking behavior, anger, aggression, acute insomnia with agitation, acute psychosis); 4) environmental circumstances (e.g., loneliness, social isolation, negative life events, access to lethal means, family conflict, contagion, bullying); 5) identification as lesbian, gay, bisexual, transgender, or queer/questioning (LGBTQ); 6) genetic factors (family history of suicide); and 7) gender (male individuals are more likely to die by suicide) and age (suicide is the second leading cause of death for individuals ages 15–24 in the United States [Centers for Disease Control and Prevention 2014]). Additional risk factors may exist; however, the large number of studies and the variation across studies make it difficult to compile an exhaustive list (for reviews, see Franklin et al. 2017; Suicide Prevention Resource Center 2014).

Despite the identification of multiple risk factors, it remains impossible for clinicians to accurately predict which individuals with these risk factors will go on to attempt suicide at any given time or will ultimately die by suicide (Fowler 2012). Risk increases with the number of risk factors present; however, no algorithms exist to predict which combinations of risk factors are most likely to lead to suicidal behavior (Franklin et al. 2017). Suicide prevention efforts have logically focused on identification of individuals at risk, linkage of those individuals to mental health services, and the use of treatment approaches that directly target the reduction and/or elimination of malleable risk factors.

TABLE 20–1. Definitions of suicidal and self-harm behaviors

Behavior	Definition[a]	Risk/relation to suicide[b]
Suicide attempt	A potentially self-injurious behavior associated with at least some nonzero intent to die.	Strongest predictor; method critical to understanding risk Moderate false-positive rate
Interrupted attempt	Person begins to take steps toward making a suicide attempt, but somebody else stops the person prior to any self-injurious behavior.	Unknown predictive strength
Aborted attempt	Person begins to take steps toward making a suicide attempt but stops prior to any self-injurious behavior.	Unknown predictive strength
Nonsuicidal self-injury	Self-injurious act without any intent to die. Often associated with other goals, such as to relieve distress.	Strong predictor, potentially equal to suicide attempt
Suicidal ideation	Thinking about killing self; ranges from passive (wish to be dead) to active (thoughts about killing self).	High false-positive risk

[a]Posner et al. 2009. [b]Fowler 2012.

As discussed in other chapters in this book, there are unique aspects of the lives of college students that may increase their risk for suicidal behavior via the presence or exacerbation of the risk factors described above. Students may be living away from home for the first time and coping with increased academic and social stressors as well as disruptions in their preexisting social support networks. These stressors may contribute to the onset of mental illness, as well as to an increase in risk factors such as loneliness, hopelessness, and social isolation. Moreover, students who enter college with preexisting mental health needs may be without the supervision of parents who had been closely monitoring their safety and compliance with needed mental health services. Alcohol use and substance use are also risk factors for suicidal behavior and are common among college students. In the general college population, 63.6% of students reported using alcohol and 18.6% reported using marijuana within the past 30 days (American College Health Association

2016). Finally, students may have increased opportunities to engage in suicidal behavior, as a result of the lack of close monitoring by adults.

Despite the high prevalence of mental health problems, colleges and universities have limits on their resources to help students in need. According to the National Survey of College Counseling Centers, 30% of college counseling center directors reported that (with some exceptions) students are allowed a limited number of counseling sessions, whereas 43% of the directors reported promoting their center as a short-term counseling service but not having a specific limit on the number of sessions (Gallagher 2014). In addition, it was reported that only 58% of students at 4-year colleges have access to an on-campus psychiatrist. The directors of college counseling centers reported 125 student suicides in the preceding year; 86% of these students had not sought counseling center assistance. Hence, increased availability of on-campus care is needed, in addition to strategies for identifying and linking at-risk students to these services as well as to off-campus mental health services beyond the scope of what the college counseling center can provide.

Campus Suicide Prevention Protocols

It is recommended that all universities have a protocol outlining a formal, standardized response to students at risk for suicide. These protocols must take into account an array of complicated issues, such as whether or not mental health services for students at risk are mandated by the university; when to maintain student confidentiality or inform parents; and whether or not the student can safely remain at the university or should withdraw (for a review, see Cohen 2007). Exemplary strategies for campus-wide suicide prevention have been developed by counseling centers at the University of Illinois (https://counselingcenter.illinois.edu/outreach-consultation-prevention/outreach-consultation-teams/suicide-prevention-program/suicide) and at the University of Puget Sound (www.pugetsound.edu/student-life/counseling-health-and-wellness/suicide-prevention/suicide-prevention-at-ups/marssh-protocol). At both of these institutions, students who are identified as being at increased risk for suicide are mandated to attend a minimum of four assessment sessions with a campus mental health professional or risk being withdrawn from the university. At the University of Illinois, suicide rates declined by almost half during the 21-year follow-up period since the program began, compared with the 8-year period prior to the existence of the program (Joffe 2008). Additional components of these protocols include a process for student body members, staff, and faculty to escalate concerns about student safety; an on-campus committee that reviews all concerns about potential suicide risk; an articulation of how to intervene when risk is high; and management strategies including safety planning and an array of resources for psychological treatment. Use of such protocols may be of benefit by increasing the likelihood that high-risk students receive appropriate mental health care and experience fewer disruptions in their education, while offering legal protection to the university (Cohen 2007; Joffe 2008).

Suicide Risk Assessment

All clinical contacts with potentially suicidal students should include detailed risk assessment. Core components of suicide risk assessment include inquiry about current and past history of suicidal ideation, suicide attempts, and nonsuicidal self-injury; risk and protective factors; access to lethal means; and the availability of friends, family, or residence advisors/campus staff to provide safety monitoring of the suicidal individual. Structured interviews, such as the Columbia Suicide Severity Rating Scale (CSSRS; Posner et al. 2011), the Linehan Risk Assessment and Management Protocol (LRAMP; Linehan et al. 2012), and the Collaborative Assessment and Management of Suicidality (CAMS) framework Suicide Status Form (Jobes 2006), may assist clinicians in conducting and documenting a comprehensive risk assessment.

If it is determined that a student is at high risk of imminent suicidal behavior, psychiatric hospitalization should be considered. However, decisions about hospitalization should be made conservatively, and the best interest of the student should be prioritized over concerns about liability, because there are no empirical data supporting the effectiveness of hospitalization versus outpatient care, and hospitalization may have iatrogenic effects (Pistorello et al. 2017). If the decision is that the individual does not require hospitalization but is at increased risk, the therapist should work with the patient and the individual's residence directors, friends, and family to ensure that lethal means have been removed and that someone is available to monitor safety. The therapist should also increase the frequency of contact with the patient, via additional therapy visits and phone calls (Bongar et al. 1998; Shaffer et al. 2001).

Managing Suicide Risk: Safety Recommendations

Regardless of the specific population or the treatment approach, several basic safety strategies should be used when working with all suicidal individuals. Restricting access to lethal means has been shown to be a highly effective suicide prevention strategy (Barber and Miller 2014). Firearms were the most common method used in 51% of suicide deaths between 1996 and 2010 in the United States, followed by hanging/suffocation (33.9%) and poisoning (7.9%) (Fontanella et al. 2015). Hence, it is essential that individuals who are suicidal do not have access to guns (for information about how to safely remove and/or store a firearm, see www.hsph.harvard.edu/means-matter/recommendations/families/). Indeed, the rates of suicide among college students are lower than those of age- and gender-matched control subjects, primarily owing to an approximately ninefold decrease in the availability of firearms on campus versus off campus (Schwartz 2011). Suicidal individuals should be directed to remove all lethal means (e.g., guns, pills, knives, razors) from their residences and possession. If the individual is unwilling and/or unable to do this, then it may be necessary to involve residence directors and assistants, campus security, family, friends, or other known staff and faculty to assist with this task. It may also be necessary to block access to "suicide hotspots," such as bridges, tall buildings, cliffs, and trains, if these exist in proximity to the campus (Public Health England 2015). Access to lethal means should be assessed repeatedly, in every contact with suicidal clients, because new means may be acquired between sessions or it may be revealed that they have been hiding means that they had not yet been willing to give up. We have found that using the following metaphorical question works well to illustrate the risk of impulsive suicidal behavior when means are readily available: "If you were on a diet, would you be more likely to break your diet if you did or did not have a chocolate cake in your kitchen?" Although the client can always acquire additional means for self-harm, removing the possibility of an impulsive suicide attempt may give the patient time to reconsider, seek help, and/or be interrupted by others (continuing the metaphor: "You can always go to the store to buy a chocolate cake, but that would take much more time and effort and you would have more opportunities to change your mind or for somebody else to stop you"). Unwillingness to remove lethal means can often reveal important therapeutic issues. For example, it may suggest that the client is not fully committed to giving up suicide or self-harm as an option, and this would become a critical treatment goal.

A written safety plan should also be created with the suicidal individual. Patients often find it difficult to plan and implement adaptive coping strategies in the place of self-harm when they are experiencing overwhelming distress and hopelessness. For this reason, it is important to develop a detailed, written crisis plan that can be easily accessed for use in future crisis situations (Berk et al. 2004). An example of a safety plan template identified as a best practice by the Suicide Prevention Resource Center Best Practices Registry for Suicide Prevention is shown at www.sprc.org/sites/default/files/resource-program/Brown_StanleySafetyPlanTemplate.pdf (Stanley and Brown 2012; see also www.sprc.org/resources-programs/safety-plan-treatment-manual-reduce-suicide-risk-veteran-version-0 and www.sprc.org/sites/default/files/SafetyPlanningGuide%20Quick%20 Guide%20for%20Clinicians.pdf). The client should be instructed to keep copies of the safety plan easily accessible at all times. In our clinics, we also give suicidal individuals and families wallet-sized cards that they can keep with them at all times with the phone numbers for local emergency departments, mobile crisis teams, 24/7 crisis hotlines, and 911.

As a companion to the safety plan, we suggest having the suicidal individual create a "hope box," which includes tangible reminders of the coping skills listed in the safety plan, as well as materials needed to utilize them (see Berk et al. 2004). The hope box can be a box or other container in which the individual places items and mementos that elicit positive feelings, cue the use of coping skills (e.g., distraction and self-soothing), and serve as reminders of reasons to live. For example, items placed in the hope box might include photographs of favorite people and places, postcards, letters, gifts, a scented candle, paper and pencils for drawing, puzzles, and books. Copies of the written safety plan, including the therapist's phone number and a list of other emergency numbers, can also be placed in the hope box. The client should be told to put the hope box in a place where it can be easily accessed when the client feels suicidal. There is also a "virtual hope box" mobile application that can be downloaded for free from the National Center for Telehealth and Technology, a U.S. Department of Defense Center of Excellence for Psychological Health and Traumatic Brain Injury (http://t2health.dcoe.mil/apps/virtual-hope-box).

One important consideration for campus mental health professionals is whether to notify the student's parents or caretakers if the student may be at risk of suicide. Because an 18-year-old-youth is legally considered to be an adult, a mental health professional cannot release information obtained during treatment without the patient's written consent. Although there are legal exceptions to confidentiality when an individual is an imminent danger to self or others, past suicidal behaviors and/or an increase in risk factors for suicidal behavior may not meet this bar. It is questionable whether college-age individuals, despite legally being adults, have the capacity to keep themselves safe, particularly when they are experiencing severe psychopathology. For youth under age 18, parents play a critical role in maintaining safety by providing close monitoring, restricting access to lethal means, and facilitating compliance with mental health treatment. Hence, it is recommended that mental health professionals who treat college students at risk for suicide work closely with each student to obtain consent to disclose information to parents as needed to maintain safety (unless there is reason to believe that involving parents will substantially increase risk). The role of the university in managing the safety of suicidal students is complex, and clinicians working at college counseling centers should be well informed of the policies at their university and work closely with campus risk management professionals (Cohen 2007).

Additional risk factors that are particularly relevant to college students and important targets of safety interventions are sleep disturbance, alcohol and drug use, and suicide contagion. Sleep disturbance, such as insomnia, is a risk factor for suicidal behavior (Bernert and Joiner 2007), and college students may be especially prone to sleep disturbances due to their shared living situations and late-night studying and socializing. Psychoeducation about the importance of adequate sleep and sleep hygiene should be provided as part of individual counseling sessions and via campus-wide education efforts (for a review of campus sleep education interventions, see Hershner and Chervin 2014). Similarly, because of the frequency of substance use on campus, education about the risks of substance use and suicidality (e.g., the potential for intoxication to increase impulsivity and lower the threshold for dangerous behavior, the dangers of mixing alcohol with other substances or medications) should also be provided. Finally, adolescents and young adults are particularly susceptible to contagion effects related to suicidal behavior. For example, exposure to information about suicidal behavior in the media or through social networks leads to increases in suicidal behavior and, in severe cases, to "suicide clusters" (Gould et al. 1990). Hence, students who are at risk for suicidal or self-harm behaviors should be cautioned against sharing information with peers about these behaviors, as well as receiving this information from peers, including via social networking platforms and Web sites. Guidelines for reporting on-campus suicides in a manner that reduces the likelihood of contagion are available from the Higher Education Mental Health Alliance (http://hemha.org/postvention_guide.pdf).

Treatment Recommendations

As noted in the earlier section on risk factors, college counseling center directors responding to a national survey reported that 86% of the students who had died by suicide had not sought counseling center assistance (Gallagher 2014). Hence, strategies for identifying students at risk and linking them to mental health care are critical. One strategy that addresses this goal is gatekeeper training, in which individuals who typically interact with students who may be at risk—such as other students, resident advisors, and university staff—are trained to identify suicide risk factors, increase their comfort discussing the topic of suicide, and assist with linkage to mental health services. Multiple gatekeeper training programs have been implemented and tested with college students (for reviews, see Lipson 2014; Pasco et al. 2012). Recent evaluations of the Garrett Lee Smith Memorial Act of 2004 indicate that efforts to train gatekeepers to identify individuals at risk for suicide and connect them to services can be effective in reducing suicide attempts (Godoy Garraza et al. 2015) and death by suicide (Walrath et al. 2015). However, these studies found that training efforts must be *ongoing* to yield reductions in suicide-related outcomes, because the 1-year postimplementation suicide attempt and death rates returned to preimplementation levels. It has been shown that providing gatekeepers with experiential training (e.g., role-plays, practices) leads to greater change in their subsequent behaviors toward suicidal individuals than providing didactic training alone (Pasco et al. 2012).

Another strategy has been to identify high-risk students via mass online screenings, followed by online personalized feedback and counseling. In one study, conducted by the American Foundation for Suicide Prevention, it was found that of those students who screened as being at high risk, 91% viewed the counselor's personalized feedback, 34% engaged in online dialogues with the counselor, 20% went for an in-person evaluation, and 15% entered treatment (Haas et al. 2008). In another study, which provided feedback and online dialogue using a motivational interviewing approach, 29% had some correspondence with the online counselor and, at 2-month follow-up, individuals in the intervention group reported significantly higher readiness to engage in treatment and were more likely to have received mental health treatment, compared with those in the control group, who received feedback without motivational interviewing principles (King et al. 2015).

When college students do seek services at college counseling centers, treatment length is usually brief, the most common number of annual appointments per student being 1, with a mean of 5.84 appointments (Center for Collegiate Mental Health 2017). This suggests the need for short-term treatment approaches, as well as established referral streams to off-campus services for students who need extended care (see Chapter 22, "Brief and Medium-Term Psychosocial Therapies at Student Health Centers").

A recent meta-analysis found that brief cognitive-behavioral and mindfulness-based approaches are effective at reducing anxiety and depression in college students (Regehr et al. 2013). These treatment approaches may also be effective at reducing suicide risk factors. Currently, no treatments specifically targeting suicide attempts in college students, or for adolescents in general, meet criteria for a "well-established" empirically supported treatment (APA Presidential Task Force on Evidence-Based Practice 2006). Dialectical behavior therapy (DBT; Linehan 1993) is considered to be the gold-standard treatment for chronically suicidal and self-harming adults, and there is an emerging body of evidence supporting the effectiveness of DBT with adolescents (Mehlum et al. 2014). DBT is a principle-based approach that incorporates a range of behavioral strategies, as well as practices derived from philosophy and Eastern religion (e.g., mindfulness, radical acceptance, dialectics), aimed at teaching clients emotion regulation skills (Linehan 1993). In DBT, difficulty regulating emotion is seen as the primary mechanism underlying self-injurious behaviors. Standard DBT typically incorporates four components: 1) individual therapy, 2) group skills training, 3) availability of 24/7 telephone skills coaching by the therapist, and 4) a mandatory consultation team meeting for therapists. The typical treatment length is 1 year for adults and 4–6 months for adolescents.

Pistorello and colleagues (2012) conducted a randomized controlled trial of a DBT in a college counseling center with 63 college students ages 18–25, with current suicidal ideation, lifetime history of either nonsuicidal self-injury or a suicide attempt and three or more features of borderline personality disorder. Standard adult DBT was modified for the college population by reducing the standard attendance requirements and skills group schedule to accommodate the university semesters and breaks; shortening the typical length of skills groups from 2 to 1.5 hours; and adding skills training on validation of self and others (which students had endorsed as being particularly helpful in pilot work). Compared with treatment as usual, DBT led to greater reductions in suicidal ideation; in depression; and in number of nonsuicidal self-injuries, among those who had engaged in nonsuicidal self-injury. These data highlight the feasibility of providing comprehensive DBT in college counseling centers. Multiple small studies have tested the effectiveness of providing brief DBT skills groups in college counseling centers to students presenting with emotion dysregulation and/or symptoms of borderline personality disorder. Although these studies have shown improvements in students' emotion regulation following participation in DBT skills groups, inclusion criteria have not focused on suicidality and/or self-harm, and these outcomes have not been measured in these studies (Chugani et al. 2013; Meaney-Tavares and Hasking 2013; Rizvi and Steffel 2014; Uliaszek et al. 2016).

Another approach that has been used with college students experiencing suicidality is the CAMS intervention (Jobes and Jennings 2011). CAMS is a brief, suicide-specific approach that emphasizes collaborative engagement with the client. It begins with a detailed assessment of factors contributing to suicidality and then uses problem solving to address these factors. Preliminary data suggest that this approach may be an effective intervention for reducing suicide risk in open trials with college students (Jobes and Jennings 2011; Jobes et al. 1997). Research is currently in progress examining the combined use of CAMS and DBT in college counseling centers using a sequential multiple assignment randomized trial, in which individuals who do not improve following a brief trial of CAMS or treatment as usual then receive DBT (Pistorello et al. 2017).

Case Example

Ellen is an 18-year-old first-year student at a small and competitive liberal arts college. The college was Ellen's first choice, and she was relieved when she received admittance off the wait-list. As a high school student, Ellen had experienced mild to moderate depressive symptoms, including rigid, negative beliefs about her academic ability and school performance. These symptoms were successfully treated at the time using cognitive-behavioral therapy. The first few weeks of college were exhilarating and difficult for Ellen. She began to doubt herself and her ability to achieve like her peers and experienced depressed mood, insomnia, anxiety, and a high frequency of negative thoughts about being inadequate and unworthy of being at college. Despite struggling, Ellen maintained a cheery façade, straining to keep up with course expectations and develop new social connections. At midterm, Ellen received an extremely low score on her biology exam. She took this to mean that she was less capable than others at her college, and she found the pain of being inadequate unbearable. She began to experience suicidal ideation and had thoughts that she did not deserve to live and had no reason to live if she was not going to be successful at college.

Ellen's roommate became concerned when Ellen stated to her that she had no reason to live, and the roommate talked with the residence assistant (RA) about her concerns. Consistent with the university protocol, the RA immediately brought the concern to the college counseling center. A clinician from the counseling center responded by scheduling a same-day appointment for Ellen. During this session, the clinician conducted a detailed risk assessment, during which Ellen revealed that she had been experiencing daily thoughts of suicide. However, she denied engaging in any planning for a suicide attempt or having any current intent to act on her suicidal thoughts. She also denied any prior history of a suicide attempt or nonsuicidal self-injury. Ellen and the clinician completed a written safety plan, including a list of 24/7 emergency hotline numbers. Ellen left the session with a written copy of this plan, as well as an assignment to make a hope box prior to the next session. She denied having any current access to lethal means and agreed to inform the clinician or RA, or to call a suicide hotline number, if she had urges to engage in suicidal or self-harm behavior in the future. Ellen also agreed to sign a release-of-information form allowing the therapist to speak with her parents to obtain information about prior treatment and to collaborate around any future safety concerns. The clinician reviewed with Ellen the importance of getting adequate sleep and avoiding drug and alcohol use for reducing suicidal ideation and depressive symptoms. The clinician also provided Ellen with on-campus resources for obtaining tutoring and support with her classwork. By the end of the session, the clinician and Ellen agreed to continued individual psychotherapy at the counseling center to directly target suicidal ideation, depression, and self-doubt. A second session was scheduled for later the same week, to enable the clinician to closely monitor Ellen's safety. Ellen also agreed to consider a referral to an off-campus psychiatrist for a medication evaluation if her symptoms did not improve with psychotherapy alone, as well as a referral for additional off-campus psychotherapy if her symptoms did not sufficiently improve after completion of the 10 sessions offered at the college counseling center.

Conclusion

Being a college student is associated with both risk and protective factors for suicidal behavior, and colleges and universities play a critical role in suicide prevention among students. It is recommended that mental health professionals working with college students be knowledgeable about the unique risk factors for suicide in this population, the method of conducting a thorough risk assessment, safety planning strategies, evidence-based treatment approaches, and university policies for managing risk for suicide. It is also recommended that colleges and universities utilize campus-wide suicide prevention plans based on evidence-based strategies that take into consideration complex issues regarding confidentiality, requirements for mental health assessment and treatment, and the pros and cons of allowing students at risk for suicide to remain on campus.

KEY CONCEPTS

- College students are at risk for suicide, and effective suicide prevention strategies are needed for this population.

- It is important for colleges and universities to have campus-wide suicide prevention protocols and to ensure that students have access to care both on and off campus.

- Mental health professionals treating college students should be aware of the specific risk factors for suicide in this population, conduct thorough risk assessments with all students at increased risk, and follow evidence-based safety practices. These practices include removal of lethal means, creation of a written safety plan, providing 24/7 emergency numbers, involving parents or families when possible, increasing monitoring of the suicidal individual, and linkage of the individual to ongoing mental health treatment.

Recommendations for Psychiatrists, Psychologists, and Counselors

1. Be aware of risk factors for suicidal behavior in college students.
2. Increase availability of on-campus mental health services, develop strategies for identifying and linking at-risk students to these services, and link students in need of more intensive treatment to off-campus mental health services.
3. Create or follow a campus-wide protocol for responding to students at risk for suicide.
4. In all clinical contacts with potentially suicidal students, perform a detailed risk assessment.

5. If the student is determined to be at high risk of imminent suicidal behavior, consider psychiatric hospitalization. However, be conservative in making decisions about hospitalization, and give priority to the best interest of the student over concerns about liability.
6. Reduce access to lethal means.
7. Increase monitoring of student.
8. Create a written safety plan.
9. Involve parents when possible.
10. Provide campus-wide intervention to address poor sleep and substance use, which are common in college students and increase risk for suicide.
11. Consider campus-wide gatekeeper training, which increases the likelihood that students in need will be identified and linked to care.
12. Provide students with evidence-based treatments when possible.

Discussion Questions

1. What are the risk and protective factors for suicide among college students, and how should these factors be incorporated into safety planning with this population?
2. What are the institution's roles and responsibilities in relation to suicide prevention among students?
3. What is an optimal campus-wide suicide prevention policy?

Suggested Readings

Chiles JA, Strosahl, KD, Roberts, LW: Clinical Manual for Assessment and Treatment of Suicidal Patients, 2nd Edition. Washington, DC, American Psychiatric Association Publishing (in press)

Fowler JC: Suicide risk assessment in clinical practice: pragmatic guidelines for imperfect assessments. Psychotherapy (Chic) 49(1):81–90, 2012

Joffe P: An empirically supported program to prevent suicide in a college student population. Suicide Life Threat Behav 38(1):87–103, 2008

Pistorello J, Coyle TN, Locey NS, Walloch JC: Treating suicidality in college counseling centers: a response to Polychronis. J Coll Stud Psychother 31(1):30–42, 2017

Stanley B, Brown GK: Safety planning intervention: a brief intervention to mitigate suicide risk. Cognit Behav Pract 19:256–264, 2012

References

American College Health Association: American College Health Association–National College Health Assessment II: Spring 2016 Reference Group Executive Summary. Hanover, MD, American College Health Association, 2016. Available at: http://www.acha-ncha.org/docs/NCHA-II%20SPRING%20 2016%20US%20REFERENCE%20GROUP%20EXECUTIVE%20SUMMARY. pdf. Accessed January 29, 2018.

APA Presidential Task Force on Evidence-Based Practice: Evidence-based practice in psychology. Am Psychol 61(4):271–285, 2006 16719673

Barber CW, Miller MJ: Reducing a suicidal person's access to lethal means of suicide: a research agenda. Am J Prev Med 47(3)(suppl 2):S264–S272, 2014 25145749

Berk MS, Henriques GR, Warman DM, et al: A cognitive therapy intervention for suicide attempters: an overview of the treatment and case examples. Cognit Behav Pract 11:265–277, 2004

Bernert RA, Joiner TE: Sleep disturbances and suicide risk: a review of the literature. Neuropsychiatr Dis Treat 3(6):735–743, 2007 19300608

Bongar B, Maris RW, Berman AL, Litman RE: Outpatient standards of care and the suicidal patient, in Risk Management With Suicidal Patients. Edited by Bongar B, Berman AL, Maris RW, et al. New York, Guilford, 1998, pp 4–33

Center for Collegiate Mental Health: 2016 Annual Report. Publ No STA-17-74. University Park, PA, Center for Collegiate Mental Health, Penn State University, January 2017. Available at: https://sites.psu.edu/ccmh/files/ 2017/01/2016-Annual-Report-FINAL_2016_01_09-1gc2hj6.pdf. Accessed January 29, 2018.

Centers for Disease Control and Prevention: National Center for Injury Prevention and Control: 10 leading causes of death by age group—2014. 2014. Available at: https://www.cdc.gov/injury/images/lc-charts/leading_ causes_of_death_age_group_2014_1050w760h.gif. Accessed July 21, 2017.

Chugani CD, Ghali MN, Brunner J: Effectiveness of short term dialectical behavior therapy skills training in college students with cluster B personality disorders. Journal of College Student Psychotherapy 27:323–336, 2013

Cohen VK: Keeping students alive: mandating on-campus counseling saves suicidal college students' lives and limits liability. Fordham Law Rev 75(6):3081–3135, 2007 17593588

Fontanella CA, Hiance-Steelesmith DL, Phillips GS, et al: Widening rural-urban disparities in youth suicides, United States, 1996–2010. JAMA Pediatr 169(5):466–473, 2015 25751611

Fowler JC: Suicide risk assessment in clinical practice: pragmatic guidelines for imperfect assessments. Psychotherapy (Chic) 49(1):81–90, 2012 22369082

Franklin JC, Ribeiro JD, Fox KR, et al: Risk factors for suicidal thoughts and behaviors: a meta-analysis of 50 years of research. Psychol Bull 143(2):187–232, 2017 27841450

Gallagher RP: National Survey of College Counseling Centers, 2014. Arlington, VA, International Association of Counseling Services, 2014

Garrett Lee Smith Memorial Act, Pub L 108-355, 118 Stat 1404, 2004

Godoy Garraza L, Walrath C, Goldston DB, et al: Effect of the Garrett Lee Smith Memorial Suicide Prevention Program on suicide attempts among youths. JAMA Psychiatry 72(11):1143–1149, 2015 26465226

Gould MS, Wallenstein S, Kleinman M: Time-space clustering of teenage suicide. Am J Epidemiol 131(1):71–78, 1990 2293755

Haas A, Koestner B, Rosenberg J, et al: An interactive web-based method of outreach to college students at risk for suicide. J Am Coll Health 57(1):15–22, 2008 18682341

Hershner SD, Chervin RD: Causes and consequences of sleepiness among college students. Nat Sci Sleep 6:73–84, 2014 25018659

Jobes DA: Managing Suicidal Risk: A Collaborative Approach. New York, Guilford, 2006

Jobes DA, Jennings KW: The Collaborative Assessment and Management of Suicidality (CAMS) with suicidal college students, in Understanding and Preventing College Student Suicide. Edited by Lamas D, Lester D. Springfield, IL, Charles C Thomas, 2011, pp 236–254

Jobes DA, Jacoby AM, Cimbolic P, Hustead LA: Assessment and treatment of suicidal clients in a university counseling center. J Couns Psychol 44:368–377, 1997

Joffe P: An empirically supported program to prevent suicide in a college student population. Suicide Life Threat Behav 38(1):87–103, 2008 18355111

King CA, Eisenberg D, Zheng K, et al: Online suicide risk screening and intervention with college students: a pilot randomized controlled trial. J Consult Clin Psychol 83(3):630–636, 2015 25688811

Linehan MM: Cognitive-Behavioral Treatment of Borderline Personality Disorder. New York, Guilford, 1993

Linehan MM, Comtois KA, Ward-Ciesielski EF: Assessing and managing risk with suicidal individuals. Cognit Behav Pract 19:218–232, 2012

Lipson SK: A comprehensive review of mental health gatekeeper-trainings for adolescents and young adults. Int J Adolesc Med Health 26(3):309–320, 2014 24243748

Meaney-Tavares R, Hasking P: Coping and regulating emotions: a pilot study of a modified dialectical behavior therapy group delivered in a college counseling service. J Am Coll Health 61(5):303–309, 2013 23768227

Mehlum L, Tørmoen AJ, Ramberg M, et al: Dialectical behavior therapy for adolescents with repeated suicidal and self-harming behavior: a randomized trial. J Am Acad Child Adolesc Psychiatry 53(10):1082–1091, 2014 25245352

Pasco S, Wallack C, Sartin RM, Dayton R: The impact of experiential exercises on communication and relational skills in a suicide prevention gatekeeper-training program for college resident advisors. J Am Coll Health 60(2):134–140, 2012 22316410

Pistorello J, Fruzzetti AE, Maclane C, et al: Dialectical behavior therapy (DBT) applied to college students: a randomized clinical trial. J Consult Clin Psychol 80(6):982–994, 2012 22730955

Pistorello J, Coyle TN, Locey NS, Walloch JC: Treating suicidality in college counseling centers: a response to Polychronis. J Coll Stud Psychother 31(1):30–42, 2017 28752155

Posner K, Brent D, Lucas C, et al: Columbia-Suicide Severity Rating Scale (C-SSRS). Baseline/Screening, Version 1/14/09. 2009. Available at: http://cssrs. columbia.edu/wp-content/uploads/C-SSRS1-14-09-BaselineScreening.pdf. Accessed July 21, 2017.

Posner K, Brown GK, Stanley B, et al: The Columbia-Suicide Severity Rating Scale: initial validity and internal consistency findings from three multisite studies with adolescents and adults. Am J Psychiatry 168(12):1266–1277, 2011 22193671

Public Health England: Preventing Suicides in Public Places: A Practice Resource. 2015. Available at: https://www.gov.uk/government/uploads/system/uploads/attachment_data/file/481224 /Preventing_suicides_in_public_places.pdf. Accessed July 21, 2017.

Regehr C, Glancy D, Pitts A: Interventions to reduce stress in university students: a review and meta-analysis. J Affect Disord 148(1):1–11, 2013 23246209

Rizvi SL, Steffel LM: A pilot study of 2 brief forms of dialectical behavior therapy skills training for emotion dysregulation in college students. J Am Coll Health 62(6):434–439, 2014 24678824

Schwartz AJ: Rate, relative risk, and method of suicide by students at 4-year colleges and universities in the United States, 2004–2005 through 2008–2009. Suicide Life Threat Behav 41(4):353–371, 2011 21535095

Shaffer D, Pfeffer CR; American Academy of Child and Adolescent Psychiatry: Practice parameter for the assessment and treatment of children and adolescents with suicidal behavior. J Am Acad Child Adolesc Psychiatry 40(7)(suppl):24S–51S, 2001 11434483

Shain B; AAP Committee on Adolescence: Suicide and suicide attempts in adolescents. Pediatrics 138:2–11, 2016

Stanley B, Brown GK: Safety planning intervention: a brief intervention to mitigate suicide risk. Cognitive and Behavioral Practice 19:256–264, 2012

Suicide Prevention Resource Center: Suicide Among College and University Students in the United States. Waltham, MA, Education Development Center, 2014

Uliaszek AA, Rashid T, Williams GE, Gulamani T: Group therapy for university students: a randomized control trial of dialectical behavior therapy and positive psychotherapy. Behav Res Ther 77:78–85, 2016 26731172

Walrath C, Garraza LG, Reid H, et al: Impact of the Garrett Lee Smith youth suicide prevention program on suicide mortality. Am J Public Health 105(5):986–993, 2015 25790418

Response to Survivors of Campus Sexual Assault

Helen W. Wilson, Ph.D.
Adriana Sum Miu, Ph.D.

ALTHOUGH recent public and media attention highlights concerning rates of campus sexual assault, college sexual violence is not a new problem and remains prevalent despite the recent attention. Even with extensive efforts to prevent and raise awareness about sexual assault on college campuses, the rates reported by college students have not changed much across recent decades (McCauley and Casler 2015).

Accurate estimation of the number of students impacted is not straight-forward. Nationally representative studies employing broad, inclusive definitions of assault are lacking, and reported rates vary depending on sample characteristics, definitions of assault, survey modality, and response rates. In general, higher rates of sexual assault are reported by college women than by college men (Banyard et al. 2007). In surveys using comprehensive definitions that include attempted and completed incidents involving both nonpenetration and penetration, approximately 20%–25% of female college students and 5%–10% of male college students report being victims of sexual assault (Banyard et al. 2007; Cantor et al. 2015; Krebs et al. 2007). Rates of college sexual assault reported by males who identify as gay or bisexual are similar to rates reported by college women, and students who identify as transgender, genderqueer, gender nonconforming, questioning, or another nonbinary gender report even higher rates. A straightforward estimate such as the often cited statistic of "1 in 5 college women" is overly simplistic, given findings from the recent Association of American Universities (AAU) Campus Climate Survey on Sexual Assault and Sexual Misconduct (Cantor et al. 2015) that rates of assault varied drastically across and within the 27 institutions surveyed. Nonetheless, past research suggests that campus sexual assault is a major problem affecting a great many college students, with women and transgender or nonbinary gender students identified as particularly vulnerable populations.

Contrary to myths evoking the image of a stranger emerging from the bushes and preying on a victim, most sexual assaults are committed by acquaintances in public social settings such as parties and residence halls. Surveys indicate that most sexual assault survivors know and trust their assailants. The Campus Sexual Assault study found that the prevalence of incapacitated sexual assault, likely from parties and social gatherings, was more than twice the prevalence of physically forced sexual assault (Krebs et al. 2007). Most incapacitated sexual assault victims (82%) also reported drinking alcohol before the sexual assault. These findings suggest that the risk for sexual violence is higher when students are under the influence of alcohol or drugs in a social setting. Although these substances can make someone more vulnerable to a sexual assault, it is important to emphasize that a survivor is not to blame due to being intoxicated and that alcohol or drugs are not an excuse for assault. Engaging in the use of substances is not and should never be construed as an invitation to violence, including sexual violence.

In general, survey data suggest that students are unlikely to make a report or seek help after a sexual assault. Barriers to reporting are numerous. Possibly because of fear of consequences for substance use, incapacitated sexual assault victims are less likely than other survivors to seek help or make police reports (Krebs et al. 2009). According to the AAU survey, the most common reason students did not disclose a sexual assault was because they did not believe it was serious enough; even in cases of penetration by physical force, nearly 60% of students gave this reason for not reporting (Cantor et al. 2015). Other common reasons for not reporting included feeling "embarrassed, ashamed or that it would be too emotionally difficult" and believing that nothing would be done about the assault. In addition, as discussed above, perpetrators of campus sexual assault are most often an acquaintance, friend, or dating partner, and survivors may not want to report a perpetrator who is a part of their social network. Moreover, campus messages that subtly tolerate sexual assault and harassment ("it's just something women have to put up with") or blame victims for these experiences ("you have to keep yourself safe") can make it difficult for students to share their experiences for fear of being penalized academically or professionally. Although the AAU survey found that most students who did make an official report were satisfied with the response, the most vulnerable populations (women and transgender or nonbinary gender students) were also the least likely to expect a supportive response and fair investigation (Cantor et al. 2015).

A variety of factors likely contribute to the alarming rates of sexual violence on college campuses. College undergraduates are typically within the sensitive phase of "emerging adulthood" as they transition from youth to adulthood. During this stage, college students often leave the relatively supportive, monitored parental environment for a less structured and more independent college campus environment. This experience, of course, differs across individuals, and not all students come from stable home environments or leave family homes; however, for many young people, this transition is a rather chaotic period characterized by risk-taking behaviors and identity exploration. Supporting the contribution of developmental stage, evidence suggests that undergraduates are more likely than graduate students to experience sexual violence, and first-year students report higher rates than senior students (Cantor et al. 2015).

Features of campus culture can interact with this developmentally sensitive period to create a context ripe for sexual assault. As described by Adams-Curtis and Forbes (2004), "The college experience juxtaposes the powerful motives of sex and aggression in a population that is still forming a stable identity within an environment that includes strong peer pressures for sexual activity, the ritualistic abuse of alcohol, a culture that objectifies women, and a culture that frequently views sexual intercourse as an act of masculine conquest" (pp. 91–92). Traditional sexual scripts, rigid gender roles, and campus dynamics of power and status (e.g., Greek system, athletics) likely contribute to normalizing coercive sexual interactions among college students. Moreover, when students enter this highly sexualized college context, they are often poorly prepared to recognize, resist, or prevent nonconsensual experiences due to lack of effective education and dialogue about these issues before coming to college.

Effects of Sexual Assault

Sexual assault can have significant and wide-ranging effects on the survivor. Immediate reactions often include intense emotional distress, unwanted memories of the event, nightmares, difficulty concentrating or focusing on academic work, sleep problems, and feeling jumpy or on edge. These reactions clearly can interfere with academic engagement and performance, as well as the social and extracurricular aspects of campus life. In addition, sexual assault can result in suicidal ideation, self-harming behaviors, excessive substance use, risky sexual behaviors, and other risk-taking behaviors as a way of coping with the intense distress. However, it is important to keep in mind that survivors of sexual trauma can present with a range of reactions; some individuals may feel numb and withdraw socially, whereas others may even seem to dismiss or make light of the situation. All of these are normal ways of coping with an otherwise unbearable experience. Sexual assault also increases risk for developing clinical disorders, including posttraumatic stress disorder (PTSD), depression, anxiety, and substance abuse and can ultimately lead to dropping out of school (Roberts et al. 2016). Thus, a comprehensive and effective response to survivors of sexual assault is critical for ensuring that this traumatic experience does not derail their education (see Chapter 16, "Stress and Trauma").

University Response to Sexual Assault: Understanding Title IX

The landmark Title IX of the Education Amendments of 1972 states, "No person in the United States shall, on the basis of sex, be excluded from participation in, be denied the benefits of, or be subjected to discrimination under any education program or activity receiving Federal financial assistance." In 2011, guidelines from the Department of Education interpreted

Title IX protections to include freedom from sexual violence and harassment, which can interfere with a student's ability to learn and participate in educational and extracurricular activities. This guidance obligates schools to prevent and respond to campus sexual assault. All schools that receive federal funding (most public and private institutions) are required to have a Title IX coordinator on campus and to have a clearly communicated, systematic process for handling sexual assault charges. Current guidelines also require most university employees to report disclosures of sexual assault to the Title IX coordinator. The Title IX response to sexual violence on college campuses recognizes the severe impact this violence can have on a student's ability to learn and ensures that universities respond to allegations. However, survivors of assault can be concerned about maintaining control over how they handle the experience and may feel that they have limited options for obtaining confidential support. Thus, mental health professionals working with college students play a crucial role in providing confidential support and helping survivors understand options for reporting and redressing sexual assault.

Prevention of Campus Sexual Assault

The most expansive and empirically studied efforts to address campus sexual assault to date focus on prevention of this problem. Historically, prevention programs tended to focus on teaching students safety skills to avoid becoming victims or to intervene instead of being a bystander. Bringing in the Bystander, an example of a program that provides college participants with skills about intervening in sexual violence, has shown mixed results on changing attitudes and bystander behaviors (DeGue 2014). In contrast, a promising program developed in Canada to empower college women to protect themselves from sexual violence demonstrated efficacy in reducing incidences of rape and attempted rape (Senn et al. 2015). This Enhanced Assess, Acknowledge, Act Sexual Assault Resistance program consists of four 3-hour units that cover risk assessment, acknowledging danger and overcoming emotional barriers to resisting unwanted sexual behaviors, and implementing effective verbal and physical self-defense. In a randomized controlled trial, 1-year risk of both completed and attempted rape was significantly lower for women who participated in this program compared with those in a control group. Although current evidence suggests that teaching women to protect themselves may be easier to achieve than shifting campus cultural norms that tolerate and promote sexual assault, this strategy is problematic in placing the burden on potential victims. Moreover, equivalent resistance programs have not been developed and evaluated with men or with transgender or nonbinary gender students.

Other efforts have focused on changing campus culture to promote values such as respect and affirmative consent. Indeed, broad cultural changes on college campuses are needed to eradicate norms that tolerate or promote sexual violence. The White House Task Force to Protect Students From Sexual Assault, formed in 2014 under the Obama administration, proposed guidelines for evidence-based interventions for shifting campus culture and preventing sexual assault. These guidelines suggest that interventions should be implemented broadly at individual, relationship, community, and society levels (DeGue 2014). For example, a campus may build a bystander program at the individual level, develop residence-based programs to promote healthy sexual relationships, engage leaders to foster a culture of respect and safety at the community level, and establish affirmative consent and alcohol policies at the societal level. To date, however, research has yielded mixed results regarding the effectiveness of such attempts to change campus culture. Programs appear to be most effective in changing attitudes, such as acceptance of sexual coercion or rape myths, and behavioral intentions, but findings vary widely across studies and often are not replicated. Moreover, studies examining long-term effects or changes in the actual incidences of sexual assault are few and inconclusive (DeGue 2014). Without documenting changes in sexual violence rates, it is unclear how well these interventions prevent campus sexual violence (see Chapter 7, "A Developmental Perspective on Risk Taking Among College Students").

Support for Survivors of Campus Sexual Assault

Given that sexual violence continues to be prevalent on college campuses and interventions have not yet been able to curb this problem, university-based mental health professionals play an important part in supporting the survivors of sexual trauma (Roberts et al. 2016). Limited research has evaluated interventions specifically designed for college sexual assault survivors. Thus, best practice guidelines apply evidence-based treatments and theoretical principles developed with broader populations of sexual assault survivors (White Kress et al. 2003). Survivors typically undergo two primary phases of reactions: the acute initial reactions phase and the reorganization phase. In addition, the effects of sexual assault vary greatly across individuals. Therefore, response must be sensitive to the differences, depending on the phase of reaction and

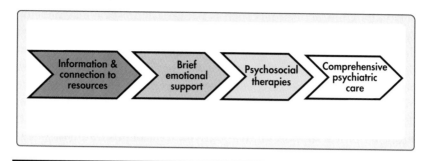

FIGURE 21–1. **Phased-based model of support for survivors of campus sexual assault.**

individual presentation. Most individuals present symptoms of acute stress immediately following a sexual assault, whereas a smaller number (typically about one-third) of survivors go on to meet criteria for PTSD, characterized by persistence of symptoms beyond 4 weeks. As these estimates highlight, most survivors benefit from support in the immediate aftermath, and a smaller proportion require ongoing intervention, including psychosocial therapies and comprehensive psychiatric care (Figure 21–1).

During the initial crisis phase, students are likely to benefit most from interventions that educate about common reactions, destigmatize symptoms, enhance positive coping, and reduce emotional distress (White Kress et al. 2003). In the immediate aftermath of a trauma, survivors may not be able to provide details or a coherent account of the event and are not likely to benefit from attempts to elicit such details. For example, a brief prevention program aimed at halting the progression of posttraumatic stress (Foa et al. 1995) was found to reduce symptoms in women who had recently (average of 15 days) experienced sexual or nonsexual assault. This brief cognitive-behavioral intervention consisted of four 2-hour sessions, beginning with psychoeducation about the common reactions to assault and skills training in breathing and relaxation, and later focusing on imaginal exposure to the assault memories, in vivo exposure to feared but safe situations, and restructuring of maladaptive cognitions related to the trauma.

For many survivors, the reorganization phase is characterized by increasing psychological adjustment, integration of the experience, and recovery from the trauma. This can happen naturally through reliance on preexisting coping capacities and social support. For others, acute symptoms persist and cause significant impairment, such as academic problems, social isolation, substance abuse, sexual risk, or self-harming behaviors. Clinical disorders such as PTSD or depression may develop. When symptoms are persistent and interfere with life functioning, students are likely to benefit from longer-term evidence-based interventions that have been effective for treating these problems in the general population. Current recommendations emphasize cognitive-behavioral treatments as first-line interventions. In particular, cognitive processing therapy (CPT) and prolonged exposure (PE) are two interventions with strong empirical support for treating symptoms of posttraumatic stress, depression, and anxiety related to sexual assault. Both treatments evidenced maintenance of treatment effects over an average of 6 years in a long-term follow-up study (Resick et al. 2012). Although theoretical underpinnings differ for these treatments, both teach survivors skills for managing distress associated with trauma memories and reminders and extinguish conditioned responses through exposure to trauma reminders by asking survivors to tell the story verbally (PE) or create a written narrative (CPT). Both treatments also involve emotional and cognitive processing, although PE emphasizes activation and processing of emotion related to the trauma, whereas CPT emphasizes identifying and restructuring cognitive "stuck points" resulting from the trauma. Thus, PE may be most suitable for survivors struggling with intense emotional reactions and avoidance of trauma reminders, and CPT is particularly beneficial when impairment is driven by maladaptive beliefs resulting from the assault.

An Innovative Approach: Support for Sexual Assault Survivors at Stanford University

In an editorial in the *Journal of Adolescent Health*, McCauley and Casler (2015) called for a trauma-informed approach to campus sexual assault whereby survivors feel more comfortable disclosing their experiences and have access to "safe spaces to share their stories." The Stanford Confidential Support Team (CST) has created this kind of trauma-informed safe space. The CST represents a unique collaboration between the Stanford Department of Psychiatry and Behavioral Sciences in the university medical center and Vaden Student Health Center. This partnership extends the expertise of academic psychiatry to the provision of specialized treatment for survivors of campus sexual assault (Roberts et al. 2016).

The CST provides a free, confidential service for all students impacted by sexual assault, as well as other forms of relationship and gender-based violence. Maintaining confidentiality, rather than reporting incidents to the Title IX office or legal authorities, allows students to regain a sense of control and mastery after a traumatic experience, which is by definition out of one's control. The CST serves as a centralized point of contact for information and guidance through university structures and processes related to sexual assault response and provides a range of supportive options to meet the varied needs of impacted students. The CST also provides support for friends, family, faculty, staff, and others who wish to support impacted students.

A student's first encounter with the CST office typically involves an initial consultation with a licensed clinician (a social worker or psychologist). During this first visit, the student can obtain information about rights, reporting options, and resources available on and off campus (e.g., medical treatment, advocacy, forensic evidence collection); education about response to trauma and normalization of reactions; emotional support; and assistance connecting with desired resources. For example, a student might want to learn more about the Title IX reporting and adjudication process in order to decide whether or not to take this step. Similarly, survivors of recent assaults may have questions about how to obtain a forensic examination (or they may not even know about this option). Others simply want to talk to a supportive person about the experience in a safe, confidential space. Following a trauma-informed approach, CST therapists remain neutral about reporting or disclosing the experience to campus or legal authorities and focus on empowering the student to determine what next steps are best for the student's unique circumstances. Clinicians engage students in a collaborative process and are available to support them in reporting, if they choose to do so, or in accessing other resources. Many students schedule only this initial consultation, because they get their needs met through this session, they are not interested in longer-term support, or they have an existing relationship with another mental health professional.

In the acute phase of response, the CST offers brief support, ranging from approximately 2 to 10 sessions. This phase extends education and resource assistance begun during the initial consultation and focuses on emotional support and coordination with other agencies and services. Many students work with the CST to make sense out of the experience, acknowledge it as sexual assault, and integrate it into a coherent personal history. This phase often includes skills training in relaxation and distress tolerance and, for some students, stabilization of suicidal ideation, self-harm, or other risky behaviors. Clinicians also work with students to identify existent coping strategies and social support and help them to engage these resources. Essentially, the CST provides a safe space in which students are able to heal from what is considered to be a normal, adaptive reaction to an undesired, unpredicted, and violating experience.

As expected from statistics available, a proportion of students do not recover after this initial phase, and in many cases students do not reach out for help until after symptoms have become entrenched. For these students, the CST offers longer-term evidence-based treatment. It is only at this point that CST therapists implement a standard mental health assessment after determining collaboratively with the student that reactions to the trauma have become impairing symptoms that significantly interfere with life goals. The assessment includes a standard set of measures to evaluate symptoms of depression, anxiety, substance use, and posttraumatic stress. Therapists also conduct a thorough clinical interview to understand a student's background and complete psychiatric history (some of which may have been gathered during the initial response phase). Consistent with best practice guidelines, clinicians implement a treatment plan drawing on the evidence base for treating symptoms associated with trauma (e.g., CPT, PE). For students presenting with complex mental health histories and more complicated symptom manifestations, CST therapists sometimes must refer them to other community professionals, such as the department of psychiatry. Similarly, the clinicians may refer students for continuing care to address additional concerns that emerge or persist after resolving trauma-related reactions and symptoms. Consistent with the number of survivors expected to develop PTSD, about one-third of students served by the CST seek ongoing therapy for impairing symptoms.

Case Examples

CASE EXAMPLE 1: BRIEF SUPPORT

Matthew, a graduate student identifying as a gay man, self-referred to a specialized program for survivors of sexual assault for support after attempted sexual assault by an acquaintance he encountered at a party. He reported that he was drinking and had at first enjoyed flirting and dancing with this person. He described feeling unsure about whether the incident counted as an assault and said that he was unsure about making an official report to the Title IX office. Specifically, he was concerned that he might not be taken seriously because of being a man and because he knew of "much worse things" happening to other people.

The initial consultation with Matthew focused on psychoeducation about consent and sexual assault and discussion of resources and reporting options. The counselor validated the student's reaction, assured the student that he was not at fault for what happened, and emphasized that what he experienced was nonconsensual and serious. The counselor shared that consent is an ongoing process and that just because Matthew enjoyed flirting and dancing did not mean that he consented to other activities. During the session, the counselor also explained the Title IX reporting process and answered the student's questions. The counselor assessed Matthew's current level of safety. Although Matthew denied concerns about current safety, the counselor provided information about making a police report and requesting a court order of protection. The counselor encouraged the student to call 911 if he were to feel in immediate danger. During the session, the counselor helped the student to explore his thoughts and feelings about these options and the pros and cons of making an official report.

The counselor talked with Matthew about how the experience was impacting him, focusing on his academic and social relationships. Matthew said that he was generally doing okay but felt more anxious than usual, particularly when he thought about the assault or encountered people who were at the party. He also said that he was having difficulty focusing on his schoolwork since the incident. The counselor helped the student to identify healthy ways of coping with his feelings and to identify social support. Matthew said that he felt relaxed when biking or hiking, so the counselor encouraged him to do these activities and helped him identify times he could schedule for pleasant activities. The counselor taught Matthew a deep breathing exercise to help him manage emotional distress elicited by thoughts or reminders of the incident. Finally, the counselor discussed options for obtaining academic accommodations.

A week later Matthew returned. He said that he had decided to report the assault to the Title IX office, which was helping him to obtain extended time for completing academic assignments because of the stress of the situation. He said that the Title IX office was conducting an investigation and that he felt good about taking action to address what happened to him. He also said that he was most concerned about whether the perpetrator harmed anyone else. He said that he had disclosed the experience to a few close friends who were very supportive. He also said that the deep breathing exercises were helpful when he felt anxious. Matthew continued to obtain support from the specialized program for survivors of sexual assault throughout the Title IX process, which resulted in sanctions placed on the accused party. Once the case was resolved, the student reported feeling that he could put the incident behind him, felt less anxious about it, and was feeling engaged in his studies again. He described taking part in regular social activities and continuing to enjoy his college experience despite this unwanted incident.

CASE EXAMPLE 2: EVIDENCE-BASED TREATMENT

Anne is a 19-year-old white college student who self-referred to a specialized program for survivors of sexual assault 2 years after ending an abusive relationship in which she experienced coerced sex and emotional abuse. She sought treatment because she wanted to better manage her emotions and have fewer intrusive memories. She presented with symptoms consistent with PTSD, including intense distress when triggered, frequent intrusive memories, and hypervigilance. The intrusive memories of her abuse interfered with her ability to concentrate in her classes. Anne described feeling disconnected and numb so as not to feel the negative emotions associated with the abusive relationship. She also believed it was her fault for being "too weak" to stop the abuse and for staying in the abusive relationship. Anne decided to seek treatment when she realized that she had changed from being an optimistic, sociable person to a depressed and isolated person.

A therapist conducted a thorough intake assessment, which included an assessment of Anne's current functioning, trauma history, developmental and social history, and symptoms of PTSD, depression, and anxiety. Intake also included several self-report measures, including the PTSD Checklist for DSM-5 (PCL-5), Beck Depression Inventory II (BDI-II), Beck Anxiety Inventory (BAI), and substance use history. Anne was diagnosed with PTSD. Given her rigid self-blame and maladaptive thoughts, the therapist provided psychoeducation about cognitive processing therapy (CPT), and Anne agreed to treatment.

During the initial CPT treatment, the therapist provided psychoeducation about PTSD and trauma. Anne learned to identify her thoughts and feelings whenever she felt triggered by memories of her trauma. At the beginning, she struggled with acknowledging and tolerating negative emotions, which resulted in minimizing the trauma and avoiding difficult topics. The therapist worked with Anne in discussing the purpose of emotions and taught her coping skills (e.g., grounding, breathing) to help her tolerate negative emotions. Anne wrote a narrative describing the coerced sexual experience during the relationship. In session, the therapist asked clarifying questions about the context and circumstances that led to the coerced sex. After revisiting the context and her decision-making process, Anne slowly realized that she had already asserted herself, but her ex-boyfriend did not respect her decision. Furthermore, after writing about what happened, she realized that her sadness and anger were valid given the sexual abuse. After learning to validate her own emotions and having a more balanced understanding of what happened, Anne was taught cognitive restructuring skills. She completed worksheets that identified cognitive distortions and assumptions, and she gradually resolved her stuck points related to the trauma and her beliefs about herself and others.

By the end of therapy, Anne reported significant decrease in PTSD symptoms and expressed being able to trust people while also feeling confident in her ability to stand up for herself when she felt disrespected. She felt proud of herself for having overcome the trauma and reported being able to manage daily stressors with the cognitive restructuring skills she had learned in treatment.

Conclusion

Campus sexual violence is a major concern that impedes students' ability to access the academic and social benefits of a college education. Populations subject to disadvantages in terms of power and privilege—such as female, gay, and transgender students—report the highest rates of unwanted and violent sexual experiences. Cultural norms on university campuses can contribute to this unacceptable situation by creating an atmosphere in which sexual coercion is overlooked, tolerated, and reinforced. Mental health professionals working with college students, therefore, play a crucial role in shifting the culture away from these unhealthy norms and in supporting students affected by sexual violence. The most extensive research attention has gone to developing and evaluating prevention programs, which have yielded mixed and inconclusive evidence. Best practice guidelines for supporting survivors recommend the implementation of a phase-based approach and use of evidence-based models developed with broader populations. Until prevention efforts are successful in eliminating the problem of campus sexual assault, innovative evidence-based programs are needed to provide trauma-informed care for impacted students.

KEY CONCEPTS

- Campus sexual assault is a significant problem that remains prevalent despite recent attention.

- College women and lesbian, gay, bisexual, transgender, and queer/questioning (LGBTQ) students report particularly high rates of sexual violence.
- Evaluation of prevention programs has resulted in mixed or inconclusive evidence of their effectiveness.
- Best practice guidelines for supporting survivors of sexual assault suggest the implementation of a phase-based approach and use of evidence-based models developed with broader populations.

Recommendations for Psychiatrists, Psychologists, and Counselors

1. Best practice guidelines for supporting survivors of campus sexual assault apply evidence-based treatments developed with broader populations of sexual assault survivors.
2. An effective response is sensitive to the phase of reaction (initial or reorganization) and individual presentation.
3. During the initial crisis phase, students are likely to benefit most from interventions that educate about common reactions, destigmatize symptoms, enhance positive coping, and reduce emotional distress.
4. Current recommendations emphasize cognitive-behavioral treatments as first-line interventions for clinical symptoms that develop during the reorganization phase. Cognitive processing therapy and prolonged exposure are two interventions with strong empirical support for treating symptoms of posttraumatic stress, depression, and anxiety related to sexual assault.

Discussion Questions

1. What characteristics of college life contribute to the prevalence of sexual violence?
2. What unique role can mental health professionals play in addressing and responding to campus sexual assault?
3. How can existing interventions for sexual assault be applied to college populations using the framework of trauma-informed care?

Suggested Readings

Know Your IX: Empowering students to stop sexual violence: campus resources. Available at: https://www.knowyourix.org/college-resources/ (for information about federal guidelines for university sexual assault response)

McCauley HL, Casler AW: College sexual assault: a call for trauma-informed prevention. J Adolesc Health 56(6):584–585, 2015

RAINN: Campus sexual violence: statistics. Available at: https://www.rainn.org/statistics/campus-sexual-violence (for data on prevalence and impacted populations)

Roberts LW, Dority K, Balon R, et al: Academic psychiatry's role in addressing campus sexual assault. Acad Psychiatry 40(4):567–571, 2016

White Kress VE, Trippany RL, Nola JM: Responding to sexual assault victims: considerations for college counselors. Journal of College Counseling 6:124–133, 2003

References

Adams-Curtis LE, Forbes GB: College women's experiences of sexual coercion: a review of cultural, perpetrator, victim, and situational variables. Trauma Violence Abuse 5(2):91–122, 2004 15070552

Banyard VL, Ward S, Cohn ES, et al: Unwanted sexual contact on campus: a comparison of women's and men's experiences. Violence Vict 22(1):52–70, 2007 17390563

Cantor D, Fisher B, Chibnall S, et al: Report on the AAU campus climate survey on sexual assault and sexual misconduct. Association of American Universities, 2015. Available at: https://www.aau.edu/sites/default/files/%40%20Files/Climate%20Survey/AAU_Campus_Climate_Survey_12_14_15.pdf. Accessed July 21, 2017.

DeGue S: Preventing Sexual Violence on College Campuses: Lessons from Research and Practice. Report prepared for the White House Task Force to Protect Students From Sexual Assault, 2014

Foa EB, Hearst-Ikeda D, Perry KJ: Evaluation of a brief cognitive-behavioral program for the prevention of chronic PTSD in recent assault victims. J Consult Clin Psychol 63(6):948–955, 1995 8543717

Krebs CP, Lindquist CH, Warner TD, et al: The Campus Sexual Assault (CSA) Study, Final Report(NIJ Grant No 2004-WG-BX-0010), December 2007

Krebs CP, Lindquist CH, Warner TD, et al: College women's experiences with physically forced, alcohol- or other drug-enabled, and drug-facilitated sexual assault before and since entering college. J Am Coll Health 57(6):639–647, 2009 19433402

McCauley HL, Casler AW: College sexual assault: a call for trauma-informed prevention. J Adolesc Health 56(6):584–585, 2015 26003573

Resick PA, Williams LF, Suvak MK, et al: Long-term outcomes of cognitive-behavioral treatments for posttraumatic stress disorder among female rape survivors. J Consult Clin Psychol 80(2):201–210, 2012 22182261

Roberts LW, Dority K, Balon R, et al: Academic psychiatry's role in addressing campus sexual assault. Acad Psychiatry 40(4):567–571, 2016 27052505

Senn CY, Eliasziw M, Barata PC, et al: Efficacy of a sexual assault resistance program for university women. N Engl J Med 372(24):2326–2335, 2015 26061837

White Kress VE, Trippany RL, Nola JM: Responding to sexual assault victims: considerations for college counselors. Journal of College Counseling 6:124–133, 2003

CHAPTER 22

Brief and Medium-Term Psychosocial Therapies at Student Health Centers

Michael Haberecht, M.D.

THE evolution of therapeutic modalities in college counseling centers mirrors the development of treatment strategies in the overall community. Greater experience with different types of therapy and an increasing number of medication options have led to a movement toward evidence-based treatment modalities that are time limited and adaptable to a variety of clinic settings. In college counseling centers, these therapies include cognitive-behavioral therapy (CBT), time-limited dynamic psychotherapy (TLDP), dialectical behavior therapy (DBT), and acceptance commitment therapy (ACT). College counseling clinicians have identified fundamental building blocks common to many of these therapies that can be adapted to the needs of university students.

These strategies must work with the societal trends, institutional expectations, and developmental experience of late adolescents and young adults. The approach of selecting certain tools and excluding others, as well as adapting the treatment style from university to university, creates challenges for assessing overall effectiveness of the therapy provided in counseling centers and for establishing more general guidelines for the field of university mental health. In this chapter, I identify the societal trends and developmental challenges facing students and discuss how they impact the provision of short-term therapies in a student health center; I also discuss the building blocks of treatment in a university mental health system and the therapies from which they are derived.

Societal Pressures

In recent years, parents, teachers, and community institutions (e.g., media, medical groups, social support agencies) have increasingly focused on the mental health and emotional well-being of university students as well as on the campus climate at universities across the country. High-profile events throughout the nation have highlighted the potential tragedy associated with emotional instability in a group of individuals just beginning their adult lives. High-visibility incidents have shone a light on the wide impact of mass shootings at several universities; of clusters of suicide (up to five or six students) at high-pressure residential universities; and of problem drinking leading to increased medical transports and behavior problems. Recent attention also has focused on the increase in sexual assaults and how they are handled at universities. Furthermore, there has been an increase in more typical psychiatric problems for students on college campuses, with a greater prevalence of depression, anxiety, attention-deficit/hyperactivity disorder (ADHD), and eating disorders.

Significant changes also have occurred in the demographics of university students. In recent decades, there has been an overall increase in the number of students and, with that, an increase in the diversity of students. A primary change has been a wider range of many demographic cohorts, including those based on age, gender, race/ethnicity, and socioeconomic status, as well as an increasing number of international students attending university in the United States. One way of adapting to such diversity has been the establishment of colleges catering to particular populations, including liberal arts colleges, technical schools, religious institutions, and state schools. This heterogeneity has made it difficult to formulate a common framework for providing psychotherapy in student health clinics.

Developmental Trends

In addition to the demographic and cultural diversity that is changing the student population and universities, a more distinct stage of development is being recognized for late adolescents and young adults who are attending university. The developmental trajectory of students can be described based on what their age is, where they are in their academic curriculum, and what their other life experiences have been.

On the developmental trajectory, undergraduate students are generally late adolescents. One of the major developmental tasks facing younger college students involves individuation from the family of origin and reliance on relationships with peers. Of particular importance to this age group is coming to terms with sexual orientation, gender identity, religious identification, and political affiliations. Late adolescents are less likely than older peers to seek care from mental health caregivers, who may represent the parent from whom the student wishes to create space. The decision to access psychological or psychiatric help also varies based on gender, with a greater percentage of first-year women seeking help than first-year men. Unpublished data from Vaden Health Center at Stanford University, for example, suggest that the difference between the percentage of male students and female students seeking care decreases as students progress through school.

The importance of the developmental process is that when a student decides to seek care either on their own or by recommendation of another, "a moment in time" is available in which to plant a seed about the experience of mental health care that may grow in the current work or flower at some time in the future. Deciding how to optimize the potential for engaging a student in treatment at that first or second visit is very important.

Graduate students are a less developmentally distinct group than undergraduates (see Chapter 30, "Graduate Students and Postdoctoral Fellows"). These students may have just completed undergraduate studies and may have more in common with younger peers, or they may have functioned as young adults before returning to graduate school. Graduate students who have just completed undergraduate studies have, nonetheless, completed a significant developmental task—graduation—and likely will have attained a level of independence. A significant portion of graduate students will be older and will have held jobs, lived independently, and paid their own bills. They also may have a spouse or partner and perhaps children. At schools with graduate students, services at health centers must be flexible to accommodate young adults who are no longer late adolescents. A developmental model acknowledging the formation of adult relationships, occupational endeavors, and formation of community is useful with this population.

Problems Presented by Students at University Counseling Centers

The types of problems for which students come to the university counseling center often differ from the ones that bring individuals to psychiatric clinics focusing on either pediatric or adult issues. Young adults who are still in the process of learning emotion regulation and *mentalization* (the process of keeping differing perspectives in mind) often present with "stress" around interpersonal or academic disappointments. The acute presentation of "stress" is the anxiety that results from the struggle to regulate emotions and the difficulty of being able to hold the fear in mind with a more stable perception of the reality.

Also, a large number of students present to counseling centers with chronic or acute exacerbations of chronic illness, such as major depressive disorder, generalized anxiety disorder, bipolar disorder, or ADHD. Compared with the students with the stresses mentioned above, these students present with more typical symptom clusters, including depressed mood, enjoyment, or motivation; paranoid ideation; and mania. These students may have had previous exposure to mental health care or may be presenting with such symptoms for the first time (because such disorders often have their onset during adolescence and young adulthood). The expectations for assessment and treatment of these students are different compared with the students with the stresses described above. Students with chronic illness may require more frequent visits, coordinated care with therapists and psychiatrists, case management, or a higher level of care with regard to acuity.

Students in a third group seek care for psychosocial stressors embedded in the mores of the community. For instance, more students are coming forward now than in the past for help with their experiences with sexual harassment, sexual assaults, acts of intolerance, and problem drinking. Such problems may be addressed through a combination of psychological interventions at the counseling center and community-based interventions for creating a safe environment for learning.

Treatment Modalities in University Counseling Centers

After an initial phone screening by a staff clinician to check for suicidality and therapeutic needs, most students are referred to an in-person appointment for a full assessment of the manifesting problem in the context of biological, psychological, and community factors. This assessment leads to a formulation of the student's goals and an agreement on a therapeutic strategy, taking into account the diversity of manifesting problems, cultural and ethnic identities, and levels of acuity. The typical approach to treatment of college students is individually tailoring therapy to the goals of each student using a set of therapeutic building blocks that share commonalities with aspects of most evidence-based therapies. Potential modalities include modifications of CBT, ACT, DBT, and TLDP for both individuals and groups. The following subsections summarize the therapies that contribute to the fundamental building blocks used in college counseling therapy.

COGNITIVE-BEHAVIORAL THERAPY

A connection can be seen between the basic components of CBT and several of the building blocks of brief therapy in the college counseling center (Beck et al. 1979). First, CBT is the primary influence on how the therapeutic frame is viewed. The most defining and consistent element of the frame is that treatment is typically time limited (5–10 sessions). The frequency or length of sessions may change depending on each student's therapeutic needs. For example, acute stressors may lead to the student's being seen twice weekly immediately after the event and then every week for some time. If the student improves and needs only intermittent check-ins for consolidation of skills learned, the student may be scheduled for an appointment once monthly or for a 30-minute rather than 1-hour appointment. The therapist has the responsibility to monitor the impact of such choices and changes in treatment. This adaptable frame can be kept in mind and monitored by the therapist for and with the student. Concerns on which the therapist can focus include the capacity of the student to tolerate change and the impact of frequency and intensity on meeting the student's goals. Other challenges to a rigid frame are inherent in university settings: summer break, academic scheduling, and university administrative requirements. For example, a student being seen just prior to summer break may require a plan for checking in by phone over the summer. As another example, a student may be seen after a sexual assault and may receive ongoing psychotherapy outside the typical limitations of the service. In summary, the therapeutic frame in college counseling centers is flexible and adaptable, with the therapist actively engaging and guiding the student toward the established therapeutic goals.

The second building block adapted from CBT is the structure of the therapy overall, as well as the structure of each session as an individual unit within the therapy. The therapist establishes a collaborative and transparent approach by including in the first session an explicit overview of the therapeutic setting (number of sessions, potential utilization of campus partners to enhance therapy or mental health treatment, and potential referrals to other clinicians or clinics once therapeutic goals are met). Students and therapists engage in goal setting, with attention to the amount of time a student has in treatment as well as to the emotional input required by the goal. Each session may have its own goal, encouraging progress to be measured from session to session. Some therapists ask students to provide written feedback at the end of each session that states what the student wished for coming into the session, how well the therapist connected with the student, and what was accomplished during the session. An alternative approach to monitoring progress and keeping to a schedule involves setting up phases of treatment for the anticipated time of working together. For example, an initial phase may involve identifying the problem, with an intermediate phase of working through, and a termination phase dedicated to synthesis.

A third building block is the development of skills for addressing automatic negative thoughts and irrational beliefs in which the therapist works with the patient to identify and defuse such thoughts about himself or herself or the world. In the first step, the patient learns how to identify emotional states and then link them with negative thoughts and irrational beliefs. The patient then learns how to challenge those thoughts and assess their validity. If the patient feels that the belief is not valid, the patient then learns how to substitute alternative rational thoughts for the irrational or negative beliefs. This process aims to give the patient the skills to pursue this process of behavioral modification on their own.

ACCEPTANCE COMMITMENT THERAPY AND DIALECTICAL BEHAVIOR THERAPY

The building block of skill acquisition through homework assignments is elaborated in the behavioral strategies, ACT and DBT, to include more holistic approaches to skill development. Just as the campus and greater community are considered learning environments, therapy can be thought of as a therapeutic process that occurs in and out of session. Each hour can be thought of as an anchor for making an emotional connection with a therapist, learning something new emotionally or psychologically, and receiving support. Much of the learning, however, necessarily happens in relationships and situations external to the session. For example, students may learn in session that they feel anxiety and self-doubt in certain circumstances. One homework assignment may be to notice day-to-day situations and the attendant emotion and then generate alternative thoughts. The student then brings this information back to the next session for discussion. This process of learning and implementing in everyday living prepares the student for what happens once the brief therapy is over.

Mindfulness and relaxation skills are other skills common to ACT and DBT that are often taught in session and meant for everyday use. Inclusion of these skills is a helpful augmentation strategy for students with acute anxiety or emotional dysregulation. For the student to learn these techniques, it is important for the student to experience the process of relaxation techniques, such as deep breathing, progressive muscle relation, or visualization, in the office or in another structured venue. Therapists often walk the student through the process of the technique, observing the student and giving the student a chance to ask questions. Such skills are then practiced in many venues across campus—such as a relaxation room in the student union or a mindfulness meditation group that meets in the dorm. Ultimately, the mission and the functioning of the counseling center overlaps with these other venues on campus.

A significant number of students contact the student health center during a moment of crisis, and management of these situations is one of the most critical building blocks of the work done in a college counseling center. The most important of these crisis situations involves suicidal students. When suicidal ideation comes up at initial presentation, the student is evaluated on the same day or as soon as possible depending on the situation. Such an evaluation has a different purpose and structure when compared with a typical evaluation. The focus of the appointment is to assess the nature of the suicidal ideation, the potential for a plan or intent to carry through with the ideation, and the risk for the student. If the risk is elevated, a transfer to a higher level of care, such as intensive outpatient or inpatient services, may be indicated. If the student is suitable for outpatient treatment, DBT skills for distress tolerance and emotion regulation may be used to help the student through the crisis.

Because a crisis is defined by the student's experience of urgency, students with a variety of problems may want a same-day appointment for acute environmental stressors such as relationship problems, academic failure, housing concerns, and academic accommodations. These students are seen as soon as possible because this is another opportunity to make key educational and supportive interventions.

GROUP THERAPY

Group therapy has become an integral component of the major behavioral strategies, including CBT, ACT, and DBT. In particular, DBT skills groups for interpersonal effectiveness, distress tolerance, and emotion regulation were found to be effective (Meaney-Tavares and Hasking 2013; Pistorello et al. 2012; Rizvi and Steffel 2014). The use of groups also fits well with the developmental requirements for young adults to identify with their peers and build social connections with peers rather than parents or authority figures. To this end, group therapy is a treatment strategy in which students can find support for their problems and feel that they are not alone. Students with a psychological problem with which a stigma is associated particularly benefit from working in groups. Successful groups have addressed students with a diverse range of problems, such as eating, anxiety, and depressive disorders. These groups often follow the format of a therapeutic group with the clinical considerations discussed above: frame, structure of session, and assignments. Other groups have focused on issues of cultural, racial/ethnic, sexual, or gender identity. These groups have a less-defined structure, may take place in dorms or community centers, and may be driven by students rather than facilitators. These groups share the commonality of providing peer support under the guidance of sensitive, trained clinicians.

An integral part of group therapy is the use of psychoeducation, which is valuable for teaching students about emotional well-being from a psychological perspective. Although psychoeducation is used to some degree in most treatment modalities, it is particularly prominent in group work at college counseling centers focusing on the development of emotional well-being.

TIME-LIMITED DYNAMIC PSYCHOTHERAPY

A significant number of students seek help with interpersonal issues and are in the process of learning about their relational styles and attachment patterns. In addition to behavioral therapies, these students may benefit from TLDP, a different approach to therapy, in which the therapist and student focus on working with the student's feelings toward the therapist (*transference*) and the therapist's reactions to the student (*countertransference*) as a template for understanding emotional stressors in client-other relationships. The student who develops a better understanding of transference and countertransference in work with the therapist often learns about how to better navigate other relationships. The client and therapist work collaboratively to examine the cyclical maladaptive patterns that impact the student's relational interactions.

Brief therapies often use principles of TLDP, including openly discussing planned treatment termination. The consideration of a student's reaction to termination as the therapy progresses allows the termination to serve a therapeutic purpose—mirroring the student's own developmental stage of individuation and separation. Limited evidence validating psychodynamic approaches to treatment for college students exists.

Clinical Studies Defining Best Practices

A review of the literature shows that few studies have examined the utility and effectiveness of various behavioral and psychodynamic therapeutic modalities in the treatment of students in university mental health centers. This absence is based in part on the unique administrative and academic structure of student health centers. Administratively, college counseling centers are often funded by student fees or allocations from an endowment and do not support research or academic endeavors. In addition, clinicians often report through an office of student affairs or through a dean of students and therefore are not affiliated with medical schools or larger health centers; this lack of connection decreases the potential for finding financial, administrative, and intellectual collaboration. Although a number of surveys such as those by the American College Health Association (www.acha-ncha.org) and the Healthy Minds Study (www.healthymindsnetwork.org/research/hms) characterize the emotional well-being of students as well as the campus climate, few clinical trials have examined the application of various evidence-based therapies to the problems afflicting students in the settings in which they live and learn.

Uliaszek and colleagues (2016) examined the addition of DBT or positive psychotherapy to individual therapy in a group of 54 students and found that augmentation strategy with group therapy, particularly DBT, enhanced effectiveness of treatment. Daltry (2015) presents a case study of an ACT stress management group that discusses the effectiveness of

ACT in increasing distress tolerance and decreasing avoidance behaviors in the face of unwanted emotional experiences. Other studies investigating Web-based applications showed equivocal results regarding effectiveness for mental health prevention for a broad range of problems from alcohol abuse, eating disorders, and hostility (Levin et al. 2016). Carlson (2004) discusses the techniques used in intensive short-term dynamic psychotherapy and ways they may be used in college counseling centers, with a presentation of clinical material to support the findings.

Case Example

Sam is a 20-year-old sophomore man who is struggling with long-standing depressed mood and a recent worsening of his grades, social isolation from friends, and a breakup with a romantic partner. His friends and an instructor are concerned for his well-being and walk him over to the university counseling center.

Sam is embarrassed because of the stigma of being brought to the counseling center, is ashamed because in his family he should not be the one asking for emotional support, and is expressing guilt because he carries the hopes of the family to become the first college graduate. The approach that was applied to this situation involves many of the treatment building blocks discussed in the chapter. The first step is to provide emotional support by hearing his story. In spite of being surrounded by people in the dorms and in class, this opportunity may be the first Sam has to fully and emotionally express himself. The therapist will engage Sam in a conversation about his physical and emotional safety from a crisis management perspective. Sam and the therapist together come up with a safety plan that reinforces skills for tolerating distress, calming down physical symptoms, and using more effective skills for managing distress. These dialectical behavioral strategies will be assessed and reinforced for effectiveness.

Sam and the therapist may end the first session with a review of goals for treatment and psychoeducation about how treatment may proceed. The therapist will work with Sam to address the current symptoms of depression from biological and psychotherapeutic perspectives. This approach may involve the use of cognitive behavioral strategies to address automatic negative thoughts, using worksheets that help with identifying and thinking through cognitive distortions. Medication will likely be considered to address long-standing depressive symptoms that began in childhood. Another treatment modality is group therapy, which provides an opportunity to connect with peers who have similar problems and to give/receive support from his peers.

As therapy visits continue, Sam may become more aware of his role in the family and his reliance on his substantial intellectual capacity to manage his deep-seated anxiety. The therapist may have an opportunity to reflect on the transference/countertransference communications that may lead to a bit more curiosity on Sam's part about his internal emotional states. The combination of these multiple approaches leads to a significant improvement in Sam's symptoms. The next step for Sam and his therapist is to consider medium- to longer-term treatment given Sam's overall situation. This care will likely be provided outside the university counseling center and may be pursued immediately or later in his academic career.

Conclusion

Therapeutic modalities for treatment of a broad range of problems presented by students in college counseling centers have been substantially derived from behavioral strategies such as CBT, ACT, and DBT. In addition, there has been a long-standing but less pronounced contribution from time-limited psychodynamic approaches. A panoply of societal and developmental influences has led therapists in college counseling centers to apply aspects from multiple psychological theories. A consensus is emerging, but more evidence regarding essential techniques is needed. Useful building blocks of the behavioral treatments described above include frame setting, structure of therapy and goal development, cognitive-behavioral skills, mindfulness and relaxation skills, crisis intervention, psychoeducation, and use of groups. Given the diversity described in this chapter and the individualized use of various techniques, the few studies that have been conducted are limited in providing broad applicability. A concerted effort to elucidate the best practices would include testing the usefulness of these modified strategies as adapted from the original therapeutic paradigm.

KEY CONCEPTS

- In recent years, parents, teachers, and community institutions (e.g., media, medical groups, social support agencies) have placed an increasing focus on the mental health and emotional well-being of university students as well as the campus climate at universities across the country.

- Common building blocks derived from various therapeutic strategies, including cognitive-behavioral therapy (CBT), acceptance commitment therapy (ACT), dialectical behavior therapy (DBT), and time-limited dynamic psychotherapy (TLDP), have been modified for brief interventions in college counseling centers.

- For a number of clinical and administrative reasons, few clinical studies have been conducted to support "best practices" for treating students in university counseling centers.

Recommendations for Psychiatrists, Psychologists, and Counselors

1. A full assessment is recommended for most students to establish a context for creating a therapeutic alliance and setting therapy goals.
2. Students benefit from a flexible approach to therapy incorporating elements of different psychotherapy techniques (e.g., crisis management and CBT skills, CBT followed by a psychodynamic intervention).
3. It may be helpful to conceptualize the brief intervention as "the planting of seed" that may grow in the student's experience at a later point long after the therapy is over.

Discussion Questions

1. A number of societal trends and demographic changes have influenced the provision of services in university mental health. Identify and discuss the impact of these developments.
2. Discuss the essential techniques for brief therapy and compare the treatment paradigms from which they arise.
3. Identify the contributing factors that impede the study of specific treatment modalities in university mental health.

Suggested Readings

Grayson PA, Meilman PW (eds): College Mental Health Practice. New York, Routledge, 2015
Iarovici D: Mental Health Issues and the University Student. Baltimore, MD, Johns Hopkins University Press, 2014
Kadison R, DiGeronimo TF: College of the Overwhelmed. San Francisco, CA, Jossey-Bass, 2004

Wright JH, Brown GK, Thase ME, Ramirez Basco M: Learning Cognitive-Behavior Therapy: An Illustrated Guide, 2nd Edition (Core Competencies in Psychotherapy series; Gabbard GO, series ed.). Arlington, VA, American Psychiatric Association Publishing, 2017

References

Beck AT, Rush AJ, Shaw BF, Emery J: Cognitive Therapy of Depression. New York, Guilford Press, 1979

Carlson TM: A short-term dynamic psychotherapy approach for college students. Journal of College Student Psychotherapy 18(3):47–67, 2004

Daltry RM: A case study: an ACT stress management group in a university counseling center. Journal of College Student Psychotherapy 29(1):36–43, 2015

Levin ME, Hayes SC, Pistorello J, Seeley JR: Web-based self-help for preventing mental health problems in universities: comparing acc0eptance and commitment training to mental health education. J Clin Psychol 72(3):207–225, 2016 26784010

Meaney-Tavares R, Hasking P: Coping and regulating emotions: a pilot study of a modified dialectical behavior therapy group delivered in a college counseling service. J Am Coll Health 61(5):303–309, 2013 23768227

Pistorello J, Fruzzetti AE, Maclane C, et al: Dialectical behavior therapy (DBT) applied to college students: a randomized clinical trial. J Consult Clin Psychol 80(6):982–994, 2012 22730955

Rizvi SL, Steffel LM: A pilot study of 2 brief forms of dialectical behavior therapy skills training for emotion dysregulation in college students. J Am Coll Health 62(6):434–439, 2014 24678824

Uliaszek AA, Rashid T, Williams GE, Gulamani T: Group therapy for university students: a randomized control trial of dialectical behavior therapy and positive psychotherapy. Behav Res Ther 77:78–85, 2016 26731172

CHAPTER 23

Innovation, Technology, and Student Well-Being

Rachael Flatt, B.S.
Mickey Trockel, M.D.

IN this chapter, we introduce the opportunities available for universities to develop and integrate digital tools into currently existing mental health care services. We begin by outlining the need for technology-based resources. Recent studies and examples of advancements in digital tools and modes of delivery are discussed within the scope of the most common psychological problems among university students: anxiety, depression, alcohol misuse, sleep disorders, suicidal ideation, and eating disorders. We then present an adapted transdiagnostic, stepped-care model that integrates screening, personalized feedback, and prevention and intervention program recommendations. Finally, we present one case example, demonstrating the possible benefits of utilizing technology in mental health care.

The Need for Technology-Based Mental Health Care

The prevalence of mental health disorders among college students is high. A national epidemiological study of college students reported that almost half of all college students met criteria for DSM-IV psychiatric disorders in the previous year (Blanco et al. 2008). Unfortunately, most students with mental health problems do not receive treatment; between 15% and 36% of college students with probable disorders receive some method of treatment (Blanco et al. 2008; Eisenberg et al. 2011a), and roughly 10% of students seek out at least one therapy or counseling session (Eisenberg et al. 2007). In a nationwide survey of colleges, the ratio of college counselors to students was 1:2,081, and 70% of colleges reported a concern about "[t]he growing demand for services without an appropriate increase in resources" (Gallagher 2009). Considering the low percentage of students seeking counseling, the low counselor-to-student ratio, and the growing concerns of counseling centers, it is unlikely that college counseling centers would be able to treat all students who experience psychiatric disorders during their time at college with traditional in-person mental health care.

Other significant problems among college students are the lack of knowledge surrounding mental health services and the barriers to service uptake among students. At some universities, one-quarter to one-half of students do not know where to access psychological counseling on campus (Eisenberg et al. 2007; Saitz et al. 2007). In addition, although approximately half of students have a mental health disorder, a lower proportion (roughly 30%) of students perceive a need for mental health care (Eisenberg et al. 2007). Other common barriers to pursuing treatment include stigmatization of psychological disorders, lack of perceived urgency, unknown or high cost of treatment, lack of time and availability of treatment, cultural differences, and skepticism of treatment efficacy, among others (Benton et al. 2003; Givens and Tjia 2002; Mowbray et al. 2006; Saitz et al. 2007).

The various barriers and a lack of specialized treatment options outside of in-person therapy often prevent students from resolving their symptoms in a timely and effective manner. Expanding development of computer, online, and smartphone technology–based intervention tools may help overcome these barriers on the path toward adequate delivery of and access to student mental health care. In 2014, Dahlstrom and Bichsel reported that 90% of students owned a laptop and 86% of undergraduate students owned a smartphone, and these numbers are expected to increase. The tremendous accessibility of technology across college student populations demonstrates great opportunity to reach a majority of students through scalable and affordable models of treatment. Established uses of mobile technology for prevention and treatment include assessing symptomatology, delivering psychoeducational materials, and self-monitoring of situational stressors and treatment progress (Bang et al. 2007; Luxton et al. 2011). Additionally, a growing number of online and mobile phone application–based prevention and treatment programs have already been developed or are currently being evaluated. These digital treatment programs aim to deliver care to those suffering from psychiatric disorders, particularly to those who do not currently receive care because of barriers that can be readily remedied with these convenient, low-cost programs. Continued development and evaluation of mobile phone and online mental health interventions promise to increase the proportion of students who receive evidence-based treatment among those who are likely to benefit from these interventions.

Benefits and Applications of Mobile Mental Health Technology Across Disorders

A growing number of mobile phone and online–based interventions address specific mental health issues that are common among college students. The most prevalent mental health problems among college students include anxiety, depression, alcohol misuse, sleep disorders, suicidal ideation, and eating disorders (these problems are also addressed individually in separate chapters of this book).

ANXIETY

In the 2015 American College Health Survey, about 58% of college students reported feeling overwhelming anxiety at least once in the previous year, and more than one in five students reported that anxiety affected their academic performance (American College Health Association 2016). Leading stressors driving students' situational anxiety include academic performance, plans following graduation, and the pressure to succeed (Beiter et al. 2015). Traditionally, college students seeking to treat their anxiety could visit a mental health care professional by visiting their campus counseling center or accessing off-campus community resources. However, evidence-based online and mobile application–based programs make it possible to effectively treat anxiety symptoms through the adaptation of traditional therapeutic approaches that may make accessing treatment more convenient and more affordable.

Many evidence-based online cognitive-behavioral therapy (CBT)–based treatment programs developed to address anxiety have been shown to be effective (Davies et al. 2014). Although most online CBT-based anxiety programs generally consist of similar content and techniques (Saddichha et al. 2014), variations on secondary therapist support for online programs have been tested to determine approaches that may achieve a similar, if not better, outcome when compared with face-to-face treatment. A meta-analysis conducted by Saddichha et al. (2014) compared the efficacy of guided self-help anxiety programs, in which a therapist or coach provides additional support outside of the program, with face-to-face treatments. The analysis included 18 studies, which addressed a variety of anxiety disorders including social anxiety disorder, generalized anxiety disorder, and mixed anxiety disorders. Although the content and length of intervention varied across the studies, most therapist-assisted online self-help programs were as effective as—or, in some cases, more effective than—face-to-face therapy. Additionally, therapists who provided support in the guided self-help programs spent significantly less time treating participants while achieving similar outcomes compared with face-to-face treatment. Therefore, integrating similar types of programs into current university mental health care models may allow counseling centers and therapists to reach a greater proportion of the student population. Recommending guided self-help programs should not be considered as a substitute for offering mental health services on campuses; rather, guided self-help programs are a way of expanding availability of effective care and a strategy to help clinicians maximize their time.

DEPRESSION

In college populations, between 17% and 30% of students exhibit clinical depression (Eisenberg et al. 2013; Ibrahim et al. 2013). Additionally, over 35% of students reported feeling so depressed that it was difficult to function at least once in the previous year (American College Health Association 2016). To address this high prevalence, numerous online depression prevention and intervention programs have been developed and evaluated or are currently in the process of evaluation. The majority of online programs for depression deliver CBT, as it is the leading and most popular treatment for anxiety and depression in terms of long-term relapse prevention and symptom management (Grist and Cavanagh 2013; Luxton et al. 2011). Like similar programs for anxiety disorders, online CBT-based depression programs can be as effective as face-to-face treatment (Saddichha et al. 2014). Researchers are now testing modes of delivery through various technology media to determine the most effective medium.

In a recent study, the efficacy of a CBT-based depression program delivered through a Web site was compared with that of a mobile phone application (Watts et al. 2013). Participants were randomly divided into two groups: one group completed a six-session CBT-based program on an online platform, and one group completed the same program through a mobile phone application. Participants from both groups achieved similar reductions in symptoms, and less than half of the participants met criteria for depression after completing the program. The results suggest that previously developed online programs can be adapted for delivery through mobile phone applications and achieve similar results in efficacy. This is especially pertinent to on-the-go college students, who spend an estimated 7.5–10 hours on their mobile phones daily (Roberts et al. 2014). Flexibility in the mode of delivery may make interventions for students experiencing depression more user-friendly by allowing students to choose their preference in mode of delivery. Although comparable efficacy across modes of delivery is less established for mental health disorders other than depression, it is likely that both online programs and mobile phone applications will achieve relatively similar efficacy across other disorders.

ALCOHOL MISUSE

Heavy drinking on college campuses is a chronic problem. At least 40% of students report having drunk five or more drinks in a row in the previous 2 weeks (O'Malley and Johnston 2002), and approximately 20% of students have an alcohol abuse or dependence disorder (Blanco et al. 2008). Men engage in unhealthy alcohol use more frequently than women (O'Malley and Johnston 2002; Saitz et al. 2007), and white men tend to lead all demographic groups in heavy drinking (O'Malley and Johnston 2002). Greek student organization involvement also significantly predicts alcohol use and problems, ranging from unwanted sexual encounters, neglecting responsibilities, feeling physically sick from drinking, or drinking and driving, during the first 2 years of college (Capone et al. 2007). It is apparent that gender, social, and demographic differences particularly affect alcohol misuse; therefore, mobile technology–based programs should address these personal identifiers similarly to the way in which tailored in-person treatments address these attributes.

In one study, first-year college students were randomly assigned to receive either brief "minimal" or "more extensive" online interventions after reporting unhealthy alcohol use (Saitz et al. 2007). Compared with those who received the minimal intervention, men who received the more extensive intervention reported greater intention to seek help, and women reported a greater increase in readiness to change. After 1 month, there was no significant difference between the brief and more intensive interventions, and 33% of women and 15% of men with unhealthy alcohol use at the start of the trial no longer had unhealthy alcohol use. This study highlights the ability of a brief online program to both reduce unhealthy alcohol use and identify unique characteristics of men and women in their help-seeking behaviors and motivation to change. If generalizable, the results of this study indicating greater efficacy among women suggest the need for tailoring interventions for specific demographic groups rather than adoption of one-size-fits-all programs.

SLEEP DISORDERS

Pulling an occasional all-nighter may seem normative among college students, yet frequent erratic sleep patterns and poor sleep quality are pervasive and problematic across college campuses (Brown et al. 2002). Up to 89% of college students report poor sleep quality (Buboltz et al. 2001), and one study found 27% of students to be at risk for a sleep disorder (Gaultney 2010). Poor sleep quality has potentially negative consequences, including daytime sleepiness, challenges in performing normal daytime tasks, and poor academic performance (Gomes et al. 2011; Hershner and Chervin 2014; Trockel et al. 2000). With the particularly high rates of reported poor sleep quality and the associated risks and consequences of poor sleep quality, perhaps the importance of consistent sleep patterns is not communicated or emphasized enough to college students. To reach the almost 90% of students suffering from poor sleep quality, a broad and low-cost approach would be essential.

One study tested a cost-effective and useful delivery system for a CBT-based sleep intervention program (Trockel et al. 2011). First-year college students at a large private university were offered one unit of course credit to participate and were randomly assigned to receive Refresh, an intervention to improve sleep, or Breathe, a more generic health promotion program designed to help students cope with stress and to improve their emotional health. Both programs were delivered as PDF documents via e-mail over 8 weeks. Students with poor sleep who received Refresh demonstrated greater improvement in their sleep quality in comparison with those who received Breathe. The results indicate that Refresh was effective in improving sleep even when delivered through e-mail documents, thus demonstrating the utility of a no-cost and easily accessible technology platform.

Utilizing e-mail to deliver care may not be the most effective way to treat all psychiatric disorders; however, e-mail may be extremely useful in delivering helpful information and tools to promote healthier behaviors to a large number of students struggling with common problems, such as sleep. E-mail intervention, or similar low-cost interventions, may be more feasible for reaching low-risk subpopulations compared with potentially more effective, but more resource-intensive, approaches.

SUICIDAL IDEATION

Social media is ubiquitous among adolescents and college students. Whereas photos posted to social media platforms such as Instagram can chronicle changes in physical appearance, messages posted to Twitter and Facebook have the potential to illuminate psychological changes. Additionally, linguistics software can analyze trends and changes over time, and machine learning can predict certain behaviors of social media users. Businesses often use linguistic software to their benefit by promoting products when users are exhibiting behaviors indicating that they may purchase an item or a service. This technology may also be used to predict harmful thoughts or behaviors, such as suicidal ideation, in the hopes of reaching a user before harm is done.

In a recent study, linguistics software was used to analyze the composition, authenticity, and emotional tone in Twitter messages from 135 users to screen for suicidality (Braithwaite et al. 2016). Machine learning and predictive algorithms were then used to identify users currently experiencing suicidal ideation. This method proved to be effective in classifying and predicting the nonsuicidal and suicidal users. This study highlights the potential for application of modern technologies to identify students at risk of suicide and predict those who may become suicidal. Universities may choose not to monitor the social media accounts of their students for a variety of reasons, particularly out of respect for students' privacy. However, it is important for universities to provide effective resources to ensure the well-being of their students, especially those who are seriously considering suicide. Thus, earlier identification of students struggling with suicidality through analysis of social media postings may allow campus counselors to reach students sooner with more relevant and personalized resources.

EATING DISORDERS

College-age students demonstrate a high prevalence rate of eating disorders (Smink et al. 2012). An estimated 13% of college students screen positively for an eating disorder, and of students who screen positive, less than 20% report receiving any treatment (Eisenberg et al. 2011b). Frequent dieting, restrictive eating, sociocultural factors, and concern over weight and body shape are significant risk factors for developing an eating disorder (Fitzsimmons-Craft et al. 2012; Jacobi et al. 2004). These risk factors are particularly relevant to female college students, who may experience common triggers such as an unanticipated weight gain (the "freshman 15"), peer pressure to diet with a group of friends, or the internalization of the thin body ideal. College women in particular may benefit from prevention programs before clinical symptoms emerge.

In a meta-analysis, Beintner and colleagues (2012) reviewed trials using StudentBodies, an online, CBT-based, 8-week eating disorder prevention program. A total of 10 randomized controlled trials were included. Eating disorder attitudes and behaviors of American and German high school and college students were assessed to determine the students' risk of developing an eating disorder. The prevention program was associated with reductions in negative body image and desire to be thin, and the program was determined to be moderately effective immediately postintervention and at follow-up. Online indicated preventive programs, such as StudentBodies, may be cost-effective ways of reducing incidence of eating disorders in large populations of college students.

If programs that prevent mental health problems continue to be developed and evaluated, it is possible that effective primary prevention programs can be implemented to address the full range of mental health problems common in college student populations. Such broad implementation of evolving evidence-based preventive interventions may significantly reduce the number of students developing clinical disorders. In turn, this may relieve the caseload for campus counseling centers and therapists while concurrently reducing morbidity attributable to mental health problems.

Models and Suggestions for the Future

On the basis of the data presented thus far, it is clear that technology-based mental health care can be effective for students in need. However, college campuses have yet to implement effective and affordable treatment models using technology to adequately address the growing percentage of students at high risk for developing a mental disorder or those with clinical symptoms. Wilfley et al. created a novel technology-based stepped-care model to prevent and treat eating disorders, which has been shown to be cost effective (Kass et al. 2017; Wilfley et al. 2013). The investigators used an online screening tool to determine risk and symptomatology. Students then received personalized feedback and/or an optional referral followed by an offer to begin their personalized program. Students at a lower risk for developing an eating disorder received access to a wellness and health maintenance program, whereas those at higher risk received access to a prevention program. Students who screened positive for anorexia nervosa or suicidality were only offered a referral for clinical evaluations and treatment. Students who screened positive for another eating disorder (e.g., bulimia nervosa, binge-eating disorder) were offered the treatment program in conjunction with a referral for clinical evaluation.

This stepped-care model can be adapted and expanded by employing a transdiagnostic screen and by including CBT-based prevention, treatment, and maintenance programs for multiple disorders (Figure 23–1). Electronic intake forms, which are currently offered at only 6% of college campuses (Gallagher 2009), may reduce the time counseling centers use to evaluate students. Another particular advantage to this model is the algorithmically determined program offerings, which allow for flexibility in integrating treatment programs. For instance, if a student screens positive for anxiety and depression, treatment programs can be seamlessly integrated to best serve the individual's needs. This model also has the potential to provide evidence-based, affordable, and easily accessible care to students at risk for developing a mental health disorder. By providing support to at-risk populations, campus counseling centers may find increased time to provide treatment to the more severe clinical cases, while also possibly preventing the onset of new clinical cases. Meanwhile, students who are at low risk of developing clinical symptoms will have access to beneficial educational materials that help them maintain and build on their previously established healthy habits.

As this model is implemented, data can be collected to create improved iterations of programs and resources. As highlighted earlier in this chapter, socially and demographically sensitive treatments are an important component of efficacy. At this point, interventions have not yet been adapted for smaller subpopulations. However, with the use of machine learning and treatment of large populations, algorithms will be able to analyze trends in program usage and subgroup cultural differences in efficacy. From there, investigators and content developers will be able to fine-tune programs for subpopulations to create evidence-based tailored content. Collecting the vast amount of data necessary to

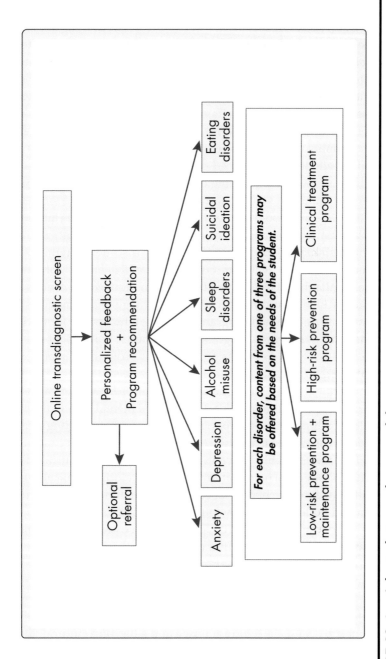

FIGURE 23–1.   **Adapted stepped-care model.**

create more personalized mobile treatments will take time and significant resources. Nonetheless, crafting, testing, and disseminating iterations of socially and demographically personalized interventions may allow technology-based treatments to further improve overall outcomes. While this model cannot be a substitute for on-campus counseling services, it is valuable as an adjuvant, sustainable, and cost-effective strategy with the potential to stretch resources currently in place, thereby addressing many of the most common mental health problems that college students experience.

Additional resources can be created in tandem to strengthen this model. These resources may consist of, but are not limited to, videos, articles, discussion forums, lists of online peer support groups, microinterventions and basic coping strategies, free screening tools, recommendations for evidence-based phone applications, and lists of therapeutic options available to students on campus and nearby. For instance, counseling centers could provide access to an interactive digital mental health handbook presenting basic strategies for a few common psychological problems experienced by a large percentage of the student population. Using weekly e-mail or text campaigns highlighting these tools and including links to the available resources can be an effective dissemination strategy, as illustrated by the success of the Refresh sleep health improvement program (Trockel et al. 2011).

Finally, more research in the field of mobile mental health technology can be conducted, ranging from the most effective way to destigmatize mental health disorders among college students to individual program tailoring and mode of delivery optimization. Use of machine learning to develop individualized predictive algorithms may render programs capable of delivering to students more relevant interventions components, tools, or treatment suggestions rather than a set of preassigned program components. This development may provide more effective and timely care to an individual, possibly preventing a negative event such as suicide, or may uncover behavior characteristics unique to specific subpopulations. Campuses may seek to integrate digital mental health programs with traditional counseling center services to ease the caseload burden, to provide accessible and affordable care to a greater percentage of the student population, and to conduct more evaluation research for iterative improvement of treatment and treatment outcomes.

Case Example

Susan was completing her third year of medical school when she learned about cognitive-behavioral therapy (CBT)–based mobile- and technology-assisted treatment programs for anxiety disorders. She had been struggling with significant anxiety for over a year and had been reluctant to seek treatment. She feared she would face potential stigmatization from peers and medical school faculty if she took time to attend weekly in-person CBT appointments at her university counseling center. Susan noticed that her intense anxiety during her internal medicine clerkship was beginning to interfere with her ability to remember and communicate clinical information during morning treatment rounds with her team. She was happy to learn from a colleague interested in specializing in psychiatry that online treatment of anxiety can be as effective as in-person treatment. Susan did some online research and found a few programs that seemed interesting to her, but she had a hard time determining which programs had been tested adequately in clinical trials. She tried three before finding a fourth that seemed to work for her, somewhat. She decided to continue her CBT during a 6-week research rotation that was flexible enough to make in-person treatment feasible. Susan felt that her online introduction to CBT for anxiety accelerated her progress during in-person treatment and noted much-reduced anxiety during her fourth-year medical clerkships.

Conclusion

There is compelling potential for integration of technology-based interventions in stepped-care models to increase access and cost-effectiveness of college student mental health services. Systematic development, evaluation, and iterative improvement of technology-based interventions may lead to optimally tailored programs that further augment effectiveness of stepped-care models. During the critical developmental years in college, students are preparing for their professional careers, establishing relationships, and transitioning into their roles as community leaders. It is imperative that students are given opportunity to flourish, unimpeded by preventable or treatable mental health problems.

Developing and compiling these resources may take a significant amount of time, and it is important to consider using evidence-based and high-quality materials. Of the thousands of digital programs from which to choose, few have substantial research to support their utility and efficacy, and some may exploit student data (Torous and Roberts 2017). Many students may unknowingly turn to poorly constructed digital programs out of ease, frustration, or the lack of stigma associated with such programs instead of using existing university services. Therefore, similar to choosing from in-person therapy options, selecting evidence-based, technology-assisted interventions improves risk-to-benefit ratio of treatment. We suggest careful vetting of programs, such that students are offered high-quality technology-based care. Tools that may be useful in determining the quality, evidence, safety, and usability of online and mobile phone application programs include PsyberGuide (https://psyberguide.org), which provides reviews of applications, and the American Psychiatric Association's model for evaluating products (American Psychiatric Association 2017). Moving forward, universities may contribute to improvements in technology-based mental health interventions by conducting rigorous research on the efficacy and quality of existing programs, thereby informing students, counseling centers, and therapists, in addition to developing novel innovative programs.

KEY CONCEPTS

- Technology provides a tremendous opportunity to aid counseling centers and mental health care professionals in supporting at-risk and clinically symptomatic college students.

- College mental health services should develop and disseminate free resources on counseling center Web sites rather than limiting information to referrals and contact information.

- College mental health services should provide technology-based prevention and treatment strategies and implement stepped-care models as alternatives for students seeking immediate assistance, alternatives to face-to-face therapy, or additional support to supplement in-person treatment.

- More research in the field of mobile mental health technology is necessary in order to optimize assessments, programs, modes of delivery, and implementation models.

Recommendations for Psychiatrists, Psychologists, and Counselors

1. Develop and disseminate free resources through schoolwide communications (e.g., e-mail, text). Consider launching quarterly or weekly electronic newsletters with embedded materials or attachments.
2. List available online resources through the counseling Web site, and consider developing a downloadable or interactive online mental health handbook for students.
3. Integrate a confidential, evidence-based, online screening tool for students to assess anxiety, depression, suicidality, substance abuse, and sleep, eating, and alcohol disorders. If students screen positively for any of these disorders, provide personalized feedback, provide a list of available resources on campus, and recommend technology-based programs to target those who are reluctant to seek treatment.
4. Implement a stepped-care, technology-based model for students at risk and students exhibiting clinical symptoms to support those who do not have access to or cannot afford traditional in-person therapy.

Discussion Questions

1. What types of online resources does your counseling center currently provide for free? Are they easily accessible to students? Are there gaps in the information or tools currently available to students? If so, what are those gaps, and how could you address them through the use of technology?
2. How would you address outreach and use technology tools to address destigmatization of mental health disorders among college students?
3. If you were to design a mobile program for one of the more common mental health disorders you see, what would this program look like? What psychoeducation or therapeutic techniques would you include? How would you disseminate this program to the student population?
4. How can you work with other key stakeholders to implement an online, evidence-based model at your institution?

Suggested Readings

Hsin H, Torous J, Roberts L: An adjuvant role for mobile health in psychiatry. JAMA Psychiatry 73(2):103–104, 2016

Schueller SM, Washburn JJ, Price M: Exploring mental health providers' interest in using Web and mobile-based tools in their practices. Internet Interventions 4(2):145–151, 2016

Wilfley DE, Agras WS, Taylor CB: Reducing the burden of eating disorders: a model for population-based prevention and treatment for university and college campuses. Int J Eat Disord 46(5):529–532, 2013

References

American College Health Association: American College Health Association–National College Health Assessment II: Fall 2015 Reference Group Executive Summary. Hanover, MD, American College Health Association, 2016. Available at: http://www.acha-ncha.org/docs/NCHA-II%20Fall%202015%20Reference%20Group%20Executive%20Summary.pdf. Accessed May 16, 2017.

American Psychiatric Association: Mental health app evaluation model. Available at: https://www.psychiatry.org/psychiatrists/practice/mental-health-apps/app-evaluation-model. Accessed July 21, 2017.

Bang M, Timpka T, Eriksson H, et al: Mobile phone computing for in-situ cognitive behavioral therapy. Stud Health Technol Inform 129(Pt 2):1078–1082, 2007 17911881

Beintner I, Jacobi C, Taylor CB: Effects of an Internet-based prevention programme for eating disorders in the USA and Germany—a meta-analytic review. Eur Eat Disord Rev 20(1):1–8, 2012 21796737

Beiter R, Nash R, McCrady M, et al: The prevalence and correlates of depression, anxiety, and stress in a sample of college students. J Affect Disord 173:90–96, 2015 25462401

Benton SA, Robertson JM, Tseng WC, et al: Changes in counseling center client problems across 13 years. Prof Psychol Res Pr 34(1):66–72, 2003

Blanco C, Okuda M, Wright C, et al: Mental health of college students and their non-college-attending peers: results from the National Epidemiologic Study on Alcohol and Related Conditions. Arch Gen Psychiatry 65(12):1429–1437, 2008 19047530

Braithwaite SR, Giraud-Carrier C, West J, et al: Validating machine learning algorithms for Twitter data against established measures of suicidality. JMIR Ment Health 3(2):e21, 2016 27185366

Brown FC, Buboltz WC Jr, Soper B: Relationship of sleep hygiene awareness, sleep hygiene practices, and sleep quality in university students. Behav Med 28(1):33–38, 2002 12244643

Buboltz WC Jr, Brown F, Soper B: Sleep habits and patterns of college students: a preliminary study. J Am Coll Health 50(3):131–135, 2001 11765249

Capone C, Wood MD, Borsari B, Laird RD: Fraternity and sorority involvement, social influences, and alcohol use among college students: a prospective examination. Psychol Addict Behav 21(3):316–327, 2007 17874882

Dahlstrom E, Bichsel J: ECAR Study of Undergraduate Students and Information Technology. Louisville, CO, EDUCAUSE Center for Analysis and Research, October 2014

Davies EB, Morriss R, Glazebrook C: Computer-delivered and Web-based interventions to improve depression, anxiety, and psychological well-being of university students: a systematic review and meta-analysis. J Med Internet Res 16(5):e130, 2014 24836465

Eisenberg D, Golberstein E, Gollust SE: Help-seeking and access to mental health care in a university student population. Med Care 45(7):594–601, 2007 17571007

Eisenberg D, Hunt J, Speer N, Zivin K: Mental health service utilization among college students in the United States. J Nerv Ment Dis 199(5):301–308, 2011a 21543948

Eisenberg D, Nicklett EJ, Roeder K, Kirz NE: Eating disorder symptoms among college students: prevalence, persistence, correlates, and treatment-seeking. J Am Coll Health 59(8):700–707, 2011b 21950250

Eisenberg D, Hunt J, Speer N: Mental health in American colleges and universities: variation across student subgroups and across campuses. J Nerv Ment Dis 201(1):60–67, 2013 23274298

Fitzsimmons-Craft EE, Harney MB, Koehler LG, et al: Explaining the relation between thin ideal internalization and body dissatisfaction among college women: the roles of social comparison and body surveillance. Body Image 9(1):43–49, 2012 21992811

Gallagher RP: National Survey of Counseling Center Directors 2008. Pittsburgh, PA, University of Pittsburgh, 2009

Gaultney JF: The prevalence of sleep disorders in college students: impact on academic performance. J Am Coll Health 59(2):91–97, 2010 20864434

Givens JL, Tjia J: Depressed medical students' use of mental health services and barriers to use. Acad Med 77(9):918–921, 2002 12228091

Gomes AA, Tavares J, de Azevedo MH: Sleep and academic performance in undergraduates: a multi-measure, multi-predictor approach. Chronobiol Int 28(9):786–801, 2011 22080785

Grist R, Cavanagh K: Computerised cognitive behavioural therapy for common mental health disorders, what works, for whom under what circumstances? A systematic review and meta-analysis. Journal of Contemporary Psychotherapy 43(4):243–251, 2013

Hershner SD, Chervin RD: Causes and consequences of sleepiness among college students. Nat Sci Sleep 6:73–84, 2014 25018659

Ibrahim AK, Kelly SJ, Adams CE, Glazebrook C: A systematic review of studies of depression prevalence in university students. J Psychiatr Res 47(3):391–400, 2013 23260171

Jacobi C, Hayward C, de Zwaan M, et al: Coming to terms with risk factors for eating disorders: application of risk terminology and suggestions for a general taxonomy. Psychol Bull 130(1):19–65, 2004 14717649

Kass AE, Balantekin KN, Fitzsimmons-Craft EE, et al: The economic case for digital interventions for eating disorders among United States college students. Int J Eat Disord 50(3):250–258, 2017 28152203

Luxton DD, McCann RA, Bush NE, et al: mHealth for mental health: Integrating smartphone technology in behavioral healthcare. Prof Psychol Res Pr 42(6):505–512, 2011

Mowbray CT, Megivern D, Mandiberg JM, et al: Campus mental health services: recommendations for change. Am J Orthopsychiatry 76(2):226–237, 2006 16719642

O'Malley PM, Johnston LD: Epidemiology of alcohol and other drug use among American college students. J Stud Alcohol Suppl, March (14):23–39, 2002 12022728

Roberts JA, Yaya LH, Manolis C: The invisible addiction: cell-phone activities and addiction among male and female college students. J Behav Addict 3(4):254–265, 2014 25595966

Saddichha S, Al-Desouki M, Lamia A, et al: Online interventions for depression and anxiety—a systematic review. Health Psychol Behav Med 2(1):841–881, 2014 25750823

Saitz R, Palfai TP, Freedner N, et al: Screening and brief intervention online for college students: the ihealth study. Alcohol Alcohol 42(1):28–36, 2007 17130139

Smink FR, van Hoeken D, Hoek HW: Epidemiology of eating disorders: incidence, prevalence and mortality rates. Curr Psychiatry Rep 14(4):406–414, 2012 22644309

Torous J, Roberts LW: Needed Innovation in Digital Health and Smartphone Applications for Mental Health: Transparency and Trust. JAMA Psychiatry 74(5):437–438, 2017 28384700

Trockel MT, Barnes MD, Egget DL: Health-related variables and academic performance among first-year college students: implications for sleep and other behaviors. J Am Coll Health 49(3):125–131, 2000 11125640

Trockel M, Manber R, Chang V, et al: An e-mail delivered CBT for sleep-health program for college students: effects on sleep quality and depression symptoms. J Clin Sleep Med 7(3):276–281, 2011 21677898

Watts S, Mackenzie A, Thomas C, et al: CBT for depression: a pilot RCT comparing mobile phone vs. computer. BMC Psychiatry 13:49, 2013 23391304

Wilfley DE, Agras WS, Taylor CB: Reducing the burden of eating disorders: a model for population-based prevention and treatment for university and college campuses. Int J Eat Disord 46(5):529–532, 2013 23658106

PART IV

Fostering Mental Health for Distinct Student Populations

CHAPTER 24

First-Generation College Students

Raziya S. Wang, M.D.
Shashank V. Joshi, M.D.

THE term *first-generation college students* most often describes students whose parents did not enroll in any postsecondary education. Some research also includes in this group students whose parent(s) enrolled in but did not complete postsecondary education. Forty-three percent of beginning college students in a national data sample from 1989–1990 were first-generation students, representing a significant portion of all beginning students and a large enough group to merit special attention from educators and college mental health professionals. In this national sample, although the first-generation college students shared many characteristics and challenges with minority and low socioeconomic status students, they experienced significant disadvantages in college even when these other factors were taken into account (Nuñez and Cuccaro-Alamin 1998).

Unique Characteristics

Studies examining national data show that first-generation college students are more likely to be female, older, and Hispanic; to have dependent children; and to come from lower socioeconomic status families than their non-first-generation peers. They are less likely to be academically ready for college than their peers (Chen 2005; Nuñez and Cuccaro-Alamin 1998; Terenzini et al. 1996) (Table 24–1). Once enrolled, first-generation students work more hours off campus and spend fewer hours studying than other students (Terenzini et al. 1996) (Table 24–2). Studies have found that first-generation students experience more posttraumatic stress disorder symptoms and report lower life satisfaction and a lower sense of belonging on campus than peers (Jenkins et al. 2013; Stebleton et al. 2014). In addition, first-generation students more often attend college part time and have higher degree noncompletion rates than non-first-generation students (Chen 2005; Nuñez and Cuccaro-Alamin 1998).

Finally, first-generation students more often endorse interdependent or community-oriented values as motivation for pursuing higher education and struggle with acculturation in the university setting, which often promotes more independent or individualistic values (Stephens et al. 2012). The term *enculturation* describes the process of learning about and potentially incorporating the societal norms of the surrounding cultural environment. For first-generation students, this process may be influenced by peers, faculty, residential staff, and other adults on campus. If the enculturation process is successful, the values and rituals of a specific university or college culture may be incorporated into the student's worldview (Grusec and Hastings 2007; Sholevar and Joshi 2017). Ideally, an optimal degree of biculturalism will be achieved, whereby the student incorporates the best of their parents' (or their own) culture of origin with those of the university (host) culture (LaFromboise et al. 1993).

Multiracial first-generation students may face a more difficult challenge than their monoracial peers. They must develop this new identity and decide how, or even whether, they can reflect positive aspects of all

TABLE 24–1. **First-generation college students: precollege statistics**

More likely to be female

More likely to be Hispanic

More likely to come from low socioeconomic status families

More likely to be older students who have delayed starting college

More likely to have dependent children

Less likely to be academically prepared for college

Source. Chen 2005; Nuñez and Cuccaro-Alamin 1998; Terenzini et al. 1996.

TABLE 24–2. **First-generation college students: on-campus statistics**

More likely to attend college part time

More likely to work more hours off campus

More likely to spend fewer hours studying

May be more likely to report symptoms of posttraumatic stress disorder

May be more likely to report lower life satisfaction and lower sense of belonging on campus

More likely to struggle with acculturation issues in the university setting

Less likely to complete a college degree

Source. Chen 2005; Jenkins et al. 2013; Nuñez and Cuccaro-Alamin 1998; Stebleton et al. 2014; Stephens et al. 2012; Terenzini et al. 1996.

heritages and cultures, while also rejecting certain societal expectations and stereotypes (Kerwin and Ponterotto 1995; Pumariega and Joshi 2010; Wehrly et al. 1999). Often by college age, multiracial youth have been made aware of any racial/ethnic differences between classmates and themselves. They may be reminded of these differences when they are asked questions such as "What are you?" by classmates puzzled by their racially or ethnically mixed appearance (Sholevar and Joshi 2017). These alienating questions may contribute to the students' feelings that no one understands them, and they may feel "stuck" between cultures (Pumariega and Joshi 2010; Root 1990). Additionally, some peers, and even a student's own parents, may pressure the student to identify with only one ethnic background, potentially raising feelings of guilt or disloyalty (Cauce et al. 1992; Pumariega and Joshi 2010; Sholevar and Joshi 2017; Wehrly et al. 1999). Similarly, these students may for the first time be attracted to cultural norms outside of their culture of origin, which can create a type of distancing from their families, known as *accultura-tive family distancing*. As first described in Latino and Asian youth, those who experience acculturative family distancing may be at higher risk for severe psychological distress, depression, and other mental health conditions (Hwang 2006; Hwang and Wood 2009). On the other hand, a sense of an integrated, bicultural self-concept may allow enculturated first-generation students to create a sense of cultural self-efficacy within the institutional structure of the college or university, along with a sense of pride in and identification with their ethnic roots (Rashid 1984; Rozek 1980; Sholevar and Joshi 2017).

The challenges faced by first-generation students are significant and overlap with challenges faced by students of color and students from low-income families. Deeper understanding of the multiple disadvantages faced by these students allows college health professionals and university administrators to provide resources and enact policies to promote greater first-generation student well-being and increased college completion. The need for collaboration across university departments to create a broad structure of support remains the most important factor in the promotion of success for these students on college campuses.

The following example illustrates many of the challenges faced by first-generation students.

A Student Narrative

DB attended an elite university as a first-generation student whose parents were Central American immigrants. During her first year, she had good academic results and made numerous social connections through the on-campus Latino community center. However, she struggled to maintain these connections during her sophomore year, after some of her friends dropped out of school. She began to expand her social connections to include many students from the dominant (white, non-first-generation) student culture and at times felt estranged from her culture of origin. She felt a loss of belongingness and also began to experience a growing acculturation stress, as she tried to live her life as a bicultural young adult. DB insightfully comments on her own experience: "What really helped me the most was being able to share my story with people who *got* me. This included not only resident fellows and counselors but also my friends (both Latino and 'other') and my former counselor from high school. Also, there were classes I took that helped me focus on my own wellness, and that honored my story."

Opportunities for the College Counseling Center

College mental health professionals have a unique opportunity to expand their traditional roles beyond treatment of mental illness to serve first-generation students well. Familiar roles for the college mental health professional may include providing outreach to the student community, offering preventive health or screening programs, and referring to primary care. An expanded role includes education of university administration and department personnel regarding first-generation students and advocacy for their needs.

Although first-generation students report requiring counseling services more than their peers, they also report utilizing them less, typically due to inconvenient location, lack of awareness of services, inconvenient hours, and limited available personal time. Outreach programming that increases awareness of counseling services and offers treatment at frequented locations such as a community center with expanded hours may promote better utilization of available resources. In addition, first-generation students may present with increased somatic symptoms compared with peers, resulting in presentation to primary care clinics rather than counseling centers (Wang and Castaneda-Sound 2008). Health services can address this potential issue with close collaboration between the services and screening for mental health issues in primary care.

When students do present to student counseling services, mental health care professionals can identify and more effectively address issues by screening for first-generation status and recognized risk factors during the initial evaluation. Because first-generation students may be at risk for multiple issues, health services may consider screening to include mental health issues, acculturation issues, and various common psychosocial stressors. For example, once first-generation status is established, a college counselor may consider asking about integration into university culture, about support from parents and family, and about financial stressors. In addition, one study found that first-generation students are less likely to disclose stressful college experiences to family and friends, thus missing out on an important way to manage college life (Barry et al. 2009). College mental health professionals can foster many ways for first-generation students to disclose stressful events and receive support. Individual counseling and support groups may be useful, and low-cost or free options may increase access and utilization of services. Support groups designated for first-generation students can normalize struggles and offer a safe venue to share distress.

Finally, in addition to having roles in prevention, screening, and treatment, college mental health professionals may serve in the role of trusted advocate to facilitate connections for students to other university services or departments (Stebleton et al. 2014). For example, the college mental health professional can strongly recommend that students enroll in free health insurance coverage provided by the university, alert students to on-campus tutoring opportunities, or refer students to a Web site describing study abroad programs.

Similarly, college mental health professionals can educate university leadership and administration regarding the challenges faced by first-generation students and advocate for campus policies that support university integration, student wellness, and college persistence. For example, mental health services staff can alert university officials regarding the need for support groups for first-generation students or advocate for student financial aid to equalize access to academic programs. This expanded liaison and advocate role for college mental health services will likely improve the life and experiences of first-generation students by addressing well-known challenges.

Opportunities for University Leadership

First-generation students may especially benefit from university leadership efforts in support of their college degree completion. Because these students may arrive on campus with varying degrees of disadvantage, many educational "bridge" programs have been developed to facilitate the transition to college by offering high school students a multitude of resources. Successful programs offer college campus visits, familiarize students with college life, offer academic resources, and provide assistance with navigating college application and financial aid processes (Hooker and Brand 2010). Universities that collaborate with bridge programs may establish strong foundations for future students. Once students are on campus, however, additional support is required to promote success. On-campus tutoring and financial aid programs can address academic and financial issues; however, improving student integration into campus culture and engagement in academic offerings can be much more challenging.

The education research literature offers evidence for psychological interventions that may support student belonging and increase alignment between student and university values. One study found that first-generation students were more likely to engage in science courses when they perceived that science might fulfill their interdependent-oriented goals, such as collaborating with others or helping communities, rather than more individualistic or independent goals (Allen et al. 2015). These types of interventions that typically connect class content to students' personal goals are referred to as *utility-values interventions*.

Values-affirmation interventions seek to address first-generation acculturation struggles by reinforcing personal values, thereby improving self-worth and self-perception. One study found that first-generation students in an introductory biology class who engaged in a values-affirming writing exercise not only had improved biology class grades but also had improved overall semester grade point averages (Harackiewicz et al. 2014).

Conclusion

First-generation students may face many challenges on college campuses and are less likely to complete their college degrees than their non-first-generation peers. Particular challenges include weaker academic preparation, financial barriers, cultural struggles with university values, a potentially decreased sense of social belonging, and decreased utilization of health services. To support first-generation students, universities must create a broad safety net, including academic and financial support, mental health and wellness programming on campus, health services that are accessible and convenient, and interventions that promote social and academic integration in the university setting.

KEY CONCEPTS

- First-generation students may face many challenges on college campuses and are less likely to complete their college degrees than their non-first-generation peers.

- First-generation students are more likely to be female, to be Hispanic, to come from low socioeconomic status families, to be older, to have dependent children, and to be less academically prepared for college.

- First-generation students often struggle with acculturation issues, may experience more symptoms of posttraumatic stress disorder than non-first-generation peers, and report lower life satisfaction and lower sense of belonging on campus than their peers.

- Among the most important factors in the promotion of success for first-generation students is the need for collaboration across university departments to create a broad structure of support.
- Values-affirmation interventions that can address acculturation struggles by reinforcing personal values may improve self-worth, self-perception, and overall academic success.

Recommendations for Psychiatrists, Psychologists, and Counselors

1. Counseling centers and mental health specialists should provide student outreach, preventive health programs, screening for first-generation student risk factors, and referral to university health services with easy access.
2. Counseling centers and mental health specialists should also educate university administration and department personnel regarding first-generation students and should advocate for their needs.
3. University administrative staff should collaborate with "bridge" programs that prepare high school students to transition successfully as first-generation college students.
4. Once students are on campus, university administration should provide ongoing academic and financial support for at-risk students.
5. Mental health professionals and university administrators should collaborate to encourage first-generation student integration into university culture and to promote completion of college degrees.

Discussion Questions

1. First-generation students share characteristics with students of color and students from lower socioeconomic status families. Should universities aim their resources and programming at all disadvantaged students together or prioritize groups separately?
2. Resources and programming aimed at supporting first-generation students may also carry the risk of stigmatizing this group. What are ways universities can support students without stigmatizing them?
3. Acculturation issues are prominent for first-generation students on university campuses. In addition to formal "bridge" programs, are

there other ways universities can facilitate the transition to college life for beginning students?

Suggested Readings

Active Minds: http://www.activeminds.org. Active Minds is the nation's only peer-to-peer organization dedicated to raising awareness about mental health among college students. The organization serves as the young adult voice in mental health advocacy on over 100 college campuses nationwide.

The JED Foundation: https://www.jedfoundation.org. The JED Foundation is a national nonprofit that focuses on emotional health and suicide prevention for teens and young adults. JED partners with high schools and colleges to strengthen their mental health, substance abuse, and suicide prevention programs and systems.

The Steve Fund: http://www.stevefund.org. The Steve Fund works with colleges and universities to promote effective programs and strategies that build understanding and assistance for the mental and emotional health of the nation's students of color.

Transition Year: http://www.transitionyear.org. Transition Year is an online resource center to help parents and students focus on emotional health before, during, and after the college transition.

References

Allen JM, Muragishi GA, Smith JL, et al: To grab and to hold: cultivating communal goals to overcome cultural and structural barriers in first generation college students' science interest. Translational Issues in Psychological Science 1(4):331–341, 2015 26807431

Barry LM, Hudley C, Kelly M, Cho SJ: Differences in self-reported disclosure of college experiences by first-generation college student status. Adolescence 44(173):55–68, 2009 19435167

Cauce AM, Hiraga Y, Mason C, et al: Between a rock and a hard place: social adjustment of biracial youth, in Racially Mixed People in America. Edited by Root MP. Newbury Park, CA, Sage, 1992, pp 207–222

Chen X: First-Generation Students in Postsecondary Education: A Look at Their College Transcripts (NCES 2005-171). U.S. Department of Education, Institute of Education Sciences, National Center for Education Statistics. Washington, DC, U.S. Government Printing Office, July 2005

Grusec JE, Hastings PD: Handbook of Socialization: Theory and Research, 2nd Edition. New York, Guilford, 2007, p 547

Harackiewicz JM, Canning EA, Tibbetts Y, et al: Closing the social class achievement gap for first-generation students in undergraduate biology. J Educ Psychol 106(2):375–389, 2014 25049437

Hooker S, Brand B: College knowledge: a critical component of college and career readiness. New Dir Youth Dev 2010(127):75–85, 2010 20973075

Hwang WC: Acculturative family distancing: theory, research, and clinical practice. Psychotherapy (Chic) 43(4):397–409, 2006 22122132

Hwang WC, Wood JJ: Acculturative family distancing: links with self-reported symptomatology among Asian Americans and Latinos. Child Psychiatry Hum Dev 40(1):123–138, 2009 18663569

Jenkins S, Belanger A, Connally ML, et al: First-generation undergraduate students' social support, depression, and life satisfaction. Journal of College Counseling 16:129–142, 2013

Kerwin C, Ponterotto JG: Biracial identity development: theory and research, in Handbook of Multicultural Counseling. Edited by Ponterotto JG, Casas JM, Suzuki LA, Alexander CM. Thousand Oaks, CA, Sage, 1995, pp 199–217

LaFromboise T, Coleman HLK, Gerton J: Psychological impact of biculturalism: evidence and theory. Psychol Bull 114(3):395–412, 1993 8272463

Nuñez A, Cuccaro-Alamin S: First-Generation Students: Undergraduates Whose Parents Never Enrolled in Postsecondary Education (NCES 98-082). U.S. Department of Education. Office of Educational Research and Improvement, National Center for Education Statistics. Washington, DC, U.S. Government Printing Office, June 1998

Pumariega AJ, Joshi SV: Culture and development in children and youth. Child Adolesc Psychiatr Clin N Am 19(4):661–680, 2010 21056340

Rashid HM: Promoting biculturalism in young African-American children. Young Child 39:13–23, 1984

Root MP: Resolving "other" status: identity development of biracial individuals, in Diversity and Complexity in Feminist Therapy. Edited by Brown LS, Root MP. New York, Harrington Park Press, 1990, pp 185–205

Rozek F: The role of internal conflict in the successful acculturation of Russian Jewish immigrants. Dissertation Abstracts International 41:2778 B. University Microfilms No 8028799, 1980

Sholevar P, Joshi SV: Cultural child and adolescent psychiatry, in Lewis's Child and Adolescent Psychiatry, 5th Edition. Edited by Martin A, Bloch MH, Volkmar FR. Philadelphia, PA, Wolters Kluwer, 2017

Stebleton MJ, Soria KM, Huesman RL: First-generation students' sense of belonging, mental health, and use of counseling services at public research universities. Journal of College Counseling 17:6–20, 2014

Stephens NM, Fryberg SA, Markus HR, et al: Unseen disadvantage: how American universities' focus on independence undermines the academic performance of first-generation college students. J Pers Soc Psychol 102(6):1178–1197, 2012 22390227

Terenzini PT, Springer L, Yaeger PM, et al: First-generation college students: characteristics, experiences, and cognitive development. Research in Higher Education (AIR Forum issue) 37(1):1–22, 1996

Wang CCDC, Castaneda-Sound C: The role of generational status, self-esteem, academic self-efficacy, and perceived social support in college students' psychological well-being. Journal of College Counseling 11:101–118, 2008

Wehrly B, Kenney KR, Kenney ME: Counseling Multiracial Families. Thousand Oaks, CA, Sage, 1999

CHAPTER 25

Students of Color

Daniel Ryu, M.S.

Allison L. Thompson, Ph.D.

HIGHER education was originally designed by and for white up-per-class individuals. Research across fields of social science has demonstrated the ways in which education is racialized and resources are disproportionately available to people of racial and economic priv-ilege. As education reform and explicit anti-oppression efforts have evolved, colleges and universities are slowly shifting to better reflect the diversity of the general population. Parallel efforts have been made within the helping fields (e.g., social work, psychiatry, psychology, counseling) to call attention to the ways in which foundational ap-proaches to treatment, research, and implementation may not be one size fits all, especially with regard to culture and race. Standards have been developed to address these concerns through specific "cultural competency" training and a focus on skills, knowledge, and attitudes to more effectively approach the spectrum of human diversity (American Psychological Association 2003).

The definition of *people of color* has shifted and evolved over time, and the term has generally been used to refer to nonwhite people in a way that highlights a common experience of racism without privileging the majority group in the way that *nonwhite* or *minority* might. This label is often centered around racial minorities; for the purposes of this chapter, this label refers to nonwhite people but includes a vast array of racial and ethnic identities and lived experiences. Over the last several decades, research related to race and culture in the context of psychological treatment has proliferated, and there is more literature than this chapter can cover. Instead, in this chapter we aim to briefly define terms and propose one conceptual approach to serving students of color. The hope is that the concepts presented in this chapter provide a framework and a series of thinking points to start a dialogue about working with racial and ethnic minority students.

Foundational Concepts

A dialogue about the role that race and identity play in the therapy room requires a conceptual foundation beginning with a loose defining of terms. The list that follows is intended to be neither exhaustive nor definitive but includes distilled descriptions in an effort to begin larger conversations around these topics.

INTERSECTIONALITY

Identity politics that organize movements around individual central characteristics can sometimes conflate or ignore intragroup differences. Intersectionality acknowledges that identities interconnect in the experiences of real people such that violence and oppression toward two intersecting identities cannot be separated into two separate forms of oppression and instead need to be appreciated as a multidimensional intersection of both (Crenshaw 1991).

OPPRESSION

Oppression can be described as "the exercise of power to disenfranchise, marginalize, or unjustly ostracize particular individuals or groups. Systematic oppression occurs through repeated integration of prejudice and discrimination into societal institutions (e.g., law, social policy, schools, language, media) and through threats of violence, removal of rights, and exclusion from decision-making processes. In addition, oppression can be intentional or unintentional and exists in any society in which there are dominant and subordinate groups" (Dermer et al. 2010, p. 326). Additionally, oppression can occur on a continuum in that it can be committed directly by a person with privilege, as a result of silence in the face of witnessing injustice, and lastly through a process during which marginalized individuals seek approval from a privileged group at the expense of others (Black and Stone 2005).

PRIVILEGE

Black and Stone (2005) summarized several definitions and described *privilege* as an unearned special advantage, entitlement, power, sanction, and/or immunity that is granted by birthright membership in certain prescribed identities and is exercised to the exclusion or detriment of others. Further, the privileged group is considered the normative group, and often individuals of this group are unaware of their privilege and may believe that they possess this power due to their own personal characteristics. This may result in viewing a nonprivileged group as deviant, unnatural, and/or lacking in effort. Black and Stone (2005) also identified privilege in those who can "look on prejudice, bigotry, and conferred dominance with detachment" (p. 246).

MARGINALIZATION

Marginalization can be described as "the social process by virtue of which individuals, groups, or communities are excluded from the center (of society) or relegated to the periphery or margins of 'a center' on the basis of some characteristic (e.g., race, ethnicity, class, gender, sexual orientation)" (Rodríguez et al. 2015, p. 224). Being marginalized implies being on the margins, considered the nonnorm, and set in contrast to the majority group (e.g., "students of color" implies a contrast to white students).

MINORITY STRESS

An abundance of empirical and theoretical attention has been paid to minority stress theory, which attributes the higher prevalence of mental illness among minority groups to the deleterious psychological impact of existing in an environment (and society) of discrimination, stigma, and oppression (Meyer 1995).

CULTURAL HUMILITY

As cultural and racial theory has evolved, approaches to communities of color have shifted. For example, the concept of color-blindness was shown to harm, disadvantage, and erase racial and cultural minorities while invalidating racist/racialized experiences (Fryberg and Stephens 2010). Several approaches have arisen as other possible approaches to difference, including cultural competence, cultural sensitivity, and cultural humility. Definitions of *cultural humility* in particular tend to center around openness, a lack of claim to competence or superiority, and a collaborative focus on the patient's understanding of their own culture and identity rather than relying on past experience with or learned information about a particular group or identity (Hook et al. 2013).

MICROAGGRESSIONS

The term *microaggressions*, which was originally coined in reference to microinteractions that dismissed and/or insulted black individuals, has expanded in definition and application. The term generally refers to subtle, often seemingly benign interactions that directly or indirectly demean marginalized communities and/or affirm stereotypes.

Conceptual Approach

The following section offers one perspective on considerations when approaching clinical work with students of color. This series of thinking points speaks directly to "you" as the clinician as a way to encourage the self-reflection that is inherent to these recommendations. This section is intended to simply begin, or continue, the construction of your own conceptual approach to this work as it fits within the context of your unique perspective and values.

THE STUDENT IN CONTEXT

By the time the student has made it to your office, they already have had to negotiate several barriers to entry. Racialized oppression is multilayered and can pervade multiple levels, including the institutional level (i.e., how higher education systems are structured) and the interpersonal level (i.e., your own socialization and biases as a helper and/or an administrator). Contextualizing the student begins by holding curiosity about what it may be like to be a person with their identities at your institution. Even further, you may consider what it would be like to be a person with their identities seeking mental health care at your institution. For instance, you might ask yourself: What sort of racial and cultural diversity do you have at your university? Does your university have resources for students of color and other marginalized groups? How does your institution support and center students of color and diversity of lived experience? Is there space and acknowledgment of intersectionality (e.g., a club/event for queer people of color)?

Beyond the barriers that may exist in accessing resources generally, extant literature has shown that symptom presentation and help-seeking behaviors may differ in individuals from various racial and ethnic backgrounds. In other words, mental health concerns may be difficult to recognize, and certain individuals may be less likely to seek treatment. One approach would be to meet the student with curiosity and an investment in understanding their conceptualization of their identities, experiences, and mental health. One nuance to keep in mind when approaching with curiosity is to be aware of the ways in which the student may be tokenized and called on to educate their peers and possibly also their professors/mentors. For this reason, when contextualizing the student, know that they may engage with their identities in a range of ways, some of which may be idiosyncratic and a part of their communication style, while others may be reflective of survival and coping strategies they may have developed in response to oppression and discrimination. These may include minimizing their experience, tokenizing themselves, and/or exhibiting racism or prejudice toward their own communities. An important part of this process includes listening to the student and allowing their conceptualization of their racial (and other) identities to integrate into the holding space of the therapy room. A crucial element of this approach is the demonstration of respect and humility. Overemphasizing or underemphasizing how and/or why an individual is impacted by systems of oppression may be microaggressive, may harm the individual and the therapeutic alliance, and may mirror harmful experiences the individual has had in other areas of life. Other more concrete barriers to be aware of that have been identified in cultural competency literature include stigma, access, shame, familial expectations, expectations for treatment, and minority stress. When contextualizing the student, let them be the expert on themselves and invite them to collaborate with you in forming the context in which you hold them.

THE CLINICIAN IN CONTEXT

In the same way that you want to approach a student of color through understanding their racialized experience, you must name and acknowledge that you as a clinician are also a racialized person in the room. Oppression and hegemony label positions of privilege and power as "neutral," when the reality is that everyone experiences racial and cultural socialization, which makes "neutrality" impossible. Further, an attempt at embodying or claiming "neutrality" highlights an existing hierarchy and power differential.

You, too, have experiences and histories as a person with intersecting identities. Your students enter the room having the experience of living and moving through the world in their racialized bodies, and so do you. When we as mental health professionals approach clinical work, we bring with us our personalities and our interpersonal and affective styles, making us not quite the "blank slates" that we sometimes aspire to be. In the same way, you bring intersectional and contextual baggage both related to your own identities and to those of the students with whom you work. It is impossible to remove yourself from that baggage and from the collective histories of people like yourself interacting with people like the student before you. Particularly with majority-identity therapists and administrators, it is important to understand the history of violence and oppression that the group you represent has enacted upon intersecting communities of color. What sorts of power and privilege differentials exist between your racial group and theirs? How does this interact with other layers of power including your position as a mental health professional and/or administrator? Alternatively, although sharing certain marginalized identities may increase the likelihood of your ability to empathize with certain aspects of lived experience, it is, nonetheless, important to remember intragroup differences and to be mindful of your own reactions and assumptions both in terms of the identities you and the student share as well as those you do not.

One way to acknowledge the sometimes overwhelming task of holding histories and collective experiences in the therapy room is to be transparent with your students and contextualize yourself. It is your responsibility to name that you have privilege blinders that may shield you from being able to fully understand the experience of someone who is different from you. Part of this requires understanding that although it is not your fault that you have blind spots, it is your responsibility to continuously do the work to uncover them. A huge part of being able to contextualize yourself and have genuine humility requires doing your own work and accepting that, regardless of your race or ethnic background, you have racialized and socialized biases. This work requires educating yourself, owning what you do not know, and not expecting others to educate you through their experiences.

EMBRACING THE UNKNOWN

Embracing the unknown may seem contradictory. You may be asking yourself, "Am I supposed to know the literature and try to be culturally competent, or am I supposed to drop the pretenses and approach with humility?" In short, the answer is both. Taking an intersectional, anti-oppressive stance requires considerable flexibility and a willingness to hold two contradictory ideas. Cultural humility requires a genuine willingness to be wrong, which necessitates taking the ethical due diligence seriously by reading literature and seeking multicultural educational opportunities and then being willing to hold what you know lightly and remain open to the reality of your students' lived experiences. This literature may describe idioms of distress shown to be specific to certain racial and ethnic minorities (e.g., somatization of symptoms) and treatment-specific cultural norms (e.g., culturally seated levels of formality or familiarity with the therapist) and may suggest specific adaptations of evidence-based treatments (e.g., emphasis on problem solving or integration of family into treatment). Although it is important to be familiar with this literature and these intervention adaptations, only the student before you can tell you what it is like to be them and to move through the world as a person at the intersection of their identities. Listen and pay attention to each individual's language and framing. Show a willingness to actively unknow and to deconstruct your preconceived notions of their experience and how that fits into mental health and illness. Part of this may include working to identify and change microaggressive language and oppressive framing that you may have internalized. As a clinician or administrator, you are asked to be the expert and provider of information and knowledge. Although this may make a position of learning feel uncomfortable, transparent not-knowing and deep investment in learning may be your most therapeutic tool in relation to the identities of your students. Be okay with making mistakes, being flexible, and holding a loose grip on what you have learned.

INTERSECTIONALITY AND RESILIENCE

Taking an intersectional approach, as mentioned in subsection "Intersectionality," requires seeing the student's intersection of identities as a sum that is greater than its parts. Approaching research and clinical work through identity groupings (e.g., focusing on specific racial identities) rather than taking each individual as a whole ties all members of the group to a common experience or history and minimizes or erases the reality of intragroup differences. A student's race is inextricably bound to other aspects of their identity. A student's identity, in turn, is linked to gender, sexual orientation, strengths, class, and immigration and/or citizenship. In the same vein, other forms of oppression such as heterosexism and transphobia are not separate from but rather informed and compounded by racism. Appreciating each individual as a whole person also requires having the understanding many identities can be invisible. It is therefore likely that there are levels of power and privilege of which you may not be aware.

Last, communities of color have been shown to suffer disproportionately due to stressors that can include emotional and physical abuse, racism, poverty, and stress caused by acculturation. Although it is important to recognize the unique stressors that people of color face, the narrative is not a tragic one. In the same way that folks of color (and any marginalized community) face unique adversity, they also harbor a unique resilience that is required for survival as a person outside of the normative hegemony. For many people, being a part of marginalized communities is a point of pride and is in and of itself an act of resilience and resistance.

Case Example

David is a 21-year-old Mexican American straight trans man who identifies as "brown." David is a biology major who hopes to eventually become a sports nutritionist. He goes to a school that has a predominantly white student body and holds a part-time job as a tutor in a predominantly white tutoring organization. David expresses feeling tokenized and erased as a trans man in campus spaces for students of color and feels similarly alienated as a man of color in queer and trans student spaces. David was referred to the student mental health clinic by his resident assistant, who suspected that David may have eating concerns after his dorm mates reported regularly hearing someone throwing up in the bathroom on David's floor. David reports that he eats only one hearty meal a day and that he feels as though his eating is normal, except when he occasionally "goes crazy on food" at his hall meetings at which free food is provided. He denies the use of laxatives and other compensatory behaviors but reports exercising several hours a day and "getting sick" after particularly large meals. He has never been in mental health treatment before and when he heard the reason for his referral, he stated that eating disorders are a "white girl problem." David denies having body image concerns but made several off-hand comments during intake about being "the fat brown trans kid" on campus. David expresses frustration with the fat-shaming jokes and racial slurs that students and friends on campus regularly make and reports that he is repeatedly told he is "too politically correct" when he tries to intervene. David recalls being told he was "too thick" in elementary school and having a complicated relationship with food in his childhood home. David states that he was often shamed for his body while simultaneously being expected to eat "what was put in front of him" and to feel lucky and grateful that his parents were able to put food on the table. David reports that his family does not acknowledge his transness and continues to use the wrong name and feminine conjugation in Spanish when referring to him. David expresses embarrassment about coming to the student mental health center and adamantly states that he doesn't think he needs to be there because he isn't "crazy."

Questions:

1. What identity intersections would you want to pay attention to in David's case? How might David's brownness and trans-masculinity play into his understanding of himself and his symptoms?
2. What do you think it would be like to be David at your mental health center? What barriers do you imagine he would have to confront to be in treatment?
3. In what ways do you share and not share his identities (brown, trans, Mexican American, student, straight)? In what ways would you hold and/or lack power and privilege in the therapy room?
4. What assumptions and beliefs do you notice coming up when you read about David's experiences? What would you imagine it being like to be in the room with him?
5. Where might you have clinical and personal blind spots?
6. How comfortable would you feel asking David about his experience and reflecting his language around brownness and transness?
7. How does David show resiliency?

Conclusion

All people (including students, clinicians, and administrators) are intersectional and therefore exist in the context of their diverse lived experiences. People are resilient and should be met with deep respect, curiosity, and humility. This requires contextualizing both the student and yourself, while holding a loose grip on your own understandings of culture and race. Anti-oppression and intersectional approaches require a willingness to experience discomfort and failure by allowing the student to be your guide on their own intersections. This includes working to open your eyes to your own blind spots and embodiments of power and privilege.

KEY CONCEPTS

- Intersectionality, oppression, privilege, marginalization, and minority stress may impact the clinical presentation, self-understanding, and treatment engagement of students with various racial and ethnic backgrounds.
- A possible therapeutic stance could be one of humility and responsiveness to the student's multilayered context and their own definition of their intersectional identities.
- Clinicians, with their unique social positioning, have the opportunity to take responsibility for attending to, and holding in mind, the different race- and identity-related dynamics involved in work with students of color.

Recommendations for Psychiatrists, Psychologists, and Counselors

1. Let students be the experts on themselves and their identities. Approach each student with curiosity, respect, and humility. Consider cultural differences in presentation and barriers to treatment in the context of multilayered systems of oppression.
2. Explore, acknowledge, and take responsibility for your own intersecting identities and how they relate to your work with students. Contextualize yourself and recognize the ways in which you are not a blank slate.
3. Be unafraid of the dialectic of knowledge. Know the relevant literature and still be willing to be flexible, make mistakes, and unlearn.
4. Think intersectionally and remember that the sum is greater than its parts when it comes to identity, oppression, and marginalization.
5. Focus on and recognize strengths, resiliency, and pride.

Discussion Questions

1. What are the resources and organizations for students of color at your university?

2. What sort of relationship does the mental health center at your university have with these organizations?

3. How do you understand your own race and intersecting identities? How do you think that your race and intersecting identities impact how you are perceived and understood in the context of the clinical (or administrative) work that you do?

4. What are biases and blind spots you have of which you are aware? What are you doing to engage and challenge them?

5. What came up for you when you read this chapter? Do you notice any defensiveness? Arguments? Reactions? Reflections?

Suggested Readings

Crenshaw K: Mapping the margins: intersectionality, identity politics, and violence against women of color. Stanford Law Review 43(6):1241–1299, 1991
hooks b: Ain't I a Woman: Black Women and Feminism. Boston, MA, South End Press, 1981
Sue DW: Microaggressions in Everyday Life: Race, Gender, and Sexual Orientation. Hoboken, NJ, Wiley, 2010

References

American Psychological Association: Guidelines on multicultural education, training, research, practice, and organizational change for psychologists. Am Psychol 58(5):377–402, 2003 12971086
Black LL, Stone D: Expanding the definition of privilege: the concept of social privilege. Journal of Multicultural Counseling and Development 33:243–255, 2005
Crenshaw K: Mapping the margins: intersectionality, identity politics, and violence against women of color. Stanford Law Rev 43(6):1241–1299, 1991
Dermer SB, Smith SD, Barto KK: Identifying and correctly labeling sexual prejudice, discrimination, and oppression. J Couns Dev 88:325–331, 2010
Fryberg SA, Stephens NM: When the world is colorblind, American Indians are invisible: a diversity science approach. Psychol Inq 21:115–119, 2010
Hook JN, Davis DE, Owen J, et al: Cultural humility: measuring openness to culturally diverse clients. J Couns Psychol 60(3):353–366, 2013 23647387
Meyer IH: Minority stress and mental health in gay men. J Health Soc Behav 36(1):38–56, 1995 7738327
Rodríguez DM, Donovick M, Straits J: Counseling the marginalized, in Counseling Across Cultures. Edited by Pedersen PB, Lonner WJ, Daguns JG, et al. Thousand Oaks, CA, Sage, 2015, pp 229–246

Lesbian, Gay, Bisexual, Transgender, and Queer/Questioning Students

Ripal Shah, M.D., M.P.H.
Neir Eshel, M.D., Ph.D.
Lawrence McGlynn, M.D., M.S.

STUDENTS who identify as lesbian, gay, bisexual, transgender, queer/questioning (LGBTQ), or elsewhere on the gender and sexuality spectrum often struggle with discrimination and marginalization, which can negatively impact mental health and sense of belonging. It is not surprising that the LGBTQ population may be skeptical or uncomfortable when utilizing mental health care, considering the mental health field's historically strained relationship with the LGBTQ community (e.g., homosexuality was listed as a "sociopathic personality disturbance" in the *Diagnostic and Statistical Manual* [DSM] as late as the 1970s, and not until 1987 were all conditions related to same-sex attraction removed [American Psychiatric Association 1987]). A slew of other issues further impede LGBTQ students' access to, and comfort with, this field of care—fear that parents or others will discover what is discussed during therapy sessions, worries about being hospitalized, lack of resources to pursue mental health treatment with or without parental support, or lack of knowledge about what services are available. Thus, it becomes evident that clinicians working with LGBTQ students must make strong efforts to normalize minority gender identities and sexualities and to become well versed in the nuances of LGBTQ culture and vernacular, in order to ensure that this population feels comfortable utilizing mental health care and to reduce the impact of anti-LGBTQ stigma on mental health. Our intention in this chapter is to address some of these knowledge gaps and improve the ability of mental health specialists to provide informed, respectful, and compassionate care to LGBTQ college students.

Terminology

The terms assigned to gender and sexuality can become quite complicated, given that it is uncommon for a single definition to be universally accepted. Additionally, terminology can vary geographically, individually, and over time. The purpose, then, in reviewing appropriate terminology for the LGBTQ community is not to attach labels but, rather, to respect and cultivate the identity and sense of self of each patient. The most important thing clinicians can do is be courteously inquisitive with patients and follow the patients' lead with regard to the language they use to characterize themselves and their behaviors. Clinicians are often taught to use gender-neutral language (e.g., "Do you have a partner?") and to avoid using language with inherent assumptions (e.g., "Are you married?"). In the clinical space, mishaps happen frequently, and if a patient is called by the wrong name, pronoun, or relationship signifier, the clinician should briefly apologize and move on with the encounter.

It is useful first to separate *gender identity* from *sexual orientation*. An appropriate way to open the discussion on gender identity is to ask the student what sex they were born as, what gender they identify with now, and which pronouns they prefer for self-identification, regardless of what is in their medical record. Gender identity is inward—describing how one sees oneself—while sexual orientation is outward—indicating whom one is sexually attracted to. For example, a person who identifies as transgender may be straight, gay, lesbian, bisexual, neither, or other, and sexual orientation can evolve over time.

In regard to sexual orientation, it is useful to keep in mind a tripartite structure of *attraction* (the colloquial implication of the term *sexual orientation*), *self-identity* (how one describes oneself), and *behavior* (i.e., sexual activity). For example, a woman may be sexually active with both men and women (and have a bisexual orientation) and yet identify as "straight" and enter into romantic relationships exclusively with men. When discussing sexual identity, it is important to consider *asexuality* (the absence of sexual attraction) and *pansexuality* (attraction to all sexes and genders or regardless of sex or gender identity) as well. These three concepts—attraction, self-identity, and behavior—exist on a continuum, much in the same way that biological sex and gender expression do.

Development of Sexual Orientation

Most people are heterosexual. The development of sexual orientations differing from this majority occurs in every culture. Multiple theories address the formation of sexual orientation in the maturation process. Although some theorists may argue in favor of environmental ("nurture") factors, studies demonstrating high concordance of homosexuality among monozygotic twins and the clustering of homosexuality in family pedigrees support a biological ("nature") model. In 2013, the American Psychiatric Association (APA) Board of Trustees approved a position statement addressing homosexuality combining APA policies previously expressed in 12 separate position statements adopted between 1973 and 2011. It states, "The American Psychiatric Association believes that the causes of sexual orientation (whether homosexual or heterosexual) are not known at this time and likely are multifactorial including biological and behavioral roots which may vary between different individuals and may even vary over time" (Scasta and Bialer 2013).

It is important that clinicians confirm to patients that sexual orientation and gender identity are not "choices" but rather emerging properties of human development. It takes time to incorporate sexual orientation into an individual's sense of self. The awareness of same-sex attraction can occur as early as age 9 or 10 years. Individuals then begin to internally accept or experiment with same-sex attraction or orientation. Because society generally accepts heterosexuality as the norm, individuals at this point may experience psychological distress. Individuals then adopt their sexual identity. If that identity aligns with their sexual orientation, the feelings of distress may begin to resolve (Everett 2015). The time to progress through these experiences can vary greatly. Thus, students entering college may be at any point in embracing their gender identity and sexual orientation awareness and acceptance.

Coming Out

The transition to college is a major life event. Newly independent, many college students find themselves in a better position than previously to explore their identities and negotiate relationships. This process can be particularly fraught for LGBTQ students. Many LGBTQ students lack the typical dating experience that their straight or cisgender peers enjoyed in high school, partly because the LGBTQ population is smaller and partly because of the stigma that still abounds about such relationships. As a result, many LGBTQ students spend high school feeling isolated, confused, and marginalized. College often provides these students the opportunity to "catch up" and experiment with what they missed earlier. This process, however, happens precisely when their former support systems are no longer in place, making college a vulnerable time for the coming out process. Students who experience distress in coming out may seek emotional support or more intensive services from the student health clinic.

Coming out is the gradual and lifelong process of becoming aware of one's own sexual or gender identity and disclosing this to others. Different people undergo this process differently, in keeping with their own backgrounds, personalities, and life experiences. Generally, however, coming out involves multiple overlapping stages: a growing realization of one's identity, a struggle with internalized stereotypes and stigma, eventual acceptance and appreciation of one's identity, and disclosure to others, either with the same or different identities (Greenfield 2015). During this process, individuals can feel vulnerable, empowered, uncertain, relieved, fearful, proud, confused, and affirmed—all at once or in waves. It is not easy to build a positive sense of self in a world still too filled with intolerance.

This is where clinicians may be helpful. A clinician can fill multiple roles for a college student in the process of coming out. First, the clinician can validate and normalize the student's experience. By mirroring the student's language, avoiding assumptions, and remaining open to flexible and nonbinary models of gender and sexuality, the clinician can communicate that the student's emerging identity is healthy, normal, and positive. Ideally, the clinician's office should be a place where students can discuss their concerns without fear of punishment or censorship.

Second, and equally important, the clinician can probe where the student is in the coming out process and predict what difficulties might lie ahead. Coming out entails both benefits and risks. Benefits include living an open and honest life, joining a vibrant community, becoming a role model for others, and dispelling prevailing myths. Risks include being victimized by hostile or even violent people, overhauling existing relationships, and losing access to a "traditional" life. There are multiple mechanisms to cope with these risks. Some people hide their identity, for example, by acting and appearing stereotypically heterosexual or cisgendered. Others simply avoid this aspect of themselves, instead focusing their energies on academics, sports, religion, or other socially accepted pursuits. Still others suppress their stress with drugs or other risk-taking and self-destructive behaviors. All of these mechanisms can take their toll and contribute to the higher risk of mental illness in the LGBTQ population.

The relative balance of these benefits and risks depends entirely on people's individual situations, as do the types of coping mechanisms that people choose. Bisexual students, for example, face particularly acute challenges, often fitting poorly into either the "LGBTQ" or the "straight" world. Depending on their current relationship, they might be assumed to be either straight or gay. This compels some bisexual students to come out repeatedly even when in a stable relationship in an attempt to assert their identity. Others respond by "passing" as either gay or straight because it is easier to fit in that way, but at the expense of their own sense of self. Alternatively, for transgender students, even a basic understanding of their identity and preferred terminology is often lacking in the world around them. As a result, even well-meaning peers can contribute to isolation and abandonment. Finally, LGBTQ people with other minority statuses face their own sets of challenges. Some ethnic minority students may feel that joining the LGBTQ community hampers their ability to associate with others of the same ethnicity. For all of these cases, informed and supportive clinicians can help students navigate these important challenges.

In particular, clinicians can be ready with a set of tools to help the college student come out. Tips for the student include the following:

- Being comfortable with your identity first before disclosing to others
- Avoiding discussions of deeply personal issues such as gender identity or sexual orientation in emotionally charged settings

- Dropping hints to investigate how accepting a person might be
- Identifying a support system ahead of time
- Developing a response to negative reactions
- Giving the other person enough time to respond before feeling hurt or judged

It can be helpful for the student to hear that coming out gets easier the more one does it and that being gay or transgender is only one part of one's identity. In fact, role-playing with a student can be an effective way to overcome that initial hurdle of telling a loved one about one's identity. The more support a student gets—the more opportunities to listen and be listened to—the more likely they are to achieve a healthy and fulfilling identity.

Incidence of Mental Illness in the LGBTQ Population

The minority stress model has provided a framework for understanding sexual minority mental health disparities. The foundation of this model is that sexual minorities (i.e., LGBTQ students) experience chronic stressors related to their stigmatized identities, including ongoing victimization, prejudice, and discrimination. These distinct negative experiences related to sexual orientation, in combination with general stressors such as transitioning to life away from home, disproportionately compromise the mental health of LGBTQ students (Russell and Fish 2016). The three minority stress processes proposed by Ilan Meyer (2003) are 1) external stressors such as institutionalized discrimination, 2) a person's expectation that victimization will occur and the vigilance related to this, and 3) the internalization of negative social attitudes (often referred to as internalized homophobia). Although the social context of entering the LGBTQ community can at times be beneficial for coping and sense of togetherness, each student's interpersonal experiences and intrapersonal resources can contribute to either risk or resilience, and these experiences and resources should be discussed fully in a therapeutic and compassionate way.

Many mental disorders show onset during or directly following adolescence, making it a critical period for mental health. Multiple studies retrospectively examining the adolescent time period of LGBTQ adults with mental health disorders have shown an increased risk of developing symptoms when distress and perceived burdensomeness are experienced in adolescence.

Decades of research on sexual minority mental health have yielded rather concerning data regarding the LGBTQ experience both during and after college, particularly when compared with mental health diagnosis rates in the general population. According to Kessler et al. (2012), 18% of lesbian and gay youth participants in the National Comorbidity Survey Replication Adolescent Supplement met criteria for major depression, compared with 8.2% in the general population; rates of posttraumatic stress disorder in the prior 12 months were 11.3% in lesbian and gay youth, compared with 3.9% in the general population. Whereas 31% of LGBT students reported considering suicide at some point in life, 4.1% of the general population had (Nock et al. 2013). The increased risk of suicide in the LGBTQ community is most pronounced during adolescence and young adulthood when the desire to conform can often override internal drives, leading to a sense of internalized oppression or even self-hatred. There are also differences among LGB youth: sexual orientation has a stronger association with suicide attempts for gay and bisexual men than for lesbian and bisexual women (Fergusson et al. 2005), whereas lesbian and bisexual women are more likely to exhibit substance use problems compared with heterosexual women or gay and bisexual men (Needham 2012). This latter discrepancy appears to dissipate with time as sexual minority males seem to "catch up" and exhibit faster accelerations of substance use in the transition to early adulthood. Racial and ethnic differences also may exist. In one early study, African American and Latino youth who identified as LGB had higher rates of suicidal thoughts and depressive symptoms than their white LGB peers (Consolacion et al. 2004). Unfortunately, compared with heterosexual or solely same-sex-attracted peers, bisexual youth have higher rates of suicidality, greater levels of depression, and worse psychological adjustment in response to bullying (Poteat et al. 2009), perhaps due to a longer and intensified internal struggle of identity or frustration with not fitting into a clear "gay or straight" identity.

Although sexually transmitted infections are a consequence of specific behaviors, not of sexual orientation or gender identity, some members of the LGBTQ community are at higher risk based on sexual practices. For example, because of high vascularity and thin membrane space, anal penetrative sex allows for a larger transfer of viral load than does vaginal or oral contact. It follows that the transfer of various communicable diseases can be increased in those engaging in anal sex. Infections may include HIV, hepatitis C, syphilis, gonorrhea, and chlamydia. While HIV is now considered treatable, some individuals may opt to take preexposure prophylaxis (PrEP), a daily antiviral medication used to reduce the likelihood of becoming infected with HIV.

Substance use can also vary in the LGBTQ community compared with the general population. Risk factors may include relying on clubs and bars for socializing and peer support, the negative psychological effects of internalized homophobia, the stress of coming out or concealing an identity, trauma from violence, and feeling unaccepted (Russell and Fish 2016). Gay and bisexual men are more likely than heterosexuals to use party or club drugs (e.g., MDMA [3,4-methylenedioxymethamphetamine or Ecstasy], ketamine, or GHB [γ-hydroxybutyric acid]), which often decrease inhibition and impair judgment, and lesbian women are more likely than heterosexual women to use marijuana and cocaine (Russell and Fish 2016). As described earlier, alcohol use rates can also be elevated in the LGBTQ community; rates are usually higher in lesbian and bisexual women during adolescence until the inflection point of adulthood, after which point rates are higher in gay and bisexual men.

In addition to the factors above, it is important to note that perceptions of body image for college-age students can already be complicated, but members of the LGBTQ community can receive conflicting social cues. Some gay men may note feeling an expectation of both the mainstream and queer communities to be stylish and muscular; some lesbian women may feel pressure to reject traditional standards of female beauty. It is important to understand students' perceptions of their bodies and if they are in line with or differ from their own personal values.

Risk and protective factors for mental health disorders in LGBTQ students are a combination of general factors and ones specific to the LGBTQ experience. Universal risk factors, such as family conflict, childhood maltreatment, and substance use, often appear in conjunction with LGBTQ-specific risk factors, such as the absence of institutionalized protections, bias-based bullying, family rejection, and lack of support in a school or faith community (Russell and Fish 2016). An LGBTQ student's perception of acceptance by the surrounding community is pivotal to psychological well-being. In one study, LGBTQ youth living in neighborhoods or campuses with anti-bullying policies inclusive of sexual orientation were half as likely to make a suicide attempt as were those living in areas with fewer sexual orientation–specific anti-bullying policies (Hatzenbuehler and Keyes 2013). LGBTQ students living in communities generally supportive of LGBTQ rights (i.e., those with more protections for same-sex couples, presence of gay-straight alliances in schools, and sexual orientation and gender identity–specific nondiscrimination and anti-bullying policies) were found to be less likely to attempt suicide, even after the study controlled for other risk factors, such as abuse history, symptoms of depression, substance use, and peer victimization (Hatzenbuehler 2011). Those LGBTQ youth who fear or face rejection from their family have higher levels of depression and anxiety, and 40% of homeless youth identify as LGBTQ (Durso and Gates 2012).

To support LGBTQ youth as they enter into adulthood, solidifying strong protective factors in existence during adolescence can be a helpful intervention by clinicians. Such efforts include affirming identities, supporting the coming out process, discussing issues around family acceptance, and navigating school policies and local programs with students. Systemically, providing students with an environment in which they can feel safe, by offering student resources such as a gay-straight alliance club or LGBTQ student space, can have benefits that are seen even at later developmental stages (Toomey et al. 2011). LGBTQ-inclusive curricula, which include historical events, people, and information relevant to the LGBTQ community, improve the sense of safety and acceptance and reduce victimization in schools (Kosciw et al. 2012), whereas LGBTQ-specific training for instructors and staff is associated with more frequent adult intervention in bias-based bullying (Greytak and Kosciw 2014). Motivating students to engage in LGBTQ-based discussions with their peers and encouraging them to create a network of LGBTQ friends also contribute to positive psychological health. Although parental support is known to provide the most benefit to positive well-being in young adulthood, sexuality-related social support from friends and community, including clinicians, can be uniquely pivotal to a student's growth.

University and Community Services

Many college mental health services (called counseling and psychological services, or CAPS, at many schools) now have designated clinicians who specialize in gender identity and sexual orientation issues or offer a specific LGBTQ community resource center. However, students may also find LGBTQ-friendly therapists or psychiatrists in their area through numerous online databases (e.g., in the Bay Area, the Psychotherapist Association for Gender and Sexual Diversity has a Web site [www.gaylesta.org] to help individuals find such a clinician). The online database of therapists through Psychology Today also lists "bisexual," "gay," and "lesbian" as a potential client focus for the clinician (https://therapists.psychologytoday.com/rms). The major limitation with databases such as these is that they often require clinicians to subscribe, so not all practitioners are listed. In addition, areas of expertise are self-determined and may not necessarily be the result of specialty training such as a dedicated fellowship or education track.

Students also may find a sense of community from joining LGBTQ groups on campus (ranging from advocacy groups to social organizations), so it is important to know what options are available. Students who feel reluctant to be public about their identity can be referred to online resources, such as the National Alliance on Mental Illness (NAMI; www.nami.org) or can participate in NAMI groups off campus. Community centers specifically for LGBTQ-identifying individuals, which organize anything from support groups to recreational activities, can be found at the CenterLink Web site (www.lgbtcenters.org). Given the discrimination often experienced in the LGBTQ community both in school and in the workplace, a referral to the American Civil Liberties Union (ACLU) or similar local advocacy agency may be appropriate, depending on the student's situation. Searching online for recovery services, support groups, social clubs, youth spaces, and counseling services specifically for the area local to the patient may also prove fruitful.

Case Example

Patricia is a college sophomore and identifies as a lesbian. She comes to the college counseling service to address her ongoing depressive symptoms that interfere with her academic performance. She has developed romantic feelings for a female classmate and reports that the feelings are mutual. Her new friend, however, refuses to engage in a relationship with someone who remains in the closet. The recognition and acceptance of LGBTQ individuals has evolved over time, but some cultures and communities may be resistant to this change. Patricia feels that coming out of the closet would mean certain rejection by her family and community of origin. "I think I just need an antidepressant," she says.

Question: What should be included in a comprehensive treatment plan for Patricia?

Conclusion

As access to mental health care at colleges and universities continues to improve, we must also remember the importance of bringing LGBTQ students from the margins and into the conversation. Not only is there a tremendous need for general mental health care due to the increased prevalence of mental illness and addiction in this population, but there is also a need for more culturally competent clinicians. Continuing to learn about the issues faced by LGBTQ students—issues unique to the queer experience as well as those in line with general adolescence and young adulthood—is essential to facilitate a healthy and productive college experience.

KEY CONCEPTS

- Being LGBTQ is not equated with having a mental disorder.
- Coming out can be a liberating but stressful process.
- Individuals who identify with more than one underrepresented group may encounter greater challenges in coming out.
- Bullying continues to be a problem for students who are (or are perceived to be) LGBTQ in some communities, including high schools, colleges, and universities.
- Students who identify as members of the LGBTQ community have higher rates of mental illness and suicide and decreased access to care.
- Some campuses and neighboring communities have dedicated LGBTQ-specific services and organizations that may be useful sources of ongoing support for the isolated or struggling LGBTQ student.

Recommendations for Psychiatrists, Psychologists, and Counselors

1. Terminology in gender and sexuality has changed over time, and is likely to continue to evolve. Health care professionals should become familiar with the basic terms and concepts, including, for example, the difference between *gender identity* and *sexual orientation*, and also remain courteously inquisitive with all patients when unfamiliar terminology or concepts are discussed.
2. Avoid making assumptions about a student's gender identity and orientation (attraction, self-identity, and behavior), and, instead, inquire about these in a nonjudgmental way.
3. Errors happen. If you make a mistake in addressing a person by the wrong name, gender pronoun, or relationship signifier, be sure to acknowledge the mistake and continue to seek to build rapport with the student.

4. Coming out is a gradual and lifelong process that may present with varying degrees of distress, but it also may be celebrated. Health care professionals should provide a nonjudgmental space for LGBTQ college students as they come to understand and accept their identity.

5. Data on mental illness, substance abuse, and suicide in LGBTQ youth are concerning. College and university health care centers must be prepared to screen, support, and treat students from these affected communities.

6. Certain health risks are greater in LGBTQ individuals, depending on their sexual behaviors. Mental health clinicians in college and university health centers must be prepared to screen and refer students for evaluation and treatment.

Discussion Questions

1. In general, mental health clinicians do not disclose much about their personal lives when caring for patients. Some opinion leaders advocate self-disclosure of sexual orientation when caring for LGBTQ individuals. What are the positives or negatives of self-disclosure?

2. What are constructive, nonjudgemental approaches to speaking with student patients about health risks associated with sexual behaviors and advocating for safe sex practices?

Suggested Readings

Consortium of Higher Education LGBT Resource Professionals: www.lgbtcampus.org

Drescher J, Roberts LW, Termuehlen G: Treatment of lesbian, gay, bisexual, and transgender patients, in The American Psychiatric Association Publishing Textbook of Psychiatry, 7th Edition. Edited by Roberts LW. Washington DC, American Psychiatric Association Publishing (in press)

The Fenway Institute: www.fenwayhealth.org

Healthy Minds Network: www.healthymindsnetwork.org

National Center for Transgender Equality: www.transequality.org

References

American Psychiatric Association: Diagnostic and Statistical Manual of Mental Disorders, 3th Edition, Revised. Washington, DC, American Psychiatric Association, 1987

Consolacion TB, Russell ST, Sue S: Sex, race/ethnicity, and romantic attractions: multiple minority status adolescents and mental health. Cultur Divers Ethnic Minor Psychol 10(3):200–214, 2004 15311974

Durso LE, Gates GJ: Findings from a National Survey of Service Providers Working With Lesbian, Gay, Bisexual, and Transgender Youth Who Are Homeless or at Risk of Becoming Homeless. Los Angeles, CA, Williams Institute True Colors Fund, 2012

Everett B: Sexual orientation identity change and depressive symptoms: a longitudinal analysis. J Health Soc Behav 56(1):37–58, 2015 25690912

Fergusson DM, Horwood LJ, Ridder EM, Beautrais AL: Sexual orientation and mental health in a birth cohort of young adults. Psychol Med 35(7):971–981, 2005 16045064

Greenfield J: Coming out: the process of forming a positive identity, in Fenway Guide to Lesbian, Gay, Bisexual, and Transgender Health, 2nd Edition. Edited by Makadon H, Mayer K, Potter J, Goldhammer H. Philadelphia, PA, American College of Physicians, 2015, pp 49–78

Greytak EA, Kosciw JG: Predictors of U.S. teachers' intervention in anti-lesbian, gay, bisexual, and transgender bullying and harassment. Teaching Education 25(4):410–426, 2014

Hatzenbuehler ML: The social environment and suicide attempts in lesbian, gay, and bisexual youth. Pediatrics 127(5):896–903, 2011 21502225

Hatzenbuehler ML, Keyes KM: Inclusive anti-bullying policies and reduced risk of suicide attempts in lesbian and gay youth. J Adolesc Health 53(1)(suppl):S21–S26, 2013 23790196

Kessler RC, Avenevoli S, Costello EJ, et al: Prevalence, persistence, and sociodemographic correlates of DSM-IV disorders in the National Comorbidity Survey Replication Adolescent Supplement. Arch Gen Psychiatry 69(4):372–380, 2012 22147808

Kosciw JG, Greytak EA, Bartkiewicz MJ, et al: The 2011 National School Climate Survey: The Experiences of Lesbian, Gay, Bisexual and Transgender Youth in Our Nation's Schools. New York, GLSEN, 2012

Meyer IH: Prejudice, social stress, and mental health in lesbian, gay, and bisexual populations: conceptual issues and research evidence. Psychol Bull 129(5):674–697, 2003 12956539

Needham BL: Sexual attraction and trajectories of mental health and substance use during the transition from adolescence to adulthood. J Youth Adolesc 41(2):179–190, 2012 22076077

Nock MK, Green JG, Hwang I, et al: Prevalence, correlates, and treatment of lifetime suicidal behavior among adolescents: results from the National Comorbidity Survey Replication Adolescent Supplement. JAMA Psychiatry 70(3):300–310, 2013 23303463

Poteat VP, Aragon SR, Espelage DL, Koenig BW: Psychosocial concerns of sexual minority youth: complexity and caution in group differences. J Consult Clin Psychol 77(1):196–201, 2009 19170465

Russell ST, Fish JN: Mental health in lesbian, gay, bisexual, and transgender (LGBT) youth. Annu Rev Clin Psychol 12:465–487, 2016 26772206

Scasta D, Bialer P: Position Statement on Issues Related to Homosexuality. Arlington, VA, American Psychiatric Association, 2013. Available at https://www.psychiatry.org/home/policy-finder?=6ecb08ea-153f-4b38-afff-58946ea7d1ef&Page=9

Toomey RB, Ryan C, Diaz RM, Russell ST: High school gay-straight alliances (GSAs) and young adult well-being: an examination of GSA presence, participations, and perceived effectiveness. Appl Dev Sci 15(4):175–185, 2011 22102782

CHAPTER 27

Transgender Students

Christina Tara Khan, M.D., Ph.D.

Inge Hansen, Psy.D.

COLLEGE is a time of intense personal growth for many students. Many find themselves in an important stage of identity development, in which individuals examine or question aspects of identity encompassing the whole person, including gender, sexual orientation, ethnicity, race, and other important components of individual and collective identity. The college years can be an exciting time in this regard but also a challenging time, as students learn to navigate the potential conflicts or incongruences between their diverse experiences and those of others. For transgender students, additional considerations may come into play as they navigate a world not always accustomed to a gender spectrum. In this chapter, we introduce readers to basic terminology and concepts for working with gender-diverse populations. We outline key aspects of the transition process. We lay out important considerations for working with transgender students and explore institutional supports to help students across the gender spectrum have an equitable and fulfilling university experience.

Definitions and Terminology: The Basics

The terminology associated with gender identity is continually changing. Although numerous terms are used to describe having a gender identity that differs from the sex one was assigned at birth, including *transgender, gender nonconforming, gender diverse*, and others, we use the term *transgender* as an umbrella term to encompass all of these variations on the gender spectrum. We present in Table 27–1 some of the most basic terms to aid in the understanding of the diverse gender spectrum and to differentiate among three terms that are commonly misused interchangeably: *gender, sex*, and *sexual orientation*.

Elements of Transition: Key Considerations

Transitioning toward one's authentic gender often involves several components, including psychological, social, medical, surgical, and legal aspects (Boedecker 2011). *Psychological transition* is a largely internal process, which often precedes other types of transition. A person may experience an internal sense of gender that is different from the sex assigned at birth. For instance, a person who was assigned male at birth may recognize that they actually experience themselves more as a girl or a woman or as a blend of gender characteristics. Psychological transition often involves exploring and experimenting with gender-role behaviors and appearance, which may include wearing clothes or engaging in activities usually associated with a different gender. A person who is transitioning psychologically may also explore what name, gender label(s), and pronouns feel appropriate given what they recognize their authentic gender to be. Once a person has a sense of their gender, they will go through a decision-making process regarding whether and to what degree to come out to others (social transition), whether to engage in medical interventions to bring their physical body more in line with their gender identity (medical and surgical transition), and whether to change

TABLE 27–1. Transgender terminology

Agender: Identifying as not having a strong gender or any gender at all.

Cisgender: A term describing an individual whose gender identity aligns with the sex they were assigned at birth.

Gender: The socially constructed roles, activities, behaviors, and attributes that a given society considers appropriate for people based on their sex.

Gender dysphoria: A feeling of stress or discomfort an individual can feel toward their assigned sex or gender, gender expression, physical body, and/or others' responses to any of these.

Gender expression: An individual's way of expressing gender-related traits through appearance, behavior, and mannerisms. It is sometimes an extension of an individual's gender identity but need not be.

Gender fluid: A gender identity that may move or fluctuate between two or more gender identities or on a continuum; alternate term: **Genderfluid**.

Gender identity: An individual's internal sense of what their gender is and what it means to them.

Genderqueer: A gender identity outside of "man" or "woman." May signify an identity in between "man" and "woman" or outside of these binary categories altogether. The term is often used in response to the societal/political conceptualization of gender. Not everyone who identifies as genderqueer identifies as transgender or nonbinary.

Misgendering: To address or refer to someone with a word or pronoun that does not accurately reflect the gender with which they identify.

Nonbinary: A gender identity outside of "man" or "woman." May signify an identity between "man" and "woman" or outside of these binary categories altogether. Not everyone who identifies as nonbinary identifies as transgender and vice versa.

Pronouns: In this context, pronouns are significant because they often communicate gender. A person transitioning genders may start using new pronouns (e.g., "she" instead of "he" or "they" as a gender-neutral pronoun).

Sex: The biological, physiological, and genetic characteristics that define individuals as male, female, or intersex.

Sex/gender assignment: The process most newborns go through whereby a doctor assigns them a sex category (male/female/intersex) and a gender (boy/girl) based on physical and reproductive characteristics such as the length of the phallus or the presence of a uterus.

Sexual orientation: An individual's personal understanding of whom they are attracted to, how they experience intimacy, and what they desire.

Transgender: An umbrella term describing an individual whose gender identity does not align with the sex assigned at birth; alternate term: **Trans**.

TABLE 27–1. Transgender terminology *(continued)*

Intersectionality: The ways in which multiple identities (gender, race, ethnicity, social class, sexual orientation, etc.) intersect to create a whole that is different from the component identities.	**Transition:** The process of moving toward living in and expressing one's authentic gender; often a lifelong process.

their legal status and identification documents to reflect their gender (legal transition). Counseling with a gender specialist can be a great support for the process of psychological transition.

Social transition is the process of communicating one's gender identity outwardly to others, a "coming out" that can look similar to disclosing one's sexual orientation but that also contains a set of unique steps and considerations. An individual who is transitioning often will start by sharing their gender identity with a small number of close confidantes. They may then expand to speaking with a wider social circle—family, professors, and so on—until most people they encounter in their day-to-day life are aware of this information. The individual may share their new name and/or pronouns and ask that these be used in the future. They may also obtain new identification documents (e.g., driver's license, passport, student ID), reflecting their gender identity (as discussed in the later paragraph on legal transition). Many students also create a new social media identity reflecting their gender. Finally, appearance and presentation are often a large part of social transition: an individual may alter clothing, hair, or other aspects of their appearance to communicate and express their gender more accurately.

Medical transition involves a variety of medical interventions to bring one's appearance and physical characteristics more in line with one's gender identity and/or desired gender expression. These interventions range from puberty-blocking medications in children to hormonal and surgical interventions in adolescents and adults. An important consideration in this step of the transition process is that many of the treatments, unlike social and psychological transitions, cannot be easily reversed. The main categories of hormones include feminizing and masculinizing treatments. The most recent Standards of Care put forth by the World Professional Association for Transgender Health (WPATH; Coleman et al. 2012) recommend documentation by a mental health professional of the following criteria for individuals to proceed to therapy with hormones: persistent gender dysphoria, capacity for fully informed consent, age of majority or parental consent, and adequate control of any physical or mental health conditions. Although there are controversies over what specific criteria should be used and whether these standards place mental health professionals in a "gatekeeping" role, many physicians who prescribe hormonal treatments prefer to adhere to the guidelines and require a mental health evaluation prior to initiation of therapy with hormones. There are many potential side effects of hormone therapies, including cardiovascular, endocrine, psychiatric, hepatic, and neoplastic risks, among others. It is crucial that students seeking therapy with hormones are aware of the potential risks and discuss these with their clinicians prior to initiation of hormonal treatments.

Surgical transition is another form of medical intervention that involves physical changes to one's body to better represent one's desired gender expression. Interventions range from simple plastic surgery procedures (e.g., facial or body contouring, breast augmentation, mastectomy) to more complex gender confirmation surgeries done by urologists, gynecologists, and plastic surgeons (e.g., vaginoplasty, phalloplasty, metoidioplasty). The goal of surgical and other medical interventions is to provide lasting comfort with one's gendered self, to maximize psychological well-being, and to increase personal safety and minimize risks associated with being misgendered. With surgical transition, as with therapy with hormones, there is a recommended pretreatment evaluation process involving assessment of readiness, capacity for consent, responsibility to follow treatment recommendations, and stability of any medical or psychological conditions. The WPATH criteria are more stringent for genital surgery than for hormones and chest surgery, requiring letters from two different mental health professionals and evidence of social transition or having lived continuously in the gender role that is congruent with the gender identity for at least 12 months. These procedures are increasingly being covered by both public and private health insurance plans.

Transgender individuals encounter misgendering, which contributes to the stigma and discrimination they face. A mismatch between gender expression and legal gender can pose serious safety risks, and legal challenges are common, as transgender individuals attempt to live in an expressed gender that may differ from what is represented on their identity documents. *Legal transition* refers to the process of changing one's legal status to more accurately reflect one's gender identity. This includes obtaining identity documents that accurately reflect one's authentic gender (e.g., birth certificate, driver's license, passport) and navigating systems that utilize gender for identification (e.g., schools, health care systems). The laws guiding changes to identity documents vary from state to state and are frequently changing. The National Center for Transgender Equality (www.transequality.org) and the Transgender Law Center (www.transgenderlawcenter.org) are good sources of information for students seeking legal transition. The benefits of legal transition are many. Reduced misgendering can contribute to an experience of greater emotional safety, a decrease in concern about potential incidental "outing," and decreased anxiety for transgender individuals while accessing health care and other public resources that require identity documentation.

Nonbinary Identities

Although many transgender individuals identify with binary gender categories, such as man or woman, a large number feel that their authentic gender falls in between or outside of these categories. These individuals may use terms such as nonbinary, gender nonconforming, genderqueer, gender fluid, or agender to describe themselves. Nonbinary individuals may also use gender-neutral pronouns such as *they/them* to refer to themselves rather than gendered pronouns such as *he* and *she*. One can support nonbinary individuals by consistently using their preferred pronouns. Also, it is important to avoid language or activities that promote a gender binary and therefore may exclude those who do not fit into a binary gender. For instance, instead of addressing an audience as "Ladies and gentlemen," one might say "Esteemed colleagues."

Institutional Considerations: Policies and Resources

STUDENT RECORDS AND INFORMATION SYSTEMS

Student records can include academic records, medical records, and general information collected by the registrar's office. It is important to document the student's preferred name as well as their legal or given name; the appropriate pronouns for the student; and a clear system for name and identification change, should the student change their name, legal gender, and/or photo during or after their time with the institution. Also, records that collect gender information should offer gender options beyond the binary (man/woman), such as a fill-in-the-blank for gender or a third gender option (e.g., "both/neither/fluid").

FACILITIES

Housing

An inclusive housing environment means offering housing options that reflect students' diverse gender identities. The current standard is to house according to a student's current gender identity rather than the sex assigned at birth, regardless of degree of medical transition. For instance, a student who was assigned female at birth but currently identifies as male would be housed as a male student. Students who identify as nonbinary or gender fluid should be offered an all-gender housing option if one is available and/or asked what feels like the most appropriate gender housing option for them. Roommates who will potentially be housed with transgender or nonbinary students should also be surveyed to ensure they are open to this option, in order to prevent potential distress on both sides.

Restrooms

It is vital to offer all-gender restrooms throughout campus. Students can feel extremely uncomfortable being forced to use a restroom facility for a gender that does not fit for them. Doing so can also be a safety issue, because others will sometimes "police" restrooms and confront or aggress against people who appear to be in the "wrong" restroom for their gender.

SUPPORT RESOURCES

Mental Health Resources

Transitioning can raise many questions and concerns, such as fears about finding a partner, concerns about disclosing to dates, impact on family relationships, fears of violence and prejudice, and concerns about legal and medical aspects of transition. Many concerns also may arise following medical transition, such as ongoing dissatisfaction with one's appearance or with the impact of hormones/surgery, postoperative pain, and emotional issues that were not previously addressed. Transgender students seek out mental health professionals for support with stressors such as these; or for other reasons, such as to help guide a gender exploration process or to obtain a support letter for therapy with hormones or surgery; or for reasons completely unrelated to gender, such as relationship issues or anxiety. Students who are seeking therapy to aid a gender exploration process will benefit most from a relaxed, open exploration of different aspects of gender to see what fits. After experimenting, a student may decide that some, but not all, of the means of expressing gender they have explored feel right for them personally.

As noted in section "Elements of Transition," letters of support from licensed mental health professionals are required before a student begins therapy with hormones or surgery. Historically, letters have been obtained through what is known as a *gatekeeper model of care*, in which the clinician has the power to determine whether and when a given person is appropriate and ready to transition and whether a certain minimum number of therapy sessions may be required before providing a letter. Now, however, most practitioners are moving into an *informed consent model of care*, where the process of obtaining letters is transparent and the person's sense of their own readiness for transition is respected. The clinician may at times still delay or deny a letter if there is a clear risk in moving forward with transition, but the process is as collaborative as possible. It is often helpful to have a sample letter of support on a central drive that all clinicians can use as a model.

A clinic or health center can benefit greatly by having a clinician on staff who is a gender specialist. This person would have attended training sessions through WPATH or a local equivalent and have extensive experience working therapeutically with gender-diverse students, including both providing general mental health care and writing letters of support.

Medical Resources

Transgender students seek out medical services for a variety of reasons, just as they do mental health services. Many of these students present with an interest in medical transition, such as therapy with hormones or surgery, to bring their physical bodies closer in line with their gender identities. Others may already be engaged in the process of medical transition and are seeking related support, for instance, around fertility, side effects of hormones, or consultation regarding hair removal. Still others will present with medical needs unrelated to their gender identity or transition. In all cases, students will have a need and desire for gender-inclusive care.

Ways in which a medical setting can be gender inclusive are to minimize gender-binary medical options or clinics (e.g., "Women's Health Clinic," "Men's Health Clinic"), to offer a "Transgender Health Clinic" option, or simply to offer options based on services ("Sexual and Reproductive Health Clinic"). The latter is preferable. Another area worthy of attention is language use. It is important that all medical forms requesting a student's gender offer options beyond the binary (see earlier subsection "Student Records and Information Systems"). Additionally, when staff call a student from the waiting area to the examination room, it is important to be sure to use the student's preferred name rather than assuming their legal name is the correct one to use.

University health clinics can serve as vital resources for students who are actively transitioning. Therapy with hormones can be offered as a part of primary care, and referrals can be made for surgery. In the case of therapy with hormones, it is important to create a detailed informed consent packet so that the student is fully clear on the effects of the intervention being undertaken. As is the case with mental health services, having a gender specialist on staff can be enormously helpful.

Educational Resources

Although not all academic courses focus on gender, all can be gender inclusive in both curriculum and classroom culture. Faculty can check syllabi, forms, surveys, and course readings to ensure that material does not rely on gender stereotypes or require students to check one of two gender boxes. In many disciplines, faculty can further seek out material that exposes students to current concepts and data regarding gender diversity. With regard to classroom culture, it is helpful to do introductions at the first class, giving students an opportunity to share both their name and appropriate pronoun(s), so that they are referred to correctly during the remainder of the course. Faculty who are uncomfortable asking for pronouns or who are concerned that students may be uncomfortable disclosing pronouns, may alternatively use "they" as a default pronoun for all students. Inclusive practices such as these may be facilitated by offering university-sponsored training for faculty to introduce them to gender-inclusive policies and transgender resources on campus.

Organizational Considerations

The experience of receiving care or service goes beyond the student's direct interaction with staff. Often, a student will gain an impression of a clinic or office where they are receiving care or service before they have even met with a staff member or clinician. Many factors, such as the following, can be considered in creating a welcoming environment:

- Does the waiting room reflect a diversity of identities through its literature, art, and brochures, or does it feel neutral and barren?
- Are front desk staff trained in gender inclusiveness?
- Do they know to check for a student's preferred name and pronouns, and do they use "they" as a default pronoun when they do not know?

- Are all-gender restrooms available and well marked?
- Do intake forms gather gender information in an inclusive manner?

DISCRIMINATION AND HARASSMENT

Unfortunately, transgender students are subject to significant discrimination and harassment. In the 2015 Transgender Survey, 24% of participants reported verbal, physical, or sexual harassment, and 16% reported that they left school because of the harassment (http://www.ustranssurvey.org) (James et al. 2016). Title IX of the Education Amendments of 1972 and its implementing regulations prohibit sex discrimination in educational programs and activities operated by recipients of federal funding. In May 2016, the U.S. Department of Justice and the U.S. Department of Education coauthored a "Dear Colleague" letter, which clarified the application of Title IX to gender identity and summarized schools' obligations to transgender students under Title IX. The letter notes,

> A school's Title IX obligation to ensure nondiscrimination on the basis of sex requires schools to provide transgender students equal access to educational programs and activities even in circumstances in which other students, parents, or community members raise objections or concerns. As is consistently recognized in civil rights cases, the desire to accommodate others' discomfort cannot justify a policy that singles out and disadvantages a particular class of students. (p. 2)

The letter then specifies how nondiscrimination applies in terms of identification documents, names and pronouns, sex-segregated activities and facilities, and privacy and education records. The full letter can be accessed here: https://www2.ed.gov/about/offices/list/ocr/letters/colleague-201605-title-ix-transgender.pdf.

Case Examples

CASE EXAMPLE 1

Eli is a 19-year-old sophomore at a large private university, who was assigned female at birth and currently identifies as nonbinary, using "they/them" pronouns. Eli reports being a fairly typical girl growing up, but was a "bit tomboyish" and never liked wearing dresses. Eli came out as queer while in high school and thought at the time that their queer identity accounted for their discomfort with traditional femininity. However, once in college, Eli learned about trans identities and met other students who were trans, which prompted Eli to question their own gender identity. Eli at first wondered if they might be a trans man, but quickly rejected that idea because there are many aspects of their femininity that they still appreciate and enjoy. Eli ultimately realized that they experience their gender as a mix of masculine and feminine. They wear their hair short and feel most comfortable in button-down shirts and men's pants and also show an affinity for the color pink and funky nail polish. In terms of physical transition, they would like to move forward with top surgery due to discomfort with their breasts, but they have no desire to go on masculinizing hormones.

CASE EXAMPLE 2

Jordyn is an 18-year-old freshman student at a small private university who was assigned male at birth and currently identifies as a lesbian woman, using "she/her" pronouns. Jordyn first came out as trans in high school, and after years of discussion, received her parents' permission to begin feminizing hormones prior to beginning college. She grew up with traditional religious practices and has struggled with discrimination within her church, experiencing anxiety since childhood and eventually disengaging from religious participation after high school, to her parents' dismay. While in college, she has continued to experience anxiety about her faith and about how she is perceived by others, and this has increased following her first semester, now having an impact on her ability to maintain friendships and engage in romantic relationships. Apart from the evaluation she had prior to starting therapy with hormones, she has not had therapy or counseling.

Conclusion

Working with transgender students requires embracing the diversity and individuality of the human experience. It is our hope that this chapter helps introduce readers to basic concepts that will facilitate supporting transgender students during their college years. Attention to where students are in their transition process will enable university staff to direct students to appropriate resources. Considering the oppression and discrimination faced by transgender persons nationally, it is vital to maintain a climate throughout the university that is welcoming, inclusive, and equitable, to minimize stigma and maximize learning for all students, regardless of gender identity or expression.

Key Concepts

- Gender identity is a fluid concept that varies from individual to individual.
- Transgender students are at increased risk for discrimination and harassment compared with their cisgender peers.
- Transgender students are at varying stages of transition, including social, psychological, medical, surgical, and legal aspects of transition.
- Institutional policies that support an inclusive and gender-affirming environment for all will help transgender students to achieve success in the university environment.

Recommendations for Psychiatrists, Psychologists, and Counselors

1. The terminology associated with gender identity is diverse and continually changing. It is important for university faculty and staff working with students on the gender spectrum to be familiar with basic concepts of transgender health.
2. It is highly recommended that universities have resources available to support transgender students at varying stages of transition, including social, psychological, medical, surgical, and legal transition.
3. The Standards of Care of the World Professional Association for Transgender Health (Coleman et al. 2012) provides guidance for health professionals to assist transgender individuals with safe and effective ways to maximize their physical and psychological health.
4. It is vital to maintain a climate throughout the university that is welcoming, inclusive, and equitable, in order to minimize stigma and maximize learning for all students, regardless of gender identity or expression.

Discussion Questions

1. Sex, sexual orientation, and gender refer to distinct aspects of an individual that are commonly misused as interchangeable concepts. How do you understand the distinctions between each term and where might they overlap? How have your understandings of these terms changed from when you first learned of them to the present day?

2. What are some important aspects of transition to consider when working with transgender students?

3. Many transgender individuals have trouble accessing health care due to stigma and discrimination they encounter in health care settings. What are some ways health care organizations can prepare their staff to provide equitable care for individuals on the gender spectrum.

Suggested Readings

Erickson-Schroth L: Trans Bodies Trans Selves. New York, Oxford University Press, 2014

Grant JM, Mottet LA, Tanis J, et al: Injustice at Every Turn: A Report of the National Transgender Discrimination Survey. Washington, DC, National Center for Transgender Equality and National Gay and Lesbian Task Force, 2011

World Professional Association for Transgender Health: Standards of Care, Version 7. Available at: http://www.wpath.org/site_page.cfm?pk_association_webpage_menu=1351&pk_association_webpage=3926. Accessed July 25, 2017.

Yarbrough E: Transgender Mental Health. Washington, DC, American Psychiatric Association Publishing, 2018

References

Boedecker AL: The Transgender Guidebook: Keys to a Successful Transition. CreateSpace Independent Publishing Platform, 2011

Coleman E, Bockting W, Botzer M, et al: Standards of care for the health of transsexual, transgender, and gender-nonconforming people, Version 7. Int J Transgenderism 13(4):165–232, 2012

James SE, Herman JL, Rankin S, et al: The Report of the 2015 U.S. Transgender Survey. Washington, DC, National Center for Transgender Equality, 2016

U.S. Department of Justice, U.S. Department of Education: Dear Colleague Letter on Transgender Students, May 13, 2016. Available at: https://www2.ed.gov/about/offices/list/ocr/letters/colleague-201605-title-ix-transgender.pdf. Accessed July 25, 2017.

CHAPTER 28

Student-Athlete Mental Health

Lisa Post, Ph.D.

Megan Kelly, Psy.D.

THE cultural and psychological experience of the student-athlete can be distinguished from that of the general collegiate population. Special demands are placed on student-athletes for balancing both academic and sport-related priorities and forming interpersonal relationships while managing the physical demands of training. A tendency toward perfectionism and the influence of a distinct athlete identity impact self-esteem and mental health, both positively and negatively. In this chapter, we outline the mental health concerns and psychological stressors unique to this population, describe how educational institutions can structure programs to address these needs, and discuss unique opportunities for intervening with this college population.

Athletic Participation: Factors Influencing Psychological Well-Being

Research into the overall health and well-being of student-athletes suggests that athletic participation may confer a protective effect against depression and may correlate with higher levels of self-esteem and social connectedness. It has been proposed that regular physical exercise and a built-in sense of connectedness and support gleaned from participation in a team sport may be responsible for these outcomes (Rao et al. 2015). Team cultures that support healthy normative behaviors and teach effective coping strategies, including timely help-seeking behaviors, can exert a positive influence on psychological well-being through group and peer dynamics. Although the potential for positive outcomes does exist, team participation and the group culture also can interact with preexisting individual vulnerabilities to increase negative stressors experienced by student-athletes. It is, therefore, important to understand the distinct and dual identities that student-athletes are navigating in their collegiate career.

The transition from high school to college can be stressful for any student, but recent evidence suggests that athletes may experience even greater levels of stress due to the dual demands of athletics and academics (National Collegiate Athletic Association Sport Science Institute 2016). At the collegiate level, student-athletes balance time-intensive travel schedules and physically strenuous training, while at the same time facing more rigorous academic demands than previously experienced. A student-athlete may struggle to prioritize academics alongside athletics and perceive that it is "not being a team player" to place importance on school over athletics. There has also been recent criticism of the National Collegiate Athletic Association (NCAA) and some university programs for not providing adequate support for the student identity and recognizing of academic achievements. This imbalance can extend to coaches as well, who have been found to ignore the 20-hour-per-week limit on practice time mandated by the NCAA (National Collegiate Athletic Association 2015). Additionally, these pressures on student-athletes can result in a significant reduction in time available to engage in non-sport-related social activity, which can put particular pressure on these students to juggle multiple commitments and to cope by deprioritizing sleep. Lack of sleep not only is correlated with reduced ability to manage stress, but it is also associated with higher risk for physical injury (National Collegiate Athletic Association Sport Science Institute 2016).

The multiple relationships in which student-athletes are engaged add to the challenge of navigating their dual identities. Whether with coaches, professors, or sports medicine staff, student-athletes are often in positions of less power or agency. They may not be prepared to balance demands from various stakeholders and authority figures and may struggle to identify and advocate for their emerging mental health needs. Internal pressure to perform, coupled with high levels of intra-team competition and outcome-oriented coaching styles, can increase the risk of negative mental health outcomes.

A common characterological trait for student-athletes that may impede effective coping is perfectionism. Student-athletes have been trained to perform at their best, expecting nothing less than perfection. Although perfectionism can be adaptive for student-athletes, driving motivation and achievement-oriented behavior, it can also be maladaptive, resulting in difficulty with tolerating mistakes or exacerbating fear of failure. These challenges may arise during the transition to collegiate sports because many student-athletes are accustomed to being the best, or a top athlete, at their sport in high school and are unfamiliar with coping with disappointment. Adjustment to one's role on a team, and potentially no longer being the most talented athlete, can prompt negative self-evaluation and can result in low mood or anxiety. Health care professionals will want to be aware of signs that perfectionism is having a negative impact on a student-athlete's experience. A student-athlete may grow to scrutinize their own physical appearance and body image, express highly self-critical beliefs or commentary toward others, or engage in behaviors of overcontrol or rigidity around training regimens or other aspects of life.

Student-athletes also may be affected by other social and environmental stressors. They may be exposed to other negative expressions of peer culture, whether in the context of athletics or in the broader collegiate environment, including experiences with substance use, hazing, bullying, sexual assault, and interpersonal violence. Exposure to or participation in these behaviors can influence the development of mental health issues for some student-athletes. Greater cultural diversity issues on campus can also impact minority athletes detrimentally by way of harassment or discrimination. Given the high value placed on peer approval and social acceptance during emerging adulthood, the team environment has the potential to serve as a protective factor against or risk factor for unhealthy individual and team behaviors. Fostering a team environment that is inclusive of all minority groups and in which concerns with discrimination or aversive team behaviors are directly addressed can provide student-athletes with a sense of security and belonging. This can be particularly beneficial for minority student-athletes who may experience environmental stressors outside of their sport and struggle to cope effectively when they return to the field or team (National Collegiate Athletic Association Sport Science Institute 2016).

Structuring a Program to Promote Student-Athlete Mental Health

Educational institutions have a number of opportunities to structure their athletic departments and sports medicine programs to address the factors impacting student-athlete mental health. The NCAA has provided Mental Health Best Practices to guide the development of programs that will support and promote services, destigmatize access of care, and increase understanding of institutional resources (National Collegiate Athletic Association Sport Science Institute 2016). Components of a sports medicine program can vary from setting to setting depending on the resources available. A good program will support the whole student by making available licensed and trained professionals for routine and emergency services, providing a clear pathway to identification and referral of student-athletes, and encouraging a health-promoting environment that supports mental well-being and resilience (National Collegiate Athletic Association Sport Science Institute 2016).

Student-athlete mental health care is best conducted within the context of an interdisciplinary care team. This team may consist of athletic trainers, coaches, sports medicine support staff, physical trainers, sports performance trainers, physicians, academic advisors, psychiatrists, and psychologists or other mental health professionals. It is often the athletic trainer who is the first point of contact in responding to mental health concerns. In most settings, the team physician is coordinating numerous aspects of a student-athlete's overall care, which will include mental health. Clearly defined and well-promoted self-referral procedures should be made available to student-athletes and the interdisciplinary care team. Written institutional procedures are recommended to distinguish procedural differences for emergency mental health situations from those for routine mental health referrals (National Collegiate Athletic Association Sport Science Institute 2016).

Creating a setting in which access to services is transparent and flexible will foster engagement and destigmatization of the use of resources. Mental health professionals are often needed outside of the traditional office session, including in the milieu, such as in the training room, at the sidelines of a game, or on the road. Programs can also aim to promote opportunities for mental health professionals to meet with students as individuals, in groups, or with coaching staff. Areas of potential conflict should be addressed with the entire interdisciplinary team. Mental health professionals may intervene through various relationships to best meet the needs of their client, the student-athlete. Lack of awareness of the role of the mental health professional can result in misunderstanding, ethical challenges, and potential stressors for the student-athlete. Clarification around topics of confidentiality, multiple relationships, role expectations, and boundaries will help in navigating these barriers to effective care (Aoyagi and Portenga 2010).

A health-promoting environment can be fostered in a number of ways. Implementation of regular meetings with the entire interdisciplinary team will promote strategic planning and communication. Circulation of information on the signs and symptoms of mental health disorders and available prevention programs to all student-athlete advisory committee representatives, student-athletes, coaches, and staff members will promote awareness and understanding. Prevention programs and peer-led interventions can address critical experiences that some student-athletes face, including sexual assault and interpersonal violence, hazing or bullying, coping with injury, and discrimination and harassment. Development of educational and group intervention programs can also provide student-athletes with mental skills to address sports performance or environmental stressors, such as injury. These programs can serve as avenues for developing cohesive team cultures and aim to promote future-oriented and preventive skills and knowledge acquisition.

Unique Opportunities to Intervene

Primary opportunities for mental health intervention exist during important periods of transition for student-athletes. The first transition occurs when a student-athlete enters into collegiate sports. The NCAA recommends implementing a preparticipation mental health screening at the initial transition to school. A mental health screening questionnaire can be included in the preparticipation examination as a procedure for identifying and referring at-risk student-athletes as well as normalizing the assessment of mental health for all participants. Common concerns include eating disorders, anxiety, depression, insomnia, substance use, trauma, attention-deficit/hyperactivity disorder, and adjustment issues (National Collegiate Athletic Association Sport Science Institute 2016).

Another important period of transition occurs when a student-athlete sustains an injury, which can result in a temporary leave from sport or a possible medical retirement. Injuries can be one of the more significant stressors in a student-athlete's career. Although most injuries can be managed with minimal disruption to the student-athlete's training and life, some can have a substantial impact on physical and mental well-being, at times triggering a serious mental health issue. Intervening with mental health services can normalize emotional reactions to injury, including shock, denial, anger, and fear, as well as provide resources to build mental resilience through the use of relaxation techniques, visual imagery, mindfulness skills, and psychoeducation about recovery.

The transition out of sports upon graduation may also be a period of distress for student-athletes. Student-athletes often have lower graduation rates than other student groups (Won and Chelladurai 2016). This can be a result of prioritizing their athlete identity over their student identity. This transition coincides with additional stressors and opportunities that accompany leaving college. For some athletes, there can be a sense of pressure or anxiety around performing at their best in their final year, achieving a competition record that the team has not yet met, or being perceived as a role model and leader for younger teammates. Additionally, this period can be a time of loss and grief as a student-athlete leaves an environment that has provided a close group of friends, a sense of community and belonging, and strong mentorship experiences. Part of this transition will involve exploring other aspects of the individual's identity during the transition to being a student who is not engaged in athletics and preparing the individual to cope with upcoming changes.

Case Example

Frances, an intelligent junior starter on the Division 1 varsity women's field hockey team, was a standout player in high school and a top recruit. She managed the transition to college well both socially and academically. Halfway through her junior season, she began to feel run-down and irritable. Her coaches noticed and referred her to her athletic trainer, but she "wasn't a quitter," and Frances downplayed her distress and continued to keep up her rigorous schedule. During the final seconds of a game, Frances slipped and tore her anterior cruciate ligament (ACL). During her ACL workup, her doctor diagnosed her with mononucleosis. Frances had surgery to repair the ACL and eventually began 2 hours of rehabilitation several days a week. Because her coach required injured athletes to attend practice, Frances sat on the sidelines or took training video of her teammates.

Frances began to feel "cut off" from teammates, whom she felt made insensitive comments. Frances also felt sad and frustrated that her coaches seemed to be less attentive than they had been when she was playing. Frances felt the coach didn't understand her when he told her to "perk up—you will be able to play again soon." Because she was less mobile and had physical therapy requirements and doctor visits that added time-intensive obligations to her already busy schedule, she also began to skip social events with friends outside of the team. Frances found that her lethargy was increasing despite her recovery from mono. She skipped classes and slept in. She skipped meals because she "was less physically active and worried about gaining weight." She had negative thoughts about her recovery and return to the team. She became anxious that she was "damaged goods" and "didn't have what it takes" and had "lost it." Eventually, her athletic trainer, noticing her weight loss, increasingly low affect, and decreasing interpersonal engagement, referred Frances to individual counseling and a support group for athletes recovering from injury. Through the group intervention, Frances was provided with education about psychological issues that athletes commonly face when recovering from injury and with connection to other student-athletes facing similar challenges. She gained perspective on how closely her identity was affiliated with her athletic success and became able to give teammates the benefit of the doubt. Frances learned important stress management strategies and communication techniques. In brief individual therapy, she explored her feelings, calibrated her expectations for recovery, and learned strategies to challenge her negative thoughts.

This case illustrates the complex interplay of developmental, environmental, and sport-related factors that can influence the emergence and progression of a mental health concern in a student-athlete. Previously thriving student-athletes can be thrown into a depressive episode due to illness; rigorous athletic, academic, and social demands; and a triggering event such as injury. It is important that coaches, athletic trainers, and medical personnel be vigilant to changes in behavior that can herald the initial stage of a mental health problem. Prompt referral to medical and psychological resources can stave off worsening of symptoms and return a student-athlete to normal functioning.

Conclusion

Participation in collegiate athletics has the potential to impact a student-athlete's mental health both positively and negatively. Factors such as the athlete identity and perfectionism, combined with a rigorous athletic and academic environment and stereotypes about the sport culture, can contribute to extraordinary demands on a student-athlete's psychological resources. Universities have a unique opportunity to intervene by developing effective multidisciplinary teams of trained athletic department and sports medicine professionals who can identify and refer students to appropriate resources. Programs can anticipate and mitigate the harmful effects of these stressors by providing accessible mental health information, support, and easy access to resources at key junctures in the student-athlete experience. In addition, prevention programs can include mental health education for coaches and staff and peer-run support interventions.

KEY CONCEPTS

- Athletic participation and a supportive team culture can protect against mental disorders and promote self-esteem, effective coping strategies, and help-seeking behaviors.
- The following are key times of stress for student-athletes: transition from high school, postinjury and recovery, and retirement from sport.
- The following are athlete-specific stressors: balancing athletic and academic demands; navigating dual identities of student and athlete; role confusion and stereotyping; group cultures that increase negative stressors or interact with preexisting individual vulnerabilities and lead to mental health issues; individual factors such as perfectionism; sleep disorders; and body image concerns.

Recommendations for Psychiatrists, Psychologists, and Counselors

1. Establish effective mental health programs that support the whole student and provide licensed professionals for routine and emergency services.
2. Provide clear procedures and pathways for identification and referral of student-athletes to confidential mental health services.
3. Provide education to destigmatize seeking help for psychological and emotional concerns. Provide education about recovery from injury and retirement from sport.

4. Promote a healthy environment by supporting peer-led programs and education regarding bullying, discrimination, hazing, sexual harassment and assault, and violence.
5. Provide positive coaching and mental health education for coaches and staff.

Discussion Questions

1. What unique aspects of the student-athlete identity are relevant to your students and institution? Which ones might exacerbate mental illness and which might serve as protective factors?
2. Can you imagine ethical dilemmas arising in your work? How might you anticipate and resolve such ethical issues?
3. How might the unique social and cultural aspects of your collegiate environment influence your student-athletes' mental well-being, resiliency, or ability to seek services?

Suggested Readings

Aoyagi MW, Portenga ST: The role of positive ethics and virtues in the context of sport and performance psychology service delivery. Prof Psychol Res Pr 41(3):253–259, 2010

National Collegiate Athletic Association: Mind, Body and Sport: Understanding and Supporting Student-Athlete Mental Wellness, October 2014. Available at: http://www.ncaapublications.com/productdownloads/MindBodySport.pdf. Accessed July 25, 2017.

National Collegiate Athletic Association Sport Science Institute: Mental Health Best Practices: Inter-Association Consensus Document: Best Practices for Understanding and Supporting Student-Athlete Mental Wellness, 2016. Available at: https://www.ncaa.org/sites/default/files/HS_Mental-Health-Best-Practices_20160317.pdf. Accessed July 25, 2017.

References

Aoyagi MW, Portenga ST: The role of positive ethics and virtues in the context of sport and performance psychology service delivery. Prof Psychol Res Pr 41:253–259, 2010

National Collegiate Athletic Association: Division I SAAC athletic time commitments study, 2015. Available at: http://www.ncaa.org/sites/default/files/DISAAC_time_commitments_summary_20160127.pdf. Accessed July 25, 2017.

National Collegiate Athletic Association Sport Science Institute: Mental Health Best Practices: Inter-Association Consensus Document: Best Practices for Understanding and Supporting Student-Athlete Mental Wellness, 2016. Available at: https://www.ncaa.org/sites/default/files/HS_Mental-Health-Best-Practices_20160317.pdf. Accessed July 25, 2017.

Rao AL, Asif IM, Drezner JA, et al: Suicide in National Collegiate Athletic Association (NCAA) athletes: a 9-year analysis of the NCAA resolutions database. Sports Health 7(5):452–457, 2015 26502423

Won D, Chelladurai P: Competitive advantage in intercollegiate athletics: role of intangible resources. PLoS One 11(1):e0145782, 2016 26731118

CHAPTER 29

Military and Veteran Students

Eric Kuhn, Ph.D.

Shannon McCaslin, Ph.D.

ASIDE from a noble desire to serve in their nation's military or to continue a family tradition of service, many young men and women are motivated to volunteer for military service to receive educational benefits to fulfill their higher education and ultimate career goals. Academic attainment can have a profound effect on career success and overall life trajectories of military service members and veterans, especially given the demand for highly educated workers in the twenty-first-century economy. Conversely, academic failure resulting from difficulty adjusting to the academic setting or untreated mental and behavioral health problems can derail such aspirations. Therefore, it is imperative for psychologists, psychiatrists, and leaders in higher education to be aware of and responsive to the unique needs of military and veteran students. In this chapter, we discuss 1) challenges many students confront when transitioning from the military to academic life; 2) common mental, behavioral, and physical health problems they may face; and 3) ways in which psychiatrists, psychologists, and leaders in higher education can help address military and veteran students' needs to optimize their academic success.

Transition From Military Service to Campus

Military and veteran students, while eager to launch a new academic chapter of their lives, may be taken aback by unexpected challenges of transitioning from the military to an academic setting. The military has a distinct culture with a unique hierarchical structure, rules, traditions, and social norms. Although military service fosters skills that are clear assets in the academic setting, including a strong sense of goal attainment (e.g., mission orientation), responsibility, perseverance, and dependability (Cate 2014), adjusting to the differences in the college setting (e.g., relative absence of structure, loss of military relationships and social network) can lead to feelings of lack of belongingness, isolation, and disconnection.

Military and veteran students may feel out of step with their traditional student counterparts, because they are typically several years older, have often had profound life experiences, and have a host of competing demands (e.g., full-time employment, children, ongoing military obligations in the case of reservists). Quite often they are the first in their family to attend college (see Chapter 24, "First-Generation College Students"). Although they do share characteristics of other nontraditional students (e.g., older age, more likely to have families, often employed full time), some may have additional challenges, including medical and mental health conditions and disabilities resulting from military service, as detailed in the next section of this chapter. Despite the additional challenges of military and veteran students, concerns that they have poorer academic achievement and lower graduation rates than traditional students are not borne out by the data; in fact, it appears that overall these students are doing as well as their nonveteran counterparts (Cate 2014), possibly attesting to their resilience in the face of multiple challenges. Regardless, the combination of their unique life experiences and nontraditional roles and responsibilities can result in their feeling out of place and disconnected from classmates. Understanding the difficulties inherent in such a major life transition can enable psychiatrists, psychologists, and leaders in higher education to ensure that support resources are available to meet these students' needs.

Common Mental, Behavioral, and Physical Health Conditions

Academic success depends on critical functional abilities such as being able to sustain attention and concentration, hear and process auditory stimuli, and read proficiently. Although most military and veteran students will not be diagnosed with an impairing physical or mental health condition, a significant number may need additional services and attention. Military, and particularly combat, service increases risk of traumatic event exposure, which consequently can result in mental and behavioral health conditions, including posttraumatic stress disorder (PTSD), depression, and alcohol and substance use disorders (Fortney et al. 2016; Whiteman and Barry 2011). In fact, higher rates of PTSD and depression have been reported among veteran students compared with nonveteran students (e.g., Fortney et al. 2016). Moreover, military training and service are inherently physically grueling (e.g., carrying heavy packs, intense physical training) and can result in degenerative or chronic health conditions (e.g., foot or back pain).

The recent wars in Afghanistan and Iraq have resulted in many combatants sustaining blast injuries resulting mostly from improvised explosive devices. Rates of traumatic brain injury (TBI) for those who have served in these conflicts have been reported to range between 10% and 23% (Sayer et al. 2015). Military-related sensory impairments, including hearing impairment and tinnitus, are also common among these veterans. For those with auditory and/or visual impairments, learning can be impacted by difficulties with listening in the presence of background noise and with following oral instructions and understanding rapid speech; blurred vision; and reading difficulties (e.g., navigation of text, sustained reading, reading comprehension). These conditions, particularly when co-occurring with mental health problems, can seriously impair social and occupational functioning, including academic performance. PTSD, depression, and TBI can lead to difficulties in attention, concentration, memory, and other areas of executive functioning. Of note, sleep difficulties can develop during military service, related to factors such as shift work and irregular sleep patterns while under threat, and these can also surface secondary to another diagnosis, such as PTSD, depression, and chronic pain. Lack of quality sleep can further compound the difficulties outlined above.

Addressing the Mental and Behavioral Health Needs of Military and Veteran Students

Psychiatrists, psychologists, and leaders in higher education all clearly have a role in addressing the mental and behavioral health needs of military and veteran students. It is important to realize that when these students experience mental health issues, they may not reach out for help for a number of reasons. The military emphasizes resilience and effective problem solving, so military and veteran students may feel that they should be able to take care of such issues on their own. Moreover, there is stigma associated with mental illness, and asking for help is often perceived as a sign of weakness. It is important for mental health professionals, with support from campus leadership, to be proactive in reaching out to these students to raise awareness of available resources. For example, an orientation day held early in the semester or quarter to provide information about campus resources, general health care, behavioral health care services, and veteran academic services (e.g., benefits information) can be an opportunity to initiate connections with military and veteran students. Mental health professionals should also work with other health care professionals to set up routine screening programs for common mental and behavioral health conditions of veterans (e.g., in primary care clinics and counseling centers on campus).

Several recommended good practices for psychiatrists and psychologists serving military and veteran students are provided at the end of this chapter. In addition, as mentioned earlier, because of these students' differences in perceptions of help seeking, it is essential that clinicians allocate adequate time to build strong rapport and promote treatment engagement. It is vital to sensitively inquire about and discuss the students' military experience and background, which can build trust as well as inform and guide treatment planning.

Psychiatrists, in particular, who are treating military and veteran students should be aware of evidence-based psychopharmacology for common mental and behavioral health conditions evidenced among some of these students (e.g., PTSD, depression, substance use problems). For example, in their practice guidelines for PTSD, the Department of Veterans Affairs and Department of Defense strongly recommend selective serotonin reuptake inhibitors (SSRIs) and serotonin-norepinephrine reuptake inhibitors (SNRIs) as first-line medications (Management of Post-Traumatic Stress Working Group 2010). The guidelines also advise against using benzodiazepines for PTSD, because the potential harms can outweigh the benefits. Of course, patient presentation, preference, and response, as well as clinical judgment, will determine which medications are employed.

Although effective medications are available to address common conditions, often a combination of medication and psychotherapy or other behavioral interventions produces the best therapeutic outcomes. In addition, because veterans often do not wish to take medication and instead prefer psychotherapy, psychiatrists should be knowledgeable of evidence-based psychotherapies, particularly those that are trauma focused (e.g., prolonged exposure therapy, cognitive processing therapy), which have the strongest evidence base for PTSD. Likewise, it is important to have knowledge of community and U.S. Department of Veterans Affairs (VA) resources, because VA medical centers can provide specialty mental health and health care services, including evidence-based psychotherapies and cognitive rehabilitation. Through VA resources along with campus services, such as counseling support, tutoring services, and student services for disabilities, students can receive comprehensive, convenient, and timely support.

Psychologists serving military and veteran students should be trained to competently deliver evidence-based psychotherapies for PTSD, depression, and other common conditions (e.g., insomnia, pain, anger). They should also be skilled in integrated treatments for PTSD and co-occurring conditions such as alcohol and substance use disorders (including nicotine dependence), because these conditions are often functionally related to PTSD. Psychologists should also routinely consider involving family members and significant others in the care of military and veteran students. Finally, because sound technology-based psychoeducational and self-help interventions are available and continue to garner evidence, clinicians should consider these resources to meet patient preferences and supplement care. Several reputable programs exist, including Web-based programs (e.g., http://afterdeployment.dcoe.mil) and mobile apps (e.g., PTSD Coach; www.ptsd.va.gov/public/materials/apps/PTSDCoach.asp).

Although not engaged in direct mental health care service delivery, leaders in higher education still have a critical role to play in helping address the needs of military and veteran students. Campus leaders should engage in a dialogue with their military and veteran students to better understand the students' needs and should share what they learn with faculty and staff.

Leaders should consider developing educational programs for faculty and staff, perhaps employing the assistance of rehabilitation counselors and veteran counselors who can share their real-world indirect and direct experiences. Providing administrative and logistical support for veteran groups and designated space for veterans to meet on campus (e.g., a veterans resource center), especially given that many may be commuters, can provide them with the essential opportunity for connection with and support from other veterans and information about relevant resources.

Given the growing numbers of veteran students on college campuses, there has been increasing attention to ensuring adequate levels of support and resources to facilitate the success of such students. Campuses vary greatly in the degree to which they provide a setting that is considered "military friendly." Military-friendly campuses have invested in supporting the presence of veteran representatives and groups on campus, ensuring a dedicated space for veterans, and providing an office with staff to facilitate successful transition to the campus setting (e.g., staff that can advise students on resources and benefits). In addition, building connections with community organizations and local VA medical centers can create a strong network of support for veteran students. These partnerships offer an opportunity to overcome barriers to mental health care by pulling in key stakeholder groups and resources.

An exemplar of this type of partnership is the VA program Veterans Integration to Academic Leadership (VITAL) (www.mentalhealth.va.gov/studentveteran/vital.asp). In the VITAL program, which currently has over 20 sites across the United States, VA staff reach out to local campuses and work with them to establish a program that brings VA staff and services directly onto college campuses. Campus administration ensures that the VA is provided with private dedicated space, and both entities work together to ensure that the partnership meets their respective requirements. On campus, VITAL personnel work closely with campus faculty and staff to ensure that veteran students are provided with necessary resources. To initiate such a partnership, campus administrators should reach out to the administrators at their local VA medical center (www.va.gov/directory/guide/home.asp).

Case Example

Recently separated from military service, Lucas, a 26-year-old Army veteran, was excited to begin a new chapter in his life by attending his local community college while residing at home with his parents to save money. He planned to finish in 2 years and then transition to a 4-year university to obtain a bachelor's degree. Lucas had served as a medic while in the Army and had been deployed to combat once in Afghanistan. During that time, he had witnessed fellow soldiers injured, had provided emergency care, and had been a go-to person for advice and support. He occasionally spoke to the chaplain, knowing that those conversations were confidential and would not be shared with other military personnel. He was determined to graduate and pursue a career that would allow him to continue to help others, perhaps in the medical field. He was unprepared for the anxiety that hit him as he walked through the crowded halls on the first day of classes. It was chaotic, and he felt vulnerable as he made his way through the crowds alone. He began to plan the time when he would arrive at the school and the ways he would get to class to avoid the crowds. Within a month of beginning classes, he received news that one of his friends with whom he had served had committed suicide. Lucas found himself being distracted during class as memories of his experiences played out in his mind and he began to have difficulty sleeping.

By the end of the semester, Lucas found himself skipping classes occasionally, and his grades were beginning to slip. He started worrying about whether he would be able to succeed in college, and at this point he reached out to a friend at the college's veterans resource center. His friend encouraged him to call the campus counseling center. Lucas was ambivalent about reaching out to the counseling center, feeling that he should be able to handle the situation on his own, and he wasn't sure that they would be able to help him. Eventually, he decided to call and to set up an appointment.

Conclusion

As military and veteran students pursue their dreams of higher education, psychiatrists, psychologists, and leaders in higher education have a responsibility to help ensure the students' academic success. It is important to understand that the transition from the military to an academic setting presents a host of adjustment challenges that can be compounded by struggles with military-related physical, mental, and behavioral health issues. Fortunately, psychiatrists and psychologists have effective treatments to help address the mental and behavioral health needs of these students. Likewise, leaders in higher education are uniquely positioned to facilitate connections and employ resources that can make a substantial contribution to the success of the military and veteran students on their campus. Collectively, these efforts can help ensure that these students can accomplish their educational and career goals so they can continue to make a great contribution to the society they have honorably served.

KEY CONCEPTS

- Transitioning from military service to the academic setting presents a host of adjustment challenges.
- Military and veteran students have many strengths that can facilitate the successful navigation of this transition.
- Common mental, behavioral, and physical health issues among these students can compound transition challenges and undermine academic success.
- Psychiatrists, psychologists, and leaders in higher education can support military and veteran students and help to address their mental and behavioral health needs to optimize their academic success.

Recommendations for Psychiatrists, Psychologists, and Counselors

1. Develop military cultural competence. Knowledge of military experiences and culture can provide context for the students' background and behavior, as well as facilitate a stronger connection with them. Information about training resources can be found on the VA Community Provider Toolkit (www.mentalhealth.va.gov/communityproviders).
2. Conduct a comprehensive assessment. A comprehensive evaluation includes attention to military experience, traumatic event exposures, and common mental and behavioral conditions in this population. Careful differential diagnoses (e.g., between anxiety, traumatic brain injury, and attention-deficit/hyperactivity disorder—all of which may impair concentration) can ensure that appropriate care will be received.
3. Use evidence-based interventions. Familiarity with current clinical practice guidelines (www.healthquality.va.gov) and evidence-based treatments for common conditions, such as PTSD related to combat or military sexual trauma, helps ensure that military and veteran students receive effective treatments.
4. Attend to social support. Military and veteran students should be helped to build social supports, because loss of military networks

can be extremely difficult during the transition to academic settings. The protective effect of social support on mental health and functioning is well established. Developing and maintaining healthy social supports and interpersonal relationships with family and friends can be helpful for academic adjustment and success.

5. Consider involving spiritually based services. During their military service, some individuals may have used chaplaincy services, which are not reported to command or included in medical records because such visits could negatively affect military or postmilitary career opportunities. Students who used these services may feel more comfortable disclosing and addressing mental health issues with these professionals. Referral to pastoral counselors or faith leaders can help smooth the path to mental health care or address issues that are more appropriately handled by these types of professionals (e.g., spiritual and faith issues, moral injury, forgiveness).

6. Be aware of on- and off-campus referral resources. Given that veteran students may be overwhelmed by having to navigate a complex new setting to get their academic career off the ground, it is important to be knowledgeable of and prepared to facilitate appropriate referrals for other needed services.

7. Prepare for academic and trauma-related stressors. Academic stress can exacerbate mental health symptoms. Stress for veteran students might increase during initial adjustment following service, at transition to college, and during typical academically stressful periods (e.g., midterms, finals). For veterans who have experienced traumatic stressors in combat or who have lost comrades, anniversary dates may trigger exacerbation of symptoms and negatively impact ability to focus on academic work.

Discussion Questions

1. Describe some strengths that military and veteran students may bring with them and challenges that they may face when transitioning to the college setting.

2. What are some common mental, behavioral, and physical health issues that military and veteran students who have been exposed to combat or other potentially traumatic stressors may be grappling with?

3. Describe best treatment practices for psychiatrists and psychologists working with military and veteran students with posttraumatic stress disorder and associated conditions.

4. What are some ways that campuses might support and promote military and veteran students' academic and life success?

5. Where might one look for information on additional training and support resources for working with military and veteran students?

Suggested Readings

Cate CA: Million Records Projects: Research from Student Veterans of America. Washington, DC, Student Veterans of America, 2014

Management of Post-Traumatic Stress Working Group: VA/DoD Clinical Practice Guideline for the Management of Post-Traumatic Stress, Version 2.0. Department of Veterans Affairs and Department of Defense, October 2010. Available at: http://www.healthquality.va.gov/guidelines/MH/ptsd/cpgPTSDFULL201011612c.pdf.

Roberts LW, Warner CH (eds): Military and Veteran Mental Health: A Comprehensive Guide. New York, Springer-Verlag, 2018.

References

Cate CA: Million Records Projects: Research From Student Veterans of America. Washington, DC, Student Veterans of America, 2014

Fortney JC, Curran GM, Hunt JB, et al: Prevalence of probable mental disorders and help-seeking behaviors among veteran and non-veteran community college students. Gen Hosp Psychiatry 38:99–104, 2016 26598288

Management of Post-Traumatic Stress Working Group: VA/DoD Clinical Practice Guideline for the Management of Post-Traumatic Stress, Version 2.0. Department of Veterans Affairs and Department of Defense, October 2010. Available at: http://www.healthquality.va.gov/guidelines/MH/ptsd/cpgPTSDFULL201011612c.pdf. Accessed July 25, 2017.

Sayer NA, Orazem RJ, Noorbaloochi S, et al: Iraq and Afghanistan War veterans with reintegration problems: differences by Veterans Affairs healthcare user status. Adm Policy Ment Health 42(4):493–503, 2015 24913102

Whiteman SD, Barry AE: A comparative analysis of student service member/veteran and civilian student drinking motives. J Stud Aff Res Pract 48(3):297–313, 2011 22328965

CHAPTER 30

Graduate Students and Postdoctoral Fellows

Amy Alexander, M.D.

Doris Iarovici, M.D.

GRADUATE school is a special opportunity for students to develop expertise in a particular field of study. Students compete academically for these positions, after having shown academic promise and accomplishment in their field of interest in their undergraduate work. A master's degree can take 1–2 years to obtain, whereas a doctoral degree can typically take 4–7 years to complete. In this chapter, we focus on working with graduate students in the United States, because there can be cultural differences when compared with students in other countries.

Aiden, a 23-year-old, first-year chemistry graduate student, presented to his school's counseling center for difficulty concentrating and studying for his preliminary exams. One of his biggest stressors is his on-again, off-again romantic relationship. Dealing with this relationship has been very time-consuming and emotionally taxing. Although he did not identify depression as a problem, he meets criteria for having a major depressive episode. He feels hopeless not only about this relationship working out but also about his future in general. He is having trouble focusing and studying, and has tried his friend's Adderall, thinking "maybe I have ADHD." However, according to Aiden, "It hasn't really helped, and I still can't study."

Population Attributes

When addressing the mental health needs of graduate students, mental health professionals should consider some of their common characteristics. Most graduate students are—almost by definition—well educated, goal directed, and intelligent. They are often accustomed to academic success, are highly competitive with peers, have high expectations for themselves, and may come from families who also have high expectations for them. These attributes potentially affect the therapeutic relationship (see section "Treating Postdoctoral Fellows").

Prevalence of Psychiatric Problems in This Population

It is difficult to obtain clear estimates of psychiatric disorders among graduate students as a group. The Healthy Minds Study is an annual Web-based survey study examining mental health issues among college students. The 2017 results aggregate data collected between 2007 and 2016, are based on more than 36,000 survey responses, and are described for graduate students in Table 30–1. In general, the Healthy Minds Study shows that graduate students as a group report lower percentages of psychiatric problems compared with undergraduate students (Healthy Minds Network 2017).

In addition, the Graduate Student Happiness & Well-Being Report (The Graduate Assembly 2014) indicated that the top predictors of depression at one state university campus involved the following factors: sleep, overall health, and academic engagement. Forty-seven percent of Ph.D. students and 37% of master's and professional degree students scored as depressed. Students in the arts and humanities were at particularly high risk, with 64% scoring as depressed. At-risk groups who re-

TABLE 30–1. Examples of mental health issues and their prevalence among graduate students in the Healthy Minds Network Study

Major depression (PHQ-9)	7%
Any depression (PHQ-9)	14%
Anxiety (GAD-7)	15%
Generalized anxiety (PHQ)	6%
Severe anxiety (GAD-7)	5%
Panic disorder (PHQ)	3%
Suicidal ideation (past year)	5%
Suicide plan (past year)	1%
Suicide attempt (past year)	0%
Nonsuicidal self-injury (past year)	11%
Eating disorder (SCOFF)	6%
Binge drinking (any in past 2 weeks)	36%
Cigarettes (any in past month)	10%
Marijuana (any in past month)	10%
Experienced discrimination in past year	30%

Note. Flourishing (positive mental health) was reported by 56% of participants. GAD-7=Generalized Anxiety Disorder 7-Item Scale; PHQ=Patient Health Questionnaire; PHQ-9=9-item Patient Health Questionnaire; SCOFF=a 5-question screening tool for eating disorders.
Source. Healthy Minds Network 2017 (http://healthymindsnetwork.org/research/data-for-researchers).

ported lower well-being included lesbian, gay, and bisexual graduate students; older students; and students of "other" race/ethnicity. Parents and married students were groups that reported higher well-being.

This study was then extended to include graduate students in 10 state university campuses within the same system; 5,356 completed responses were received, which culminated in the University of California Graduate Student Well-Being Survey Report released in 2017 (University of California Office of the President 2017). This study found that humanities students were less satisfied with their life than those in professional or STEM (science, technology, engineering, and mathematics) fields. Lesbian, gay, bisexual, and queer/questioning (LGBQ) respondents were less likely to be satisfied with their life than other respondents. There were no significant differences by race/ethnicity or gender. Thirty-five percent of students reported symptoms indicative of depression. Again, nearly half of humanities and social sciences graduate students reported symptoms of depression, higher than their peers in professional or STEM fields.

A review of the common psychiatric disorders in children, adolescents, and young adults, not only in graduate students, reveals that 75% of those who will have a mental health disorder will experience onset by age 25 (Kessler et al. 2007). Pedrelli and colleagues (2015) summarized psychiatric disorders in all college students. Anxiety disorders are the most common diagnoses, occurring in 11.9% of college students. The following are rates for other common disorders: depression, 7%–9%; bipolar disorder, 3.2%; eating disorder, 9.5%; and attention-deficit/hyperactivity disorder, 2%–8%. In one study, 47% of female individuals and 62% of male individuals had their first symptoms of schizophrenia before age 25. Autism spectrum disorders (ASD), including high-functioning ASD, are socially disabling and can be distressing. One study found 0.7%–1.9% of college students meeting criteria for high-functioning ASD. In one study of suicidality in 8,155 students, 6.7% reported suicidal ideation, 1.6% reported having made a suicide plan, and 0.5% reported having made a suicide attempt in the past year.

Substance use disorders are prevalent among college-age populations. As reported by Pedrelli and colleagues (2015), one in five college students met criteria for alcohol use disorder. Binge drinking was acknowledged by 44% of college students; one in five students acknowledged binge drinking frequently. Fewer students reported drug use; 4.2% of students met criteria for drug abuse, and 1.4% met criteria for drug dependence. Marijuana use is very common among college students. Thirty percent of college students acknowledged using marijuana prior to starting college. Among college students, 23.5% of male students and 16.1% of female students reported currently using marijuana. Some also reported abusing prescription medications, including opiates and benzodiazepines. In combination with alcohol, abuse of prescription medications can be very dangerous. Students also report abusing stimulants and taking other people's stimulants, as in the opening case example with the fictional graduate student Aiden.

Developmental Considerations

If the development of young adults in their 20s is viewed through the lens of the psychosocial stages described by Erik Erikson (1950/1993), two stages are most relevant: identity versus role confusion and intimacy versus isolation. In the stage of identity versus role confusion, young adults search for a sense of self and identity and attempt to figure out what roles they will occupy in society. This includes choice of occupation. The career path for graduate students can be quite prolonged.

One example of a career path encompasses undergraduate years, graduate school, a postdoctoral fellowship, and finally starting a first "real job." Each stage requires reexamination of goals and considering whether to continue down the set path. Students can experience a crisis when they discover that they might not want to continue. Often, therapy can be helpful in supporting and guiding students through a potential career change. Even at the end of postdoctoral fellowships, many individuals feel a lot of pressure while looking for a first job. In some fields, available jobs, especially in academia, are quite limited, and many candidates compete for each one. Fellows sometimes need support in determining whether to continue seeking a job in academia or to pursue a nonacademic job in industry or another field.

In Erikson's (1950/1993) stage of intimacy versus isolation, young adults explore relationships with others and decide whether to make long-term commitments to romantic partners. Lack of success in dating and in finding suitable romantic partners can lead to distress, low self-esteem, social isolation, and hopelessness about one's future and plans for finding a spouse or having a family. In the opening case study, Aiden experiences distress with this unresolved stage in his life. He is in an unstable relationship, which is taking a lot of his time and energy. Unfortunately, the relationship is also distracting him from his studies and graduate school and likely worsening his depression. Nevertheless, it is an important developmental task, and he may need additional support from mental health professionals during this challenging time.

Another important developmental stage to consider—separation and individuation from one's family of origin—spans the end of adolescence into young adulthood. Of note, this stage can differ based on culture. For some international students, there is less of an expectation of separation and individuation, and this difference may clash with the culture of the school they attend. The process of becoming completely independent from parents and family members typically does not happen overnight. For many graduate students, the gradual process of becoming less dependent on family started when they left for undergraduate school. Some parents, however, continue to financially support their children in graduate school. Especially with the uprooting that occurs with education, first to an undergraduate college or university and then to a graduate school, often in a different location or different state, the consistent contact with and presence of parents can be comforting to students and can reduce the isolation that can happen with all these transitions. Therefore, some graduate students may have regular contact with their parents, sometimes multiple times a week or even daily. If this type of support seems positive for a particular student, it might make sense to have parental involvement in the student's mental health care, particularly when dealing with serious illnesses such as severe depression, suicidality, psychotic depression, bipolar disorder, or schizophrenia. Of course, practitioners typically have to obtain students' signed consent to involve parents, but sometimes encouraging parent contact helps in providing comprehensive care for a student.

Sometimes there are problems with separation and individuation from one's family of origin. These can include overdependence on parents, enmeshment resulting in unhealthy and poor boundaries between parents and children, being overly consumed with problems in the family of origin, difficulty making decisions that are in opposition with the known views of the family, and high conflict with family members leading to estrangement. These problems not only can be stressful for students but also can inhibit the formation of healthy independence and healthy relationships with others.

Unique Stressors

Graduate students face common challenges in pursuing their fields of study. Their work may include a lot of reading, research, experiments, writing, and publishing. Often, the work and pressures can be cyclical. A Ph.D. student may have to pass difficult preliminary and oral qualifying exams, then work on their project and defend their dissertation to a committee, and ultimately write up and publish their work. This path can require intense periods of study and focus, often with much less imposed structure than in undergraduate settings. The fictional student Aiden cannot focus or concentrate adequately to prepare for his preliminary exams, and this is resulting in a lot of distress. If Aiden is unable to prepare adequately for his prelims, he may still have to take the exam; if he does not pass, he may have to take it again, which may slow his progression. Some graduate programs can be harsher—not passing or not getting high enough scores in qualifying exams may prevent students from continuing to pursue their doctoral degrees. If students leave their graduate program with a master's degree or no degree, they may feel shame and disappointment at not achieving their original goal. It can be difficult for these students to accept this change of plans, and it can be especially difficult to tell their families, colleagues, and professors about this change to their academic career.

In graduate school, there are high expectations and pressure to complete projects quickly, which can be stressful. Students may not have control over their schedule or may experience a lack of imposed structure in the work environment. Some students report "not doing anything for a year" while under extreme stress, and their advisors and peers may not be aware of the extent of lack of academic progress. At the other extreme, graduate school can also enable workaholic tendencies; it is not unheard of for graduate students to work 10- to 12-hour days, including weekends, and have difficulty finding work-life balance.

Financial stress is common, especially when graduate students compare themselves to their peers who are already working and receiving full-time salaries. The compensation for graduate students tends to be low and just enough to cover living expenses. It can be difficult to find additional funds to buy a car, buy a house, pay for emergency expenses, and so forth. Some of these issues have led graduate students to unionize to improve working conditions.

Both graduate students and postdoctoral fellows can experience a lack of control over their projects. At the doctoral level, students are expected to come up with something novel, for example, propose a previously untested hypothesis and perform conclusive experiments to test this hypothesis or write about a new angle on a topic, which can be very challenging. When experiments are proving inconclusive and/or nonreproducible, students may blame themselves and ruminate about perceived shortcomings. They may think, "I'm not smart enough to figure this out" and "What's wrong with me?" The situation can damage self-esteem and self-confidence, lower motivation, result in feelings of hopelessness, and potentially worsen depression. Another common scenario is believing they have done enough work to progress to the next level (i.e., progress through the different phases of obtaining their Ph.D., obtaining sufficient data to publish their writing or a paper), but their advisor disagrees and feels that more work needs to be done first. Graduate students commonly feel that their careers are held in the hands of an advisor and dissertation committee. Interpersonal conflicts with professors can be particularly stressful for students, and can exacerbate disagreements over students' progress. Students and fellows can feel very frustrated, angry, or resentful toward their advisors about not advancing along their academic trajectory.

Several groups of students, especially international and undocumented students, can be particularly affected by politics and government decisions. These groups may be reluctant or less likely to seek help in a mental health setting; however, it is important to be aware of the special needs, anxieties, and stresses these students may face. International students may have additional unmet mental health needs and may benefit from additional outreach efforts to engage them in treatment (Hyun et al. 2007). Minority students may also benefit from additional support (Williams 2000).

Student Mental Health

The reported rates for suicide have been described in the section "Prevalence of Psychiatric Problems in This Population." When addressing suicide prevention, mental health professionals need to consider access to lethal means by graduate students who work in research labs that stock dangerous chemicals, such as potassium cyanide. Although the exact rate is somewhat difficult to pin down, a number of well-publicized intentional deaths of graduate students, postdoctoral fellows, and research lab workers have been due to cyanide. One university has worked on an intervention for this issue: restricting access to laboratory cyanide, combined with mandated professional assessment after suicide attempts; this intervention was associated with reduced suicide rates (Joffe 2008).

Sexual assault and harassment have been increasingly documented on college campuses. Sexual abuse, sexual assaults, and domestic violence can involve students and their partners, friends, colleagues, acquaintances, or strangers. Substance use, especially involving alcohol, is often associated with these problems, but not always. Some students are conflicted about whether to report sexual assault or harassment, especially when another student or supervisor is involved. One of the most upsetting situations is when a student decides to forgo privacy and report an incident, and then insufficient evidence exists for any action to be taken. In these situations, students often need more support and may seek this out in a mental health setting. The experiences of reporting something this serious, dealing with the university, and potentially dealing with the police or with legal situations, can be extremely stressful and disruptive to studies for both the students reporting the incident and individuals accused of being the perpetrators. It is helpful for mental health professionals to understand their institutions' policies about sexual assault and sexual harassment, as well as when and how police get involved, because students may ask for support and guidance as they maneuver through these systems.

Universities are increasingly implementing policies that prohibit romantic and/or sexual relationships between professors and students. They may also prohibit relationships in which there is a power differential—when one person is teaching, evaluating, or supervising the other. For graduate students, this would include relationships with undergraduates whom they teach in class or supervise. There have been well-publicized sexual harassment cases between university professors and graduate students. Perhaps the large amount of time spent working together on projects, traveling to conferences, and even socializing increases the vulnerability to these problems. When professors or persons with more power do not maintain healthy boundaries with students, romantic and sexual relationships can develop in a problematic way. These problems include conflicts of interest, potential exploitation, lack of mutual agreement (students may feel unable to say "no" or feel that they will damage their careers if they turn down unwelcome advances), bias, and favoritism. In addition, there have been cases of overt sexual harassment and sexual advances made toward students, which students have felt unable to stop, even if no romantic or sexual relationship ever occurred with the professor. Such situations are extremely stressful for students and disruptive to their studies. Students may seek out mental health care during these experiences and especially when there are legal situations such as sexual harassment lawsuits. Anxiety, depression, and trauma are common issues in such situations.

Obstacles to Seeking Help

A number of obstacles exist to seeking mental health care. Graduate students cite lack of time and financial limitations as reasons not to seek or continue care. Sometimes there is a lack of family support for therapy and especially for psychotropic medications; parental views that do not support treatment can either dissuade students from seeking help or cause students to feel distressed and conflicted because they are going against parents' advice. Even when a student decides to override the parents and seek help, the conflicting feelings that ensue need to be worked through during treatment.

Graduate students and postdoctoral fellows tend to be very intelligent, resourceful, and well read. Some students may feel they are already well informed on mental health topics, having done their own searches on the Internet. Sometimes this self-confidence can become a hindrance in treatment, for instance, when students overly rely on themselves to get better and think, "I should be able to figure this out myself" and "I should be able to talk my way out of this." Broader psychoeducation can be useful in informing students about psychiatric illnesses and their common courses, as well as about the need for professional treatment for these medical disorders. Mental health professionals can also address issues related to stigma, describe how treatment works, and explain how treatment can affect and potentially help the students. Some students who value self-reliance tend to distrust medical treatment and medical advice; for these students, building good rapport and trust in the relationship becomes essential. Sometimes students will not agree to the recommended treatment plan, saying, for example, "There is no way I can come every week to talk to you." For these students, coming up with a mutually agreeable plan is also essential. The work culture of graduate school might make students balk at weekly treatment; a compromise might be effective if the student agrees to meet weekly if he or she starts to get worse.

Treating Postdoctoral Fellows

For the most part, the preceding information is also relevant to postdoctoral fellows. However, seeking mental health care can be especially challenging for postdoctoral fellows because they are often not considered students anymore and are not covered by student mental health services. They are often considered employees and sometimes have quite limited health care coverage. In addition, postdoctoral fellows are typically older, in their late 20s or early 30s; postdoctoral fellows who started graduate school late or came back to graduate school can be even older. Some fellows are already married and have children. Balancing time in fellowship with family obligations can be challenging and stressful. Postdoctoral fellows can experience more financial strain due to the pressure of supporting spouses and children and to being in school and training for an even longer period of time with limited compensation. Often postdoctoral fellows have grants and experience pressure to keep their grants and funding. There is also pressure to find a "real" job after a fellowship; this can be especially stressful for those in fields with limited job opportunities, especially in academia.

Conclusion

Working with graduate students and postdoctoral fellows can be a rewarding experience—mental health professionals help and support these students and trainees through a difficult and challenging experience that culminates in an important career achievement and milestone. Being familiar with mental health disorders and how they manifest in this population is useful, as is understanding the developmental processes of this age group. It is also helpful to be knowledgeable about the unique stressors, challenges, population attributes, and vulnerabilities in this population.

KEY CONCEPTS

- Graduate students and postdoctoral fellows encounter many of the same mental health problems as other young adults of the same age.

- Graduate students and fellows have additional characteristics, vulnerabilities, and potential challenges for practitioners to consider when working with them in a mental health setting.
- The development of rapport is particularly important, as is developing a treatment plan that the student or fellow finds acceptable and feasible.

Recommendations for Psychiatrists, Psychologists, and Counselors

1. Become familiar with the prevalence of psychiatric problems among graduate students, and be attuned to groups with additional needs, including arts and humanities graduate students, LGBTQ students, international and undocumented students, and minority students.
2. Understand the developmental tasks in this population and how they can affect and increase stress in graduate students. These tasks include identity formation, the development of romantic and intimate relationships, and separation and individuation from the family of origin.
3. Clinicians may relate easily to graduate students and their educational backgrounds; awareness of this is needed to avoid overidentification and boundary violations.

Discussion Questions

1. What are the different strategies you might use when students tell you they do not want to continue treatment for the following reasons?

   - They don't have enough time.
   - They don't have enough money or financial resources.
   - They feel it isn't helping and "nothing will help anyway."
   - Their family doesn't think they have a problem and doesn't think they need medications and/or therapy.

2. How do you help a student who is "at odds with" or has a lot of interpersonal conflict with their main professor or thesis advisor?
3. How might your identification with the issues, experiences, and cognitive style of graduate students and postdoctoral fellows facilitate treatment? How might it impede care?

Suggested Readings

Hyun J, Quinn B, Madon T, Lustig S: Graduate student mental health: needs assessment and utilization of counseling services. Journal of College Student Development 47(3):247–266, 2006

Pedrelli P, Nyer M, Yeung A, et al: College students: mental health problems and treatment considerations. Acad Psychiatry 39(5):503–511, 2015

Schmitt EN: A study on graduate students: perceptions of stress, job engagement, satisfaction, and the buffering effects of social support and coping style. Dissertation, The Chicago School of Professional Psychology, ProQuest Dissertations Publishing, 2012

Treistman DL, Lent R: Work-family conflict and life satisfaction in female graduate students: testing mediating and moderating hypotheses. Dissertation. University of Maryland, College Park, 2004. Available at: http://hdl.handle.net/1903/1702.

References

Erikson EH: Childhood and Society (1950). New York, WW Norton, 1993

The Graduate Assembly: Graduate Student Happiness & Well-Being Report, 2014. Available at: http://ga.berkeley.edu/wp-content/uploads/2015/04/wellbeingreport_2014.pdf. Accessed July 25, 2017.

Healthy Minds Network: 2017. Available at: http://healthymindsnetwork.org. Accessed July 25, 2017.

Hyun J, Quinn B, Madon T, Lustig S: Mental health need, awareness, and use of counseling services among international graduate students. J Am Coll Health 56(2):109–118, 2007 17967756

Joffe P: An empirically supported program to prevent suicide in a college student population. Suicide Life Threat Behav 38(1):87–103, 2008 18355111

Kessler RC, Amminger GP, Aguilar-Gaxiola S, et al: Age of onset of mental disorders: a review of recent literature. Curr Opin Psychiatry 20(4):359–364, 2007 17551351

Pedrelli P, Nyer M, Yeung A, et al: College students: mental health problems and treatment considerations. Acad Psychiatry 39(5):503–511, 2015 25142250

University of California Office of the President: The University of California Graduate Student Well-Being Survey Report. May 2017. Available at: http://ucop.edu/institutional-research-academic-planning/_files/graduate_well_being_survey_report.pdf. Accessed July 25, 2017.

Williams KB: Perceptions of social support in doctoral programs among minority students. Psychol Rep 86(3 Pt 1):1003–1010, 2000 10876359

CHAPTER 31

Medical Students, Residents, and Fellows

Doris Iarovici, M.D.
Amy Alexander, M.D.

YOUNG adults who decide to become physicians face a particularly extended and arduous path as students. Medical students, residents, and physicians who pursue fellowship training encounter a range of significant stressors and may have higher rates of mental health issues than age-matched nonphysician cohorts. They also face unique challenges in and barriers to receiving mental health care.

> Carlos, a 24-year-old, second-year medical student, reluctantly presented to his school's counseling center. He had been referred by his primary

care doctor after a workup for persistent fatigue indicated no abnormal results. At the counseling center, Carlos didn't complete the routine intake questionnaires or survey instruments, afraid of having any mental health issue "on his record." He agreed to feeling stressed and overwhelmed lately, but believed "I can handle it," and attributed his problems to being off-site and traveling for his past two rotations. Initially guarded and anxious, he joked, "I don't intend to be part of the thirty percent," referring to a statistic he'd heard at orientation suggesting medical students were at high risk for depression.

Many studies over the past few decades have suggested that medical students suffer from emotional distress at rates higher than age-matched control subjects. A recent meta-analysis of 183 studies from over 40 countries, comprising more than 120,000 medical students, found the prevalence of depression to be 27.2%—between two and five times higher than among similar-aged national samples (Rotenstein et al. 2016; Figure 31–1). Although previous studies associated certain moments in training (e.g., the transition from academic learning to clinical rotations) with particular vulnerability, the pooled data showed fairly constant rates across levels of training, with preclinical- and clinical-year students equally affected. Alarmingly, only 15.7% of those who screened positive for depression ever sought mental health treatment. This is particularly troubling because this and other studies have also found higher rates of suicidal ideation in medical students, residents, and physicians than in the general population; in this large meta-analysis, suicidal thinking occurred in over 10% of medical students. An earlier multi-institutional study of over 2,000 medical students and residents found higher prevalence of suicidal ideation among women physicians-in-training and those from traditionally underrepresented groups, including African Americans, Hispanic, Asian, and indigenous groups (Goebert et al. 2009). Suicidal ideation may also be more frequent among medical students than among graduate students or those in other professional school programs.

Like Carlos in the opening vignette, many medical students are aware of their greater risk for depression, but barriers persist both to admitting they personally might have a problem and to seeking help. The culture of medicine—whose business it is to take smart and empathic young adults and train them to master not only an enormous fund of information but also critical thinking, professionalism, and caring attitudes—often also presents a formidable stressor. In what has been referred to as the "hidden curriculum," attitudes encouraging "toughness" persist, with the prototypical physician viewed as intelligent, driven, capable, and resilient enough to weather any of the many challenges that medical school throws their way. Other professional school students—for example, den-

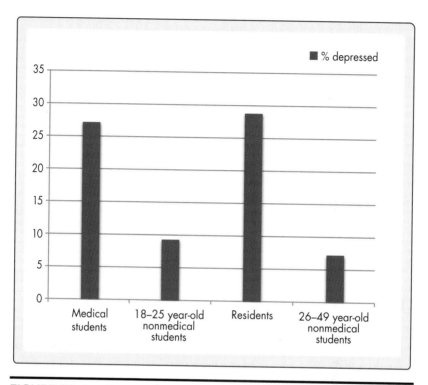

FIGURE 31–1. **Depression in medical students and residents compared with nonmedical students.**

Source. Based on data from Rotenstein et al. 2016.

tal and pharmacy students—may also have higher rates of depression than age-matched adults. However, the impact of untreated, unacknowledged emotional problems among future physicians affects not only their own quality of life—and, perhaps, their competence in generally meeting their responsibilities—but also potentially their ability to appropriately recognize and refer or treat psychiatric difficulties in their patients.

Although depression may be the best studied mental health issue that afflicts medical students at rates higher than in the general population, it is not the only one. A professional trajectory that rewards conscientiousness and checking behaviors may also exacerbate anxiety disorders such as generalized anxiety disorder, as well as obsessive-compulsive traits and obsessive-compulsive disorder, in vulnerable individuals. The experience of medical school itself, with constant exposure to illness and death in a setting that is not always supportive, may be traumatic, increasing the risk for posttraumatic stress disorder among medical students. Also, despite studying the effects of addiction during the day, many medical students turn to substances to cope with stress. They suffer from misuse of, and sometimes addiction to, not only alcohol and illicit drugs but also prescription medications, such as stimulants, to which they turn for help with academic demands—sometimes with disastrous consequences.

In addition to mental health issues, medical students and residents face high rates of burnout, a related but distinct problem that is sometimes categorized as a measure of *professional* distress (compared with the *personal* distress of depression and other psychiatric conditions). In a study measuring the burnout triad of emotional exhaustion, depersonalization, and low personal accomplishment, Dyrbye et al. (2010) surveyed over 2,200 students at seven U.S. medical schools and found that over half of the students met criteria for burnout. Those with burnout were more likely to report depression and suicidal thinking, more likely to engage in unprofessional behaviors, and less likely to hold altruistic views about physicians' responsibility to society.

Unique Stressors

To provide the best care, clinicians providing services to medical students ideally will be aware of the pressures unique to this population. Medical students, especially in clinical rotations, work very long and often irregular hours. In the past couple of decades, groups including the Accreditation Council for Graduate Medical Education (ACGME) and the Institute of Medicine (IOM) have restricted resident physician duty hours to 80 hours per week averaged over a 4-week period, but no similar universal standard has emerged for medical students. Although most medical schools have used the ACGME rules as a guideline in limiting medical student work hours to 80, students continue to have 24- to 30-hour on-call periods. Clinical rotations expose students to constant transitions, sometimes as frequently as monthly. Students must quickly adapt to different medical specialties with new funds of knowledge and different mentors, peers, and physical locations. These changes are especially challenging for those young adults who are temperamentally shy or who might have social anxiety. For everyone, however, the transitions can disrupt self-care routines and interpersonal relationships. Although university students in general are commonly uprooted from their communities and families to attend school, medical students are continuously uprooted as they progress through their education. They also often take on significant financial debt, which might limit their willingness to choose another path if they discover medicine is not a good fit.

Mistreatment and possibly even abuse of medical students and residents continue to occur within clinical settings. According to the 2015 Association of American Medical Colleges (AAMC) Medical School Graduation Questionnaire, over 38% of graduating students experienced some sort of mistreatment within their clinical settings, and nearly 20% witnessed mistreatment of a peer. Concerning behaviors that were experienced at frequencies of "occasional to frequent" include public humiliation (9.2% of students), offensive sexist remarks (8.2%), denial of opportunities for training/rewards based on gender (3.6%) or race/ethnicity (2.3%), and unwanted sexual advances (2.1%). The majority of students who noted experiencing such behaviors never reported them, either because of the perception that these incidents did not seem important enough to report or because of fear of reprisal. Also, 80% did not report mistreatment that they had experienced, and over 88% did not report such behavior that they had witnessed.

An environment that accentuates shame and secrecy is concerning when problems do arise. Medical students have unique access to medications and other potentially lethal means of self-harm. With their understanding of science, they can seek out laboratory chemicals available during research or preclinical rotations. On some clinical rotations in particular, such as anesthesiology or surgery, students have access to a variety of addictive or lethal medications.

Obstacles to Seeking Help

It is not unusual for medical students to present to counseling centers as a result of referral from a primary care physician for physical complaints, including fatigue, gastrointestinal distress, or headaches, or because the student, or a dean or professor, has noticed changes in academic performance, such as flagging concentration. Emotional complaints are less frequent. Stigma is unfortunately still alive and common in this population. Fear persists that those seeking help for mental health reasons may be seen as "weak," and students also worry that a mental health history will interfere with their professional success.

Like the medical student Carlos in the opening case example, many are particularly wary of what will be on their "record." This fear is not entirely unfounded: residency applications, and until recently, state and specialty licensing boards, have separated questions about mental and physical health in ways that suggest the two are different and implying that any past history of psychiatric health issues might need a lengthier explanation. Of course, the real question about *any* health condition is whether it causes impairment; there is scant evidence that psychiatric issues, when treated, cause any more impairment than any other health problem. The culture of medicine sometimes unwittingly reinforces stigma.

The negative distortions that can characterize depression may also exacerbate perceived stigma. One study at the University of Michigan found that depressed medical students, compared with their nondepressed peers, more frequently believed that depressed medical students' opinions would be less respected and that faculty would view such students as less capable of meeting their responsibilities (Schwenk et al. 2010). In other words, those who most needed help also had the most stigmatizing views of mental health problems.

Because most students train at the same site at which they may themselves receive care, they have many concerns about privacy and confidentiality. One study of over 1,000 medical students at nine schools found that a majority of students preferred to receive medical care outside their training site, especially for mental health concerns, and 90% wished for insurance that would cover off-site care (Roberts et al. 2001). Women and students from ethnic minority groups were more concerned than male white students about the potential for negative professional consequences if they admitted to mental health problems.

Treating Medical Students

Once Carlos was reassured that his care was confidential and that seeking help didn't imply he was any less capable of being a physician, he admitted that he had always been a worrier but that his worrying had intensified recently during a clinical rotation on which a senior resident had mocked him when he didn't answer correctly while being "pimped." He'd found himself unable to stop replaying those interactions in his mind, had had a couple of limited-symptom panic attacks, and subsequently overslept a few times, missing rounds and getting into more trouble.

Because privacy and confidentiality are such significant concerns for this population, these topics should be addressed up front. Ideally, university counseling centers would have professional staff available who do not have dual relationships—that is, staff who do not teach or mentor medical students during training. If there are psychiatry residents or fellows rotating through the counseling center, it should be made clear to medical students that they would not be assigned to them and instead would see senior staff (unless the senior staff also teach or supervise medical students in other settings). In those instances, medical students should be given the option of being referred to another clinician. When available mental health services are described to medical students, at orientation or in conversation with deans or other mentors, confidentiality and privacy should be stressed, with concrete examples of how records are protected.

Students should understand the difference between their medical and their academic records and the privacy standards that protect each. Concerns about reporting mental health issues or treatment on residency applications and for licensure should be addressed early and accurately. Students should understand that it is *untreated* mental illness and addiction that often lead to significant problems, such as impaired judgment in caring for patients, potential loss of jobs or licensure, and pain and suffering in daily life.

When psychiatrists treat medical students, certain countertransference issues may be particularly salient. The professionals may identify with the students' experiences or with their defensive or cognitive styles. The shared experience of medical school can strengthen the relationship between psychiatrist and student. The treating clinician's judicious use of self-disclosure of medical school experiences, when appropriate, can validate a student's perception of the stressors caused by the hidden curriculum and may help the student discuss inappropriate behavior, such as that of the resident who demeaned Carlos in the vignette above. Feeling validated and supported may, in turn, encourage more empathic responses from the students toward patients in their care. It is important to remain vigilant, however, to potential boundary breaches, such as overidentification, minimizing symptoms as normal because they are common among those in medical training, or attributing treatment-interfering behaviors to the students' busy schedules.

Although medical students can make great use of psychotherapy, their schedules and frequent moves from site to site often preclude ongoing weekly appointments over extended periods. However, they may benefit from psychotherapeutic techniques that are delivered episodically, even within the context of medication management appointments. A supportive therapy relationship with a psychiatric physician, or with a skilled therapist without a medical degree, may serve as a corrective emotional experience, countering negative or even abusive interactions that many students experience over the course of their training.

Residents and Fellows

Resident physicians, and physicians continuing training through fellowships, are not usually treated in traditional university counseling centers because they are not regarded as students. However, their status both as employees of university medical centers and as trainees—supervisors of students in some settings and supervises themselves in others—gives them a unique and sometimes confusing status, which can make finding appropriate psychiatric treatment challenging. Fewer studies exist on the mental health of residents compared with that of physicians or medical students. A meta-analysis of 54 studies confirms what those who treat residents might guess: resident physicians experience higher than average rates of depression and depressive symptoms, ranging from 20.9% to 43.2%, depending on the instrument used, and averaging 28.8% (Mata et al. 2015). The rates of depression and depressive symptoms seem to increase as medical students progress through training, and longitudinal studies suggest an increase in depressive symptoms over time in residency. There were no differences among medical specialties or for surgical versus nonsurgical specialties.

Residents and fellows face many of the same privacy and confidentiality concerns that medical students do. They too need access to mental health services that are separate from their work and training environment. A few universities have piloted programs for mental health care of residents, with encouraging results. For example, when the University of Michigan Health Systems designed a House Officer Mental Health Program with dedicated psychiatrists, separate from the medical staff and promising complete confidentiality, its utilization rate in the first year alone was more than double the average yearly utilization rate (from over a decade) of the faculty and staff employee assistance program, the service to which residents previously had access (Pitt et al. 2004).

Conclusion

Medical students, residents, and fellows represent a subset of the university counseling center's patient population with higher rates of emotional distress and, because of their knowledge base and access to means, higher risk for harm. Addressing their unique needs and stressors in a culturally sensitive manner benefits not only the patients themselves but also the many people these patients go on to treat in their daily work. This subpopulation is also highly motivated to improve, and they can be extremely rewarding to work with.

KEY CONCEPTS

- Medical students and residents suffer from depression at rates higher than age-matched control subjects. Other psychiatric issues, including anxiety, obsessive-compulsive disorder, and substance abuse may also be elevated in these populations.
- Stigma, fear of professional repercussions, and a culture of medicine that reinforces the stereotype of the "tough, self-sufficient" physician keep many medical students and residents from seeking mental health care.
- When confidentiality is assured, and medical trainees are given access to mental health services that are separate from their training sites, utilization rates increase significantly.

Recommendations for Psychiatrists, Psychologists, and Counselors

1. Address privacy and confidentiality up front, because these are such significant concerns for medical students and residents.
2. Attend to countertransference issues. Judicious use of self-disclosure of medical training experiences can validate the student's or resident's perception of the stressors caused by the hidden curriculum. However, be vigilant for overidentification and boundary violations.
3. Remember that the frequent geographic transitions of multiple rotation sites and very long hours may require some flexibility and more episodic patterns of treatment for medical students.

Discussion Questions

1. What are some ways to combat the stigma that many medical students feel toward reaching out for mental health services? How might you combat stigma in direct clinical work with students, compared with work at the level of the entire university community?
2. What treatment challenges arise in providing psychopharmacology to medical students? To residents?
3. How might your identification with the issues, experiences, and cognitive style of medical students, residents, or fellows facilitate treatment? How might it impede care?

Suggested Readings

Corbett BA, Love L, Yellowlees PM, Hilty DM: Taking care of yourself, in Handbook of Career Development in Academic Psychiatry and Behavioral Sciences, 2nd Edition. Edited by Roberts LW, Hilty DM. Arlington, VA, American Psychiatric Association Publishing, 2017, pp 373–383.

Gengoux GW, Roberts LW: Enhancing wellness and engagement among healthcare professionals. Acad Psychiatry 42(1):1–4, 2018.

Morris NP: If health-care providers can't overcome the stigma of mental illness, who will? Washington Post, May 20, 2016. Available at: https://www.washingtonpost.com/opinions/if-health-care-providers-cant-overcome-the-stigma-of-mental-illness-who-will/2016/05/20/993eca46-1dfd-11e6-9c81-4be1c14fb8c8_story.html?utm_term=.cd89cfe4b560.

Myers MF, Gabbard GO: The Physician as Patient: A Clinical Handbook for Mental Health Professionals. Washington, DC, American Psychiatric Publishing, 2008

Ofri D: What Doctors Feel: How Emotions Affect the Practice of Medicine. Boston, MA, Beacon Press, 2014

Trockel M, Miller MN, Roberts LW: Clinician well-being and impairment, in A Clinical Guide to Psychiatric Ethics. Edited by Roberts LW. Arlington, VA, American Psychiatric Association Publishing, 2016, pp. 223–236.

References

Association of American Medical Colleges: Medical Schools Graduation Questionnaire, 2015 All Schools Summary Report. July 2015. Available at https://www.aamc.org/download/440552/data/2015gqallschoolssummary report.pdf. Accessed February 2018.

Dyrbye LN, Massie FS Jr, Eacker A, et al: Relationship between burnout and professional conduct and attitudes among U.S. medical students. JAMA 304(11):1173–1180, 2010 20841530

Goebert D, Thompson D, Takeshita J, et al: Depressive symptoms in medical students and residents: a multischool study. Acad Med 84(2):236–241, 2009 19174678

Mata DA, Ramos MA, Bansal N, et al: Prevalence of depression and depressive symptoms among resident physicians: a systematic review and meta-analysis. JAMA 314(22):2373–2383, 2015 26647259

Pitt E, Rosenthal MM, Gay TL, Lewton E: Mental health services for residents: more important than ever. Acad Med 79(9):840–844, 2004 15326006

Roberts LW, Warner TD, Lyketsos C, et al; Collaborative Research Group on Medical Student Health: Perceptions of academic vulnerability associated with personal illness: a study of 1,027 students at nine medical schools. Compr Psychiatry 42(1):1–15, 2001 11154710

Rotenstein LS, Ramos MA, Torre M, et al: Prevalence of depression, depressive symptoms, and suicidal ideation among medical students: a systematic review and meta-analysis. JAMA 316(21):2214–2236, 2016 27923088

Schwenk TL, Davis L, Wimsatt LA: Depression, stigma, and suicidal ideation in medical students. JAMA 304(11):1181–1190, 2010 20841531

Index

Page numbers printed in **boldface** type refer to tables or figures.
Page numbers followed by *n* refer to note numbers.